POSITRON EMISSION TOMOGRAPHY OF THE HEART

Edited by

Steven R. Bergmann, M.D., Ph.D.

Associate Professor of Medicine
Cardiovascular Division
Department of Internal Medicine
Washington University School of Medicine
St. Louis, Missouri

and

Burton E. Sobel, M.D.

Lewin Professor of Cardiovascular Diseases
Director, Cardiovascular Division
Department of Internal Medicine
Washington University School of Medicine
St. Louis, Missouri

**Futura Publishing
Company, Inc.**
Mount Kisco, NY

Library of Congress Cataloging-in-Publication Data

Positron emission tomography of the heart / edited by Steven R.
   Bergmann and Burton E. Sobel.
         p.   cm.
      Include index.
      ISBN 0-87993-526-X
      1. Heart—Tomography.   I. Bergmann, Steven R.   II. Sobel, Burton
   E.
      [DNLM: 1. Heart—radionuclide imaging. 2. Myocardium—metabolism.
   3. Tomography, Emission-Computed—methods.   WG 141.5.T6 P855]
   RC683.5.T66P67   1992
   616.1'207575—dc20
   DNLM/DLC
   for Library of Congress   92-4555
                                                                  CIP

Copyright 1992
Futura Publishing Company, Inc.

Published by
Futura Publishing Company, Inc
2 Bedford Ridge Road
Mount Kisco, New York 10549

L.C. No.: 92-4555
ISBN No.: 0-87993-526-X

Printed in the United States of America

This book was printed on acid-free paper.

In addition to the contributors to this volume, many outstanding clinicians and scientists have lent their expertise to the development of cardiac positron emission tomography. This book is dedicated to them, their colleagues and ours, and to our families.

Contributors

Stephen L. Bacharach, Ph.D., *Department of Nuclear Medicine, National Institutes of Health, Bethesda, Maryland*

Steven R. Bergmann, M.D., Ph.D., *Associate Professor of Medicine, Cardiovascular Division, Department of Internal Medicine, Washington University School of Medicine, St. Louis, Missouri*

Johannes Czernin, M.D., *Visiting Assistant Professor, Department of Radiological Sciences, UCLA School of Medicine, University of California at Los Angeles, Los Angeles, California*

Edward M. Geltman, M.D., *Associate Professor of Medicine, Cardiovascular Division, Department of Internal Medicine, Washington University School of Medicine, St. Louis, Missouri*

Robert J. Gropler, M.D., *Assistant Professor of Radiology and Medicine, Division of Nuclear Medicine, Mallinckrodt Institute of Radiology, Washington University School of Medicine, St. Louis, Missouri*

Gary D. Hutchins, Ph.D., *Assistant Professor of Internal Medicine, Division of Nuclear Medicine, Department of Internal Medicine, University of Michigan Medical Center, Ann Arbor, Michigan*

Janine Krivokapich, M.D., *Associate Professor of Medicine, Division of Cardiology, Department of Medicine, UCLA School of Medicine, University of California at Los Angeles, Los Angeles, California*

René A. Lerch, M.D., *Centre de Cardiologie, Hopital Cantonal, Universitaire de Geneve, Geneva, Switzerland*

A. James Liedtke, M.D., *Professor of Medicine, Head, Cardiology Section, Department of Medicine, University of Wisconsin, Madison, Wisconsin*

Gerold Porenta, M.D., Ph.D., *Visiting Assistant Professor, Department of Radiological Sciences, UCLA School of Medicine, University of California at Los Angeles, Los Angeles, California*

Heinrich R. Schelbert, M.D., Ph.D., *Professor of Radiological Sciences, Department of Radiological Sciences, UCLA School of Medicine, University of California at Los Angeles, Los Angeles, California*

Markus Schwaiger, M.D., *Professor of Internal Medicine, Director, Cardiovascular Nuclear Medicine, Division of Nuclear Medicine, Department of Internal Medicine, University of Michigan Medical Center, Ann Arbor, Michigan*

Arooj M. Shaikh, M.D., *Division of Radiation Sciences, Mallinckrodt Institute of Radiology, Washington University School of Medicine, St. Louis, Missouri*

Burton E. Sobel, M.D., *Lewin Professor of Cardiovascular Disease, Director, Cardiovascular Division, Department of Internal Medicine, Washington University School of Medicine. St. Louis, Missouri*

Charles K. Stone, M.D., *Assistant Professor of Medicine and Radiology, Director, Nuclear Cardiology, Department of Medicine and Radiology, University of Wisconsin, Madison, Wisconsin*

Michel M. Ter-Pogossian, Ph.D., *Professor of Radiation Sciences, Division of Radiation Sciences, Mallinckrodt Institute of Radiology, Washington University School of Medicine, St. Louis, Missouri*

Donald M. Wieland, Ph.D., *Professor of Internal Medicine, Division of Nuclear Medicine, Department of Internal Medicine, University of Michigan Medical Center, Ann Arbor, Michigan*

Michael J. Welch, Ph.D., *Professor of Radiation Chemistry, Director, Division of Radiation Sciences, Mallinckrodt Institute of Radiology, Washington University School of Medicine, St. Louis, Missouri*

Contents

Preface

Myocardial imaging has helped to propel cardiology into the modern era by providing information fundamental to the understanding of the cause, pathogenesis, and diagnosis of cardiovascular disease. The cardiac silhouette seen on chest x-rays represented its beginnings. The first dynamic cardiac images were acquired by fluoroscopy soon followed by cinefluorography with contrast media from which modern ventriculography and selective coronary angiography evolved. The use of a gamma camera in conjunction with intravenously administered radioactive isotopes that accumulated in the heart or the blood pool permitted noninvasive assessment myocardial perfusion and function. These modalities facilitated objective evaluation of novel therapeutic approaches, now well established, such as coronary bypass surgery and thrombolysis.

The development of computerized axial tomography (CAT) permitted truly quantitative reconstructive tomographic imaging with high spatial resolution. Analogous algorithms combined with detection of positron-emitting radionuclides gave rise to positron emission tomography (PET). Two decades later, the horizons of PET continue to expand.

Dr. Ter-Pogossian (former Director of the Division of Radiation Sciences at Washington University School of Medicine, St. Louis, Missouri), in collaboration with Dr. Sobel (Director of the Cardiovascular Division) and their colleagues at Washington University, played a primary role in the development and application of this approach to cardiac imaging. Their multidisciplinary team effort was essential in translating a sophisticated concept into a practical procedure applicable to complex phenomena such as quantification of regional myocardial metabolism and perfusion. During the past two decades, numerous investigators from diverse institutions have contributed to the evolution of cardiac PET to its present maturity.

PET can provide quantitative information characterizing perfusion and metabolism in vivo in human subjects that cannot be obtained by any other imaging procedure. PET has provided us with the most reliable, quantitative estimates of regional myocardial metabolism and perfusion. Its application to cardiac disorders such as myocardial ischemia, myocardial infarction, and cardiomyopathies is justified not only because of its quantitative power but also because of its sensitivity and specificity. Detection of myocardial ischemia associated with modest alterations in myocardial perfusion can be accomplished much more readily than with conventional techniques.

The development of PET has made an unexpected additional contribution. It has demonstrated that conventional imaging of the heart with single photon-emitting isotopes such as thallium exhibits greater quantitative limitations than appreciated previously. As a result, conventional, single-photon imaging has been improved by development of instrumentation and novel data collection modes yielding improved sensitivity and specificity. Although single-photon imaging lacks the inherent quantitative power of PET, considerable progress has been made in optimizing single-photon scintigraphy, in part as an indirect and valuable consequence of the development of PET.

Anticipated applications for PET are impressive as well. A major objective of cardiologic research in the next ten years will involve application of the techniques used in development of recombinant DNA and molecular biology to cardiovascular disorders. Anticipated advances include gene transfer in animal and human subjects and ultimately gene replacement therapy. Through such approaches, a metabolic perturbation can be corrected through alteration of a single molecule without altering other pathways of metabolism. Detection and monitoring of such corrections of alterations in cardiac metabolism may well require the quantitative power of PET. Thus, the marriage of PET to molecular cardiology is particularly promising.

In this book, Drs. Bergmann and Sobel have brought together contributions from renowned investigators to provide the first authoritative textbook on application of PET to cardiac disorders. The background for understanding coincidence counting and the unique features of positrons that facilitate spatial localization and three-dimensional reconstructions are described comprehensively and lucidly in the initial two chapters. A detailed analysis of cardiac metabolism and the positron-emitters that can be used to characterize flux through specific metabolic pathways in the heart are discussed thoroughly to inform those new to the field as well as experienced investigators. The clarity of delineation of metabolism of fatty acids, amino acids, glucose, and of regional oxidative utilization, is particularly helpful. The analysis of methods for estimating regional myocardial perfusion, discussing limitations of conventional techniques, and advantages of PET is exemplary. The discussion on myocardial viability and its detection with PET is of seminal interest to both investigators and practicing physicians. Successful delineation of the prevalence and significance of myocardial stunning and hibernation may well depend on application of PET to quantification of the underlying alterations in regional myocardial metabolism. The use of PET to assess the integrity of the sympathetic nervous system in the heart is an attractive, rapidly developing application. The last chapter provides a comprehensive perspective on present and anticipated clinical applications of PET to the diagnosis and assessment of cardiovascular disorders.

The authors of this comprehensive, well-written, cohesive textbook are to be congratulated, particularly for their clarity. The goals stated so clearly in the editors' Foreword have indeed been met.

Robert Roberts, M.D.
Professor of Medicine and Cell Biology
Chief of Cardiology
Baylor College of Medicine
Houston, Texas

Foreword

"The work is not yours to finish; but neither are you free to take no part in it."

Ethics of the Fathers

The diagnostic potential implicit in "body section" (tomographic) radiography has been recognized for 70 years. Early efforts to develop practical approaches relied on the principle of blurring components of interest outside of the selected tomographic plane by imparting motion to the detector system, the imaged subject, or both during the imaging interval. Decades ago, such defocusing x-ray tomography (laminography) was used extensively in characterization of disorders such as pulmonary tuberculosis.

Reconstructive tomography relies on alternative principles. Multiple angles of view delineate the spatial distribution of an image forming variable in three dimensions. Reconstruction of images is accomplished with digital processing procedures and mathematical algorithms employed in modalities as diverse as computer-assisted x-ray tomography (CT scanning), nuclear magnetic resonance imaging (MRI), and positron emission tomography (PET). The evolution of reconstructive tomography coupled with advances in the understanding of the kinetics of accumulation, deposition, and disposition of radiopharmaceuticals mimicking their physiologic counterparts set the stage for the practical development of cardiac PET over the past two decades.

Progress in the application of positron emission tomography to elucidation of cardiac cellular physiology and pathophysiology, and quantification of regional myocardial perfusion has been remarkable. It provided the impetus for development of *Positron Emission Tomography of the Heart*. Considering the present maturity level of the field, serious questions confront investigators and clinicians regarding the extent to which cardiac positron emission tomography can and should be used as a primary investigative tool and as a primary diagnostic tool for resolving specific clinical dilemmas. PET centers have proliferated, particularly with the availability of generator-produced positron-emitting radionuclides that permit utilization of cardiac positron emission tomography even in centers that do not have access to an on-site cyclotron. Nevertheless, expenses associated with such installations are considerable; and accordingly, it is incumbent upon clinicians as well as investigators to be cognizant of limitations as well as strengths of cardiac PET for specific diagnostic applications so that judicious decisions can be made regarding its clinical use. Our purpose in developing *Positron Emission Tomography of the Heart* has been to provide both investigators and clinicians with the information

From *Positron Emission Tomography of the Heart* edited by Steven R. Bergmann, MD, PhD and Burton E. Sobel, MD © 1992, Futura Publishing Inc., Mount Kisco, NY.

needed for fulfillment of their responsibilities as effectively as possible without depriving patients of invaluable diagnostic procedures when indicated or unduly taxing the health care system by implementing procedures for which more cost effective alternatives are available. To this end, we have included information regarding instrumentation and physics underlying positron emission tomography in the initial two chapters prepared by Drs. Ter-Pogossian and Bacharach. We have considered myocardial metabolism and specific radiopharmaceuticals used to trace such pathways in subsequent chapters prepared by Drs. Stone and Liedtke and by Drs. Welch and Shaikh. Spatial resolution, temporal resolution, tracers employed, and processing required for quantification of regional myocardial perfusion are addressed in the following chapter prepared by Dr. Bergmann.

In the second half of the book, authorities address specific applications of cardiac positron emission tomography including delineation of regional myocardial fatty acid metabolism, assessment of myocardial viability with tracers of perfusion and metabolism, assessment of myocardial protein metabolism, and quantification of regional myocardial oxygen utilization. In the last section of the book, the utilization of cardiac positron emission tomography for assessment of the status of neuroadrenergic stimulation of the heart and for clinical diagnostic applications is addressed in detail.

Now it is not only possible but also practical to interrogate a specific region of heart muscle with a specific positron-emitting radionuclide and to obtain quantitative information regarding the flux of a specific pathway of intermediary metabolism in an individual patient under defined physiologic conditions. When this process is contrasted with classic biochemical methods for assessing metabolism in tissue slices ex vivo, it is obvious how much has been accomplished in the field of cardiac positron emission tomography. Since quantitative delineation of regional myocardial blood flow can be acquired accurately and noninvasively in brief imaging intervals with positron-emitting radionuclides, it is clear how powerfully cardiac positron emission tomography can define the physiologic significance of specific coronary vascular lesions and their response to therapeutic interventions. Because little is known regarding the etiology and pathogenesis of cardiomyopathic states whether manifested by arrhythmias in multiple members of families, hypertrophic cardiomyopathy, dilated cardiomyopathy, or right ventricular dysplasia, it is readily apparent that elucidation of derangements in specific pathways of metabolism and characterization of specific cellular biological processes with cardiac positron emission tomography offer particular promise in acquiring the information necessary to effectively mitigate manifest disease.

We appreciate the thorough, informative, rigorous, and lucid contributions that have been provided by the authors of each of the chapters in *Positron Emission Tomography of the Heart*, all of whom are authorities who have made substantial original contributions to the field and whose insights have been honed by extensive experience. We are indebted to Mr. Steven Korn and his superb staff at the Future Publishing, Co. and particularly to Ms. Lucille O'Connor who assumed major responsibilities for copy editing and compilation of the material in its final form. We thank Becky Leonard and Sue Furey for typing, and Elizabeth Engeszer for editorial assistance. Most of all, we are indebted to our colleagues, past and present, whose remarkable achievements have accounted for the maturation of quantitative cardiac positron emission tomography in a remarkably brief interval. In particular, we acknowledge the contributions of Theron Baird, James Bakke, Judy Hartman, Pilar Herrero, David Marshall, and Carla Weinheimer; the staff of the Washington University Medical Center Cyclotron; and our former Fellows: Michael Brown, Keith Fox, Stanley Hack, Gregory Henes, Robert Knabb, Donald Myears, Thomas Rosamond, Martha Senneff, Marc Shelton, and Mary Walsh.

The lay press is replete with exciting advances in molecular biology that will undoubtedly revolutionize the practice of medicine and provide powerful weapons against the toll of illness. Perhaps less widely appreciated, the advances in diagnosis made possible by cardiac PET will undoubtedly contribute to the development and assessment of novel treatments including those based on gene therapy, and facilitate early detection of disease when prevention of extensive irreversible end organ injury is still possible. The quantitative power of cardiac positron emission tomography is unequivocal. Its place in elucidation of basic mechanisms underlying disease and delineation of their response to therapeutic interventions is unambiguous. Its diagnostic utility can be invaluable. It is our hope that *Positron Emission Tomography of the Heart* will provide investigators and clinicians with the information they need to apply this powerful technology appropriately and effectively in cardiovascular research and clinical cardiology.

Steven R. Bergmann, M.D., Ph.D
Burton E. Sobel, M.D.
St. Louis, Missouri

Chapter 1

Instrumentation for Cardiac Positron Emission Tomography:
Background and Historical Perspective

Michel M. Ter-Pogossian, Ph.D.

Positron emission tomography (PET) is a noninvasive approach now widely used in biomedical research and clinical medicine. After the administration of a substrate or pharmaceutical labeled with a positron-emitting isotope, the distribution of radioactivity in a subject is assessed as a function of time and space by the generation of images of the distribution of the radioactive label by a process very similar to the one used in x-ray computed tomography. In computed tomography, however, the image-forming variable is the attenuation of x-rays in the tissue imaged, whereas in PET, it is the emitted radioactivity reflecting the distribution of the administered radionuclide.

Most biochemical processes essential to life involve one or more atoms that constitute the bulk of living matter—carbon, hydrogen, oxygen, and nitrogen. Among these, carbon, nitrogen, and oxygen exist as stable as well as radioactive isotopes, the decay of which is accompanied by secondary emission of high-energy electromagnetic radiation (Table 1-1). The radioactive isotope of hydrogen, i.e., tritium, decays only through the emission of lower energy beta particles.

The radionuclides listed in Table 1-1 share two physical features: They decay through the emission of positrons and they are relatively short-lived. The fact that these decay through the emission of positrons greatly enhances their value for imaging. Positrons are positively charged electrons that exist only fleetingly in our environment. After its emission from the nucleus, a positron loses energy in matter through ionizations and excitations. After traveling through matter (typically over a few millimeters dependent on the energy of the positron and the density of the absorber; Table 1-1), the positron interacts

Table 1-1
Physical Characteristics of Commonly Used Positron-emitting Radionuclides*

Radionuclide	$t_{1/2}$ (min)	β⁺ Energy (Max, MeV)	β⁺ Energy (Ave, MeV)	FW 0.5 M Positron Range in H_2O (mm)	FW 0.1 M Positron Range in H_2O (mm)	FW 0.1 M Positron Range in Air (mm)
Cylotron-produced						
oxygen-15	2.1	1.72	0.70	1.5	3.6	11.8
nitrogen-13	10.0	1.20	0.43	1.4	2.8	9.3
carbon-11	20.3	0.96	0.33	1.1	2.2	7.2
fluorine-18	110	0.64	0.20	1.0	1.8	5.4
Generator-produced						
rubidium-82	1.3	3.4	1.39	1.7	5.8	19.4
copper-62	9.7	2.93	1.28	n/a	n/a	n/a
gallium-68	67.8	1.90	0.78	1.7	4.0	13.0

Abbreviations: β⁺ energy = positron energy; max = maximum, ave = average; FW 0.1 M, FW 0.5 M = full width at 1/10 maximum or full width at 1/2 maximum resolution; $t_{1/2}$ = physical half-life. n/a = not available.
* Adapted from Cho et al.[21] and Graham and Lewellen.[22]

with an electron, and the masses of the 2 particles are converted into 2 photons traveling nearly collinearly in opposite directions. Each of these so-called annihilation photons carries an energy of 511 keV equivalent to 50% of the total energy corresponding to the mass of the 2 particles. The collinear, simultaneous emission of the 2 photons in opposite directions permits not only the detection of the presence of positron-emitting radionuclides by the detection of the "annihilation" radiation outside the subject, but also the imaging of the three-dimensional distribution of positron-emitting radionuclides within the body.

The radionuclides listed in Table 1-1 all decay relatively quickly, with half-lives shorter than those of the majority of radionuclides used in conventional nuclear medicine. These very short half-lives were once thought to represent formidable impediments to the utilization of these isotopes in tracers of physiologic processes because of difficulties entailed in labeling compounds of physiologic importance and limitations encountered in characterizing physiologic processes over time. It is now clear, however, that a very large number of compounds of physiologic importance can be labeled with these nuclides and that the short physical half-lives do not represent, in most instances, a serious impediment to their use. In many instances, the short half-lives have been found to be desirable because of the relatively low radiation burdens they entail in the course of imaging and because the rapid decay permits sequential studies under diverse conditions. Because the chemical properties of traced substances are unaltered, these nuclides can be incorporated into substrates and radiopharmaceuticals with physiologic behavior. Because positron decay is accompanied by emission of penetrating radiation, PET can noninvasively characterize the biochemical processes in which the radiolabeled substrates participate.

Historical Considerations

Although the physics of the positron-emitting radionuclides was studied intensely in the first half of this century, only after the development of detector systems that permitted recording of the emission of the short half-lived isotopes did the developments leading to whole-body PET imaging occur.[1,2]

Historically, the use of the physiologic radionuclides evolved in 2 phases. Initially they were used because more flexible, longer-lived radionuclides were not available. As cyclotrons and radiation of stable elements became assessable by the medical community, carbon-11 (^{11}C), nitrogen-13 (^{13}N), and fluorine-18 (^{18}F) were recognized as particularly useful radioactive tracers for biological studies. During the 1930s and 1940s, such tracers were used to characterize diverse processes such as carbon dioxide utilization in plants, carbon monoxide metabolism in man, nitrogen fixation by plants, and absorption of fluorides by dentine and bone.[1] Because of the very short half-life of oxygen-15 (^{15}O), early investigators deemed this particular nuclide to be impractical for biological studies—a point of view later proved to be unduly pessimistic.

Interest in ^{11}C, ^{13}N, and ^{18}F waned in the middle 1940s and early 1950s because of the discovery of ^{14}C, a tracer that provided the scientific community with a more flexible label than ^{11}C for tracing organic compounds. As the availability of reactor-produced radioelements grew, so did interest in other radionuclides, such as iodine-131.

Interest in the biological applications of the short-lived, cyclotron-produced radionuclides with chemical properties suitable for tracing physiologic processes was revived in the middle 1950s when Ter-Pogossian et al. revisited the concept that compounds labeled with positron-emitting radionuclides could be used to trace processes of importance in biology and medicine, and that they offered a particularly attractive tool for this purpose.[3] This was demonstrated by the use of radioactive ^{15}O in the study of oxygen distribution in neoplasms in mice, in which distribution of ^{15}O was assessed ex vivo by autoradiography. These early efforts led to the utilization of ^{15}O-labeled oxygen and other gases in respiratory and metabolic studies in animals and human subjects.

The first cyclotron installed at a medical center was commissioned in 1955 at the Hammersmith Hospital in London and used for providing radionuclides for nuclear medicine studies, radiation therapy, and radiobiological studies. The Hammersmith group was particularly active in studies of respiratory physiology carried out with radioactive gases labeled with short-lived radionuclides. In the early 1960s, a small cyclotron, specifically designed for preparation of positron-emitting radionuclides, was installed at the Washington University Medical Center, in St. Louis.

After initial studies (1950 to mid-1970s), the use of cyclotron-produced radionuclides increased as cyclotrons dedicated to production of positron-emitting nuclides were installed at the Massachusetts General Hospital in Boston and at the Sloan Kettering Institute in New York. In other centers, specifically Ohio State University and The University of California in Berkeley, existent cyclotrons were used for production of short-lived nuclides for medical applications. Three main factors contributed to the growing acceptance of the usefulness of positron-emitting nuclides and are contributing to the proliferation of the use of these nuclides today:

1. the recognition that in spite of their very short half-lives, radionuclides can be used in imaging a large number of physiologic processes
2. the successful labeling of a large number of compounds of physiologic importance with short-lived radionuclides as a result of the efforts of imaginative chemists
3. the recognition by physicists and engineers that penetrating annihilation radiation exhibited many highly desirable characteristics for imaging.

The major events leading to development of whole body PET imaging were the demonstrations by Anger that 2 static scintillation cameras could detect annihilation photons and produce images without conventional lead collimation,[4] by Kuhl and Edwards of the utility of back projection in the reconstruction of transverse sections using single photon transverse tomography[5], and by Hounsfield who pioneered tomographic reconstruction algorithms for x-ray computed tomography.[6] The final push came when a single-plane prototype PET device was built. PETT (positron emission transaxial tomography) II, built by Ter-Pogossian and colleagues at Washington University consisted of 24 sodium iodide detectors in a hexagonal array and was used for phantom studies.[7] The first scanner to be used for human studies, PETT III, was completed in 1974.[8] The first multislice whole-body machine designed and used specifically for cardiac studies was PETT IV, completed in the late 1970s.[9] The development of these early PET devices was followed by the introduction of numerous improvements to the imaging system, facilitating acquisition of data from multiple transverse sections simultaneously, improved spatial and temporal resolution, increased sensitivity, and better reconstruction algorithms.[1,10,11] More recently, several groups developed PET devices incorporating the information provided by the difference in the time of arrival of the 2 annihilation photons at each of the opposing detectors operated in coincidence into the image reconstruction process.[12,13]

Subsequent development of tomographs by commercial companies has led to further refinements of whole-body PET technology with current imaging devices collecting 15 to 30 image planes simultaneously with spatial resolutions of 5 to 8 mm (Table 1-2). Three-dimensional image display is now readily available.[14]

Specific Requirements for PET of the Heart

The effective utilization of PET for studies of the heart requires an understanding of the imaging procedures that yield data in the form of images. Knowledge of the capabilities and particularly the limitations of specific PET systems is important because none can be regarded as optimal for all applications. For example, PET devices for cerebral studies are designed usually to

Table 1-2
Selected Characteristics of Currently Available Cardiac PET Scanning Systems*

Manufacturer/Model	Crystal Type	Number of Rings	Crystals/ Ring	Number of Slices	Slice Separation (mm)	Patient Aperture (cm)	TFOV (cm)	AFOV (cm)	FWHM (mm)	Sensitivity (c/s/μCi/cc))
CEA-LETI Model TTV03	BaF$_2$	4	324	7	12.0	54	45	9	4.5	90,000
GE Medical Systems Model 4096	BGO	8	512	15	6.0	57	55	10.3	5.0	94,000
Hitachi Medico Co. PET 3600W	BGO	8	352	15	7.0	56	51.2	10.5	4.7	30,000
PETT Electronics SP-3000-E	CsF	4	192	7	14.2	52.5	52.8	10.7	8.5	136,000
Positron Corp. POSICAM	BGO	11	120	21	5.1	53.4	43.5	11.5	5.8	165,000
Shimadzu Corp. Headtome IV	BGO	4	768	7	13	50	51.2	10.4	4.5	14,000
Siemens ECAT 951/31	BGO	16	512	31	3.4	56.2	56.2	10.8	5.0	110,000
UGM Model 240H	NaI	1	6	64	2.0	50	50	12.8	5.2	120,000

Abbreviations: AFOV and TFOV = axial and transaxial field of view; FWHM = full-width at half-maximum spatial resolution; sensitivity is expressed in Counts per second per μCi per cubic centimeter for a uniform 20 cm phantom.
* All data were supplied by respective manufacturers.

encompass short distances (about 30 cm) between the detectors and aperture, whereas such instruments cannot accommodate a patient's torso for cardiac studies. This extreme example is typical. In the history of the development of PET devices, optimization of factors for certain applications are often optimized at the expense of features needed for other applications.

All existing PET devices include the following components:

1. a gantry supporting the detectors and often providing the needed mechanical motion to achieve proper sampling for reconstruction of the desired PET data along with a patient support couch and devices for calibration of the machine
2. radiation detectors and associated electronic circuitry suitable for the recording of annihilation radiation
3. a computer system with associated software and peripheral devices for collection of data and for display and analysis.

Modern PET devices incorporate gantries that provide physical support of the detectors and imaged subject, and when needed, motion required for increasing the number of angles of data acquisition. Some systems optically couple each detector to a single photomultiplier tube. To decrease tomograph expense and provide increased resolution, other tomographs have coupled several small detectors to a single photomultiplier tube with identification of the specific crystal in which the scintillation event occurs and is achieved by a logic similar to that used in conventional Anger cameras.

Detection of Radiation

Photons arising as a result of the interaction between emitted positrons and electrons in tissue are of high energy and therefore penetrate the body with less attenuation than that observed with lower energy emissions. The fact that annihilation radiation events comprise 2 photons traveling collinearly in opposite directions permits convenient collimation of radiation. Two radiation detectors suitable for sensing annihilation radiation are connected in an electronic circuit that registers an event only when both detectors are triggered simultaneously (actually within a given, brief, coincidence interval). Under such circumstances, a system consisting of 2 detectors and a coincidence circuit is sensitive to the radiation originating from the annihilation events occurring within the volume joining the 2 detectors. All PET devices use this very efficient method of collimation, but incorporate many more than 2 detectors. Most modern systems incorporate detection schemes whereby each detector forms coincidence lines with multiple opposing detectors, and multiple rings of detectors are used to obtain emission data simultaneously from several sections of tissue, thereby widening the axial field of view.

For radiation detectors, the very early PET devices used scintillation counters consisting of crystals capable of emitting a scintillation of light when struck by ionizing radiation interfaced to a photomultiplier tube that converts

Table 1-3
Selected Physical Characteristics of Scintillation Crystals Used in PET

	Sodium Iodide NaI (Tl)	*Cesium Fluoride CsF*	*Barium Fluoride BaF$_2$*	*Bismuth Germanate Bi$_4$Ge$_3$O$_{12}$*
Density (gm/cm^3)	3.67	4.64	4.89	7.13
Effective atomic number	50	52	52	72
Linear attenuation coefficient at 511 keV (1/cm)	0.34	0.44	0.47	0.92
Wavelength of emission (nm)	410	390	225/310	480
Decay constant (ns)	230	5	0.8/620	300
Light yield with respect to NaI (Tl)[a]	1	0.05	0.05/0.16	0.12
Index of refraction	1.85	1.48	1.57/1.55	2.15

[a] Some of these values are not entirely reliable. Reprinted with permission from Ter-Pogossian, 1985.[1]

the light into an electronic signal. The first scintillation detectors incorporated activated sodium iodide crystals. Since then, several other scintillators exhibiting different qualities have been used (Table 1-3).

Four types of crystals are used currently in commercial PET devices: sodium iodide (NaI), cesium fluoride (CsF), barium fluoride (BaF$_2$), and bismuth germanate (BGO).[1] Each has particular advantages and limitations (Table 1-3). NaI is the least expensive and is a reliable scintillator. However, it suffers from a long scintillation dead time that limits the temporal resolution of the scanner and limits the amount of radioactivity that can be administered and recorded faithfully. BGO is used in most of the commercially available scanners but as with NaI, it has a long decay time limiting count rate and temporal resolution. CsF and BaF$_2$ have much faster scintillation decay rate, but have less sensitivity than either NaI or BGO. However, these fast crystals have been used recently in cardiac PET scanners in which high temporal rates and high count rates are necessary for dynamic imaging.

Spatial, Contrast, and Temporal Resolution

The quality of a PET image can be defined in terms of the faithfulness with which the image reflects the distribution of the positron-emitting nuclides in the field of view. The data used in the reconstruction of the PET image are recorded by the camera's radiation detectors. Quality of PET images is always limited by statistical variations affecting recorded counts;[1,10,11] (also see chapter 2). The amount of radioactivity that can be safely administered is limited, and because the data acquisition time of the camera is determined by temporal variations in the distribution of activity in the camera's field of view and by radioactivity decay, the number of counts recorded in the overwhelming majority of studies is less than optimal, usually limiting the quality of the PET image.

Spatial resolution in PET imaging is limited most markedly by the geometry of the gantry and detector design. In addition, spatial resolution is limited by the fact that emitted positrons travel some distance before annihilation, causing blurring of the image.[15] The localization of annihilation events by coincidence detection is imperfect since the 2 photons in each pair of annihilation photons are not generally emitted exactly collinearly because conservation of momentum is required, and the positron is annihilated in motion. This divergence from collinearity also introduces blurring that is, in general, less significant than that resulting from the positron range.

Clearly, the amount of blurring is dependent on the particular energy of the administered radionuclide (Table 1-1). The ability of a PET system to precisely identify the location of a coincidence line depends on the dimension of a detector element. Typically, the resolution achieved is somewhat less than the physical dimensions of the crystal used. To enhance spatial resolution, recent scanners have used smaller crystals. Although some experimental PET devices are capable of resolution between 2 and 3 mm, commercial devices typically have resolutions of between 4 and 6 mm (Table 1-2). It should be noted, however, that because of statistical fluctuations in the data recorded, the practical resolution in PET studies rarely is better than 8 mm.

Contrast resolution is the extent to which the image accurately reflects contrast between two areas with different distributions of positron-emitting radionuclides. Two types of data recorded by PET cameras can vitiate contrast resolution: random coincidences, and coincidences generated by scattered radiation (see detailed discussion in chapter 2). Random coincidences are events recorded by the camera as coincidence lines that do not arise from the same annihilation event. They are generated when 2 radiation detectors operating in the coincidence mode record 2 independent events that are sensed simultaneously or within a short time interval (the coincidence window). The width of the coincidence window is determined primarily by the decay time of the crystals used (Table 1-3), by characteristics of the electronic components such as photomultiplier tubes, and by the balance of the electronic circuitry. Because the timing resolution of the coincidence detection is not infinitely narrow, a certain number of events will be recorded as coincidences even though they are produced by radiation originating from unrelated annihilation events. The number of such random coincidences increases linearly with the width of the electronically set coincidence window and quadratically with the amount of radiation detected. Because random coincidences occur solely on the basis of single unrelated events in physically large uncollimated detectors, their contribution to the reconstructed PET images is relatively amorphous and degrades contrast in the image.

Scattered radiation is another factor that can reduce contrast resolution. The origin of scattered radiation is identical to that in conventional nuclear medicine imaging, but its influence on the reconstructed image is somewhat different. Between the time of the annihilation event and its detection, annihilation photons have a high probability of interacting with electrons in the tissue. Most of these interactions are by the Compton effect, and the amount of energy transferred from the photon to the electron is relatively low. Under these circumstances, the photon is diverted only slightly from its original direction. Unless a large number of scattering events occur in PET imaging, it is more difficult to remove scatter by pulse-height analysis than in conventional nuclear medicine. However, because scattered radiation with PET is relatively modest, on the order of 10% to 30%, and because it is relatively amorphous with respect to the distribution of activity in the imaging structure, several correction schemes have been incorporated into the reconstruction algorithm.

In many PET studies performed, images must be acquired over a very short period of time. Thus, the imaging system must be capable of high temporal resolution. This requirement may result either from the use of a short-lived radionuclide such as ^{82}Rb or ^{15}O, or from the need to acquire data over short intervals to fulfill requirements of the mathematical model used, which is the case in myocardial perfusion studies. The incorporation of high temporal resolution in the design of a PET camera imposes stringent demands on the performance of its detectors. In the coincidence detection of 2 annihilation photons, the raw counting rate of any detector is approximately 2 orders of magnitude greater than the number of coincidence events delineated. This imbalance is in contrast to the case with conventional single-photon imaging. When PET studies are performed at high counting rates, the radiation detectors and their associated electronic circuitry are subjected to relative rates that typically exceed 100,000 counts per detector. Such high counting rates exert a deleterious influence on the quality of the image in two ways: 1) at increasing count rates the PET camera exhibits an increasing loss of counts that, in the extreme case, results in saturation because of the system's dead time, and 2) increasing count rates are paralleled by increasing percentages of random events resulting in degradation of contrast resolution in the image. The number of random coincidences is highly predictable based on the detector's counting rate and on the width of the coincidence windows. Thus, the contribution of random coincidences can be subtracted provided these factors are known. However, subtraction always adds noise to the image, and the contribution of noise increases with the percentage of randoms subtracted. Indeed, any subtraction of randoms results in the concomitant removal of "true" counts. In the extreme case with very fast PET studies, subtraction of randoms becomes ineffective because of the intolerable contribution of noise.

The deleterious contribution of dead time in the randoms can be minimized effectively by incorporating crystals with short decay times. However, the use of such fast crystals is accompanied by a loss of some desirable characteristics, particularly density. Thus, PET cameras generally fall into one of two disparate categories: 1) slower, high-resolution and high-sensitivity devices, and 2) faster, lower resolution systems. The two categories exist because at this time no scintillation crystal has yet been discovered that combines the optimal features of both the fast and slow crystals.

Time-of-flight PET

In conventional PET imaging, the information obtained when a coincidence event is recorded by 2 detectors defines the occurrence of an annihilation event somewhere along a straight line joining the detectors. Under such circumstances, no information is provided by the system delineating the site along the coincidence line at which the annihilation event occurred. It is possible, however, to gain information about the position of the event by measuring the difference in the time of arrival of the 2 annihilation photons at the 2 detectors. Since the 2 annihilation photons are generated simultaneously and travel with the velocity of light, the time of their arrival at the opposing detectors depends on the distance separating the site of the annihilation event from each one of the detectors. If the annihilation event occurs in a position equidistant between the 2 detectors, then the 2 annihilation photons will be detected simultaneously. If the annihilation event is closer to one of the detectors, that detector will be triggered first, and the delay in triggering the second detector will provide a measure of the relative distance between the annihilation event in the 2 detectors. Time-of-flight PET uses measurement of such distances. In general, a PET device with time-of-flight capabilities operates in the same manner as a conventional device but includes electronic circuitry that allows the camera to use information in the reconstruction process relevant to the position of the annihilation event along the coincidence lines. Because annihilation photons travel with the velocity of light, measurement of the difference in the time of arrival of signals at each of 2 detectors in a pair is difficult to measure with precision. Typically, time-of-flight devices are capable of providing a temporal resolution of approximately 500 ps, an interval sufficient for localization of the annihilation event along the coincidence with a precision of approximately 7.5 cm. The additional localization information provided to the reconstruction process appreciably improves the signal-to-noise ratio.[16,17]

A particularly important feature in time-of-flight PET is that it provides short effective coincidence resolving times, typically on the order of 1 ns, as opposed to the more conventional PET cameras that exhibit a coincidence resolving time of about 10 to 20 ns. From the technical standpoint, PET devices incorporating time-of-flight capabilities must use particularly fast scintillating crystals and photomultiplier tubes exhibiting very low jitter in their conversion of light to electronic signals.

Desirable Features for Cardiac PET Scanners

A PET system used for imaging of the heart should have a longitudinal field of view sufficiently large to obviate the need for multiple data acquisition with axial translation. A longitudinal field of view of 10 to 14 cm will usually fulfill this requirement with a margin to allow for suboptimal placement of the patient. High sensitivity is desirable. High spatial resolution is particularly difficult because of movement of the heart secondary to cardiac and respiratory motion. Although gating data acquisition with the electrocardiogram can compensate for cardiac motion,[18] this technique is not used widely because of consequent loss of count information. The longitudinal displacement of the heart caused by respiratory motion presents an even more difficult problem because such motion is extensive (about 2 cm for the cardiac apex) and because its magnitude varies in different segments of the heart.[19] Gating for respiratory motion is extremely difficult and has not yet been well addressed. Thus, the spatial resolution of PET images of the heart is considerably poorer than that of images of an immobile organ such as the brain.

Methods for measuring myocardial perfusion quantitatively with methods relying on rapidly changing tracer concentrations require very high data acquisition rates. The measurement of perfusion relies on defining the kinetics of tracer in the blood and myocardium and requires that images be obtained in intervals as short as possible, typically, 2 to 5 s. This demands a PET imaging device with particularly high temporal resolution that minimizes the contribution of random coincidences and has only brief dead time, generally requiring fast crystals. Because of these considerations, several PET imaging devices specifically optimized for "fast" cardiac studies have been developed.[20]

Conclusions

The now well-recognized utility of PET in cardiovascular research and in clinical cardiology results from its quantitative power and applicability to assessment of the kinetics in tissue of physiologic, labeled substrates and tracers. Its development was predicated, in part, on the fact that a handful of radionuclides possesses chemical characteristics that are particularly desirable for studies of physiologic processes. They decay through the emission of positrons in a process amenable to highly efficient collimation of the annihilation radiation by coincidence detection with characteristics that are particularly desirable for the application of reconstruction of tomographic images. Because of its quantitative power and the nature of the image forming variables employed, PET provides information delineating biochemical and physiological processes that is not available by any other means.

References

1. Ter-Pogossian MM. Positron emission tomography instrumentation. M.Reivich, A. Alavi, Eds. *Positron Emission Tomography*, Alan R. Liss, Inc.: New York, 1985; pp. 43–61.
2. Tilyou SM. The evolution of positron emission tomography. J Nucl Med 1991; 32(4):15N–23N.
3. Ter-Pogossian MM, Powers WE. The use of radioactive oxygen[15] in the determination of oxygen content in malignant neoplasms. In: *Radioisotopes in Scientific Research*. Volume III: Research with Radioisotopes in Human and Animal Biology and Medicine. Extermann RC, Editor. Pergamon Press, New York:1957; pp. 625–636.
4. Anger HO. Sensitivity, resolution and linearity of the scintillation camera. IEEE Trans Nucl Sci 1966; 13(Suppl 3):380–392.

5. Kuhl DE, Edwards RQ. Image separation radioisotope scanning. Radiology 1963; 80:653–661.
6. Hounsfield GN. Computerized transverse axial scanning (tomography): Part 1. Description of system. Br J Radiol 1973; 46:1016–1022.
7. Ter-Pogossian MM, Phelps ME, Hoffman EJ, Mullani NA. A positron emission transaxial tomograph for nuclear imaging (PETT). Radiology 1975; 114:89–98.
8. Phelps ME, Hoffman EJ, Mullani NA, Higgins CS, Ter-Pogossian MM. Design considerations for a whole body positron emission transaxial tomograph (PETT III). IEEE Nuclear Science 1976; NS–23:516–522.
9. Ter-Pogossian MM, Mullani NA, Hood J, Higgins CS, Currie CM. A multislice positron emission computed tomograph (PETT IV) yielding transverse and longitudinal images. Radiology 1978; 128:477–484.
10. Budinger TF, Rollo FD. Physics and instrumentation. Prog Cardiovas Dis 1977; 20:19–53.
11. Volkow ND, Mullani NA, Bendriem B. Positron emission tomography instrumentation: An overview. Am J Physiol Imag 1988; 3:142–153.
12. Mullani NA, Markham J, Ter-Pogossian MM. Feasibility of time-of-flight reconstruction in positron emission tomography. J Nucl Med 1980; 21:1095–1097.
13. Ter-Pogossian MM, Ficke DC, Yamamoto M, Hood JT, Sr. Super PETT I: A positron emission tomograph utilizing photon time-of-flight information. IEEE Trans Med Imag 1982; 3:179–187.
14. Miller TR, Starren JB, Grothe RA, Jr. Three-dimensional display of positron emission tomography of the heart. J Nucl Med 1988; 29:530–537.
15. Phelps ME, Hoffman EJ, Huang S-C, Ter-Pogossian MM. Effect of positron range on spatial resolution. J Nucl Med Instrum Physics 1975; 16:649–652.
16. Budinger TF. Time-of-flight positron emission tomography: Status relative to conventional PET. J Nucl Med 1982; 24:73–78.
17. Wong W-H, Mullani NA, Philippe EA, Hartz R, Gould KL. Image improvement and design optimization of the time-of-flight PET. J Nucl Med 1983; 24:52–60.
18. Hoffman EJ, Phelps ME, Wisenberg G, Schelbert HR, Kuhl DE. Electrocardiographic gating in positron emission computed tomography. J Comput Assist Tomogr 1979; 3:733–739.
19. Ter-Pogossian MM, Bergmann SR, Sobel BE. Influence of cardiac and respiratory motion on tomographic reconstructions of the heart: Implications for quantitative nuclear cardiology. J Comput Assist Tomogr 1982; 6:1148–1155.
20. Bergmann SR, Ficke DC, Beecher D, Hood JT, Ter-Pogossian MM. Design parameters and initial testing of Super PET 3000-E: A whole body PET designed for dynamic cardiac imaging. J Nucl Med 1991; 32:1838 (abstract).
21. Cho ZH, Chan JK, Ericksson L, Singh M, Graham S, MacDonald NS, Yano Y. Positron ranges obtained from biomedically important positron-emitting radionuclides. J Nucl Med 1975; 16:1174–1176.
22. Graham MM, Lewellen TK. PET and its role in metabolic imaging. Mayo Clin Proc 1989; 64: 725–727.

Chapter 2

The Physics of Positron Emission Tomography

Stephen L. Bacharach, Ph.D.

Interest in positron emission tomographic (PET) imaging is related in part to its capacity to measure regional physiologic function by tracing the biological fate of compounds that have been tagged with positron-emitting isotopes.

Making accurate measurements with PET requires great care. Attenuation, scatter, accidental coincidences, and dead time, among other factors, may distort images and thus affect the accuracy of the physiologic information to be extracted from them. Often, physiologic information is obtained with the use of mathematical models (discussed in Chapters 5, 7, and 9) that describe how biochemical concentrations change with time. Depending on how these models are used, certain factors potentially causing distortion of data may be minimized, whereas others may become important. To acquire and analyze cardiac PET data accurately, one must be aware of the origins and nature of such distorting factors, most of which can be well understood without extensive knowledge of physics or mathematics. This chapter addresses the principles needed to identify important factors in the performance of PET studies of the heart.

Although it might be assumed that corrections for potentially distorting factors would be incorporated in commercial PET scanners and that such factors therefore could be ignored, such a conclusion would not be justified. For cardiac imaging in particular, the inaccuracies and magnitude of the corrections required often limit the amount of isotope that can be injected, distort the fit of the data to the physiologic models used, or interfere with the proper interpretation of the data.

The Basics of Positron Decay

Most radioactive decay results when the nucleus of an atom emits either an electron or a positron (so-called beta particles). Except for their opposite

From *Positron Emission Tomography of the Heart* edited by Steven R. Bergmann, MD, PhD and Burton E. Sobel, MD © 1992, Futura Publishing Inc., Mount Kisco, NY.

charges, positrons (positively charged beta particles) are nearly identical to electrons (negatively charged beta particles): they have the same mass, and behave similarly. Positrons are the "antimatter" of electrons. When a positron and an electron are in close proximity for more than the briefest interval, both will disappear (called "annihilation"), and their masses will be converted into energy in the form of 2 gamma rays traveling in almost exactly opposite directions. When the nucleus of a positron emitter located in myocardial tissue decays, a fast-moving, high-energy positron is emitted. Initially the positron is moving so fast that it doesn't spend sufficient time near any electron to trigger annihilation. After traveling a few millimeters in tissue, however, the positron slows down as it loses energy and eventually remains close to one of the great number of electrons surrounding the atoms making up the tissue. The positron and the electron annihilate, being converted into 2 gamma rays that possess 0.511 MeV of energy each (the energy equivalent of the mass of each beta particle). Figure 2-1 illustrates this process. Although the annihilation photons are shown traveling in exactly opposite directions, 180° apart, occasionally photons are emitted a few tenths of a degree more or less than 180° apart.

PET scanners detect pairs of gamma rays resulting from annihilation. By determining where these 2 gamma rays (and all other pairs of gamma rays) originated, the PET scanner can produce an image showing where the decaying

POSITRON EMISSION AND ANNIHILATION

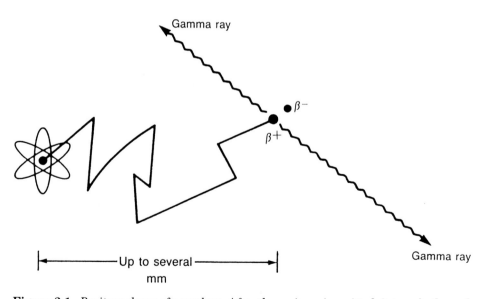

Figure 2-1. *Positron decay of a nucleus. After the positron is emitted, it travels through the surrounding tissue, bouncing off nearby atoms, and losing speed until finally it comes to rest near an electron. The electron and positron annihilate, giving off, in their place, 2 photons of energy (gamma rays), each traveling in opposite directions, and each with exactly 511 keV of energy.*

Table 2-1
Positron Energies and Ranges (in tissue)

Isotope	Max. Energy (MeV)	Avg. Energy (MeV)	Avg. Distance Positrons Travel (mm)	Max. Distance Positrons Travel (mm)
^{18}F	0.635	0.250	0.35	2.3
^{11}C	0.96	0.386	0.56	4.1
^{13}N	1.19	0.492	0.72	5.2
^{15}O	1.72	0.735	1.1	8.1
^{68}Ga	1.90	0.836	1.1	9.4
^{82}Rb*	3.35 (83%)	1.52	2.4	16.7

* Rb emits two different positrons. Eighty-three percent of the time it emits a 3.35 MeV maximum energy positron, and 12% of the time a 2.57 MeV positron.

atoms were located. However, if the positron has traveled far from its parent atom, the image will be inaccurate—the locus of the annihilating positron will not correspond to the locus of the parental radioactive atom. For this reason the initial speed, or energy, of an emitted positron will affect the capacity of the PET scanner to accurately define the position of radioactive atoms within the myocardium. This in turn affects the ultimate spatial resolution of the images that can be obtained with a PET scanner.

Positrons are not emitted with a single characteristic energy as are gamma rays. Instead they have a range of possible energies from 0 up to a characteristic maximum energy. Nevertheless, each positron-emitting radionuclide has its own characteristic maximum and average energy of positron emission, as shown in Table 2-1.[1,2] Because of this, and because the path of the positron as it slows down is quite tortuous, not all the positrons emitted by a given type of atom travel the same distance—some travel quite far and others do not. Table 2-1 shows the maximum and average energies for several common positron emitters used in PET studies, as well as the average distance from the parent atom each positron travels in tissue. The positrons emitted by fluorine-18 (^{18}F) have a very low energy. Thus, on average they travel only a very small distance away from the parent atom (about 0.35 mm). In contrast, oxygen-15 (^{15}O) emits positrons that are considerably more energetic and travel an average of 1.1 mm. Positrons from rubidium-82 (^{82}Rb) travel an average of 2.4 mm. Because the spatial resolution in a typical cardiac PET image is about 7 mm, the extra blurring caused by the range of travel in tissue can be significant for isotopes such as ^{82}Rb, and to a lesser extent, ^{15}O.

Tomograms and Positron Emission

Before it's possible to understand how factors like scatter, attenuation, and the like can alter the tomographic image, it is necessary to understand how tomographic images are made—how they are "reconstructed" from the radioactivity seen by the ring of detectors surrounding the patient. Many treatises have been written dealing with the mathematical steps necessary to produce cross-sectional images with emission tomographs.[3-6] This chapter is limited to a physical, rather than a mathematic description of the process.

To define the three-dimensional shape of an object, one must first be able to look at the object from all sides. This may be an evolutionary advantage of binocular vision (two eyes, not one). Each eye's slightly different view of the same object, when processed by the brain, allows formation of a three-dimensional image of the object's surface. Because our eyes are not placed very far apart we cannot see all sides of an object at once, and so we must extrapolate (often incorrectly) using the information from the side we can see in order to visualize the object's full appearance. In a similar manner, a physician may wish to examine several planar thallium (Tl) scans, each taken at a different angle, in an effort to mentally reconstruct the three-dimensional distribution of Tl in the myocardium. The situation in this case is more complex because nuclear medicine images portray not just the surface of an object, but its interior as well. That is, the object is transparent (except for attenuation) to its radiation.

Just as all sides of an object must be seen to appreciate its three-dimensional surface, many planar views, taken at many angles, are necessary to allow determination of the interior activity concentration of an object. Each of these views at a particular angle is referred to as a "projection." An infinite number of projections are necessary to define the three-dimensional distribution of activity in an object. In practice, cardiac PET images are reconstructed usually from 100 to 200 different views, each at a different angle.

Once the PET scanner has collected data from all these projections, or views, two steps are necessary to create a tomographic slice. The details of these steps are unimportant for understanding the rest of this chapter. They may be considered simply as two mathematical operations that convert the many projections into a single tomographic section or slice. It is important, however, to understand the general idea upon which the "reconstruction" of a tomographic slice is based.

If a person were to examine an object from all sides (i.e., collect all projections), he would be able to describe the three-dimensional shape of the object. It is reasonable to assume that a computer, given this same information (i.e., all the projections) could also be programmed to describe the object. The two steps performed by the computer to do so are "filtering" (which will be described in another context later) and "back-projection." The process of reconstructing a tomographic image by use of these two steps is often called "filtered back-projection."

PET scanners can simultaneously obtain all the views necessary to reconstruct a tomographic image with the use of a ring (or multiple rings) containing hundreds or thousands of detectors that encircle the patient. The mechanical assembly holding all these selectors is called the "gantry." The means by which the ring of detectors acquires data for the many views required can be explained in terms of another analogy to human vision. Each eye is able to form an image of an object from the many rays of light that emanate from that object. To form the image, the eye must be able to determine the direction from which each ray comes. The eye does this by use of a lens to focus each ray of light, at each angle, onto a different spot on the retina. Similarly, each "eye" or crystal detector of the PET camera must be able to define the direction from which each gamma ray that it "sees" (detects) comes. In conventional (as opposed to PET) nuclear imaging, this is done with the use of a lead collimator, which permits only gamma rays that are perpendicular to the crystal face to reach the crystal. Such a scheme blocks out a huge percentage of the gamma rays emitted by the object. In PET imaging, no collimator is needed. Instead, PET makes use of the unique property of positron decay—every positron emitted annihilates and is converted into 2 gamma rays moving in exactly opposite directions. The gamma rays travel at the speed of light. Each may strike and be detected by the 2 members of an opposing pair of detectors in the ring, as shown in Figure 2-2. When this happens, each of the 2 detectors produces an electronic pulse at almost exactly the same time. The 2 detectors record a "coincident event." Detection of a coincident event in a pair of detectors usually implies that the annihilation event occurred somewhere along the line between the 2 detectors. It is further assumed that the radioactive atom that decayed is located along the same line.

COINCIDENCE DETECTION

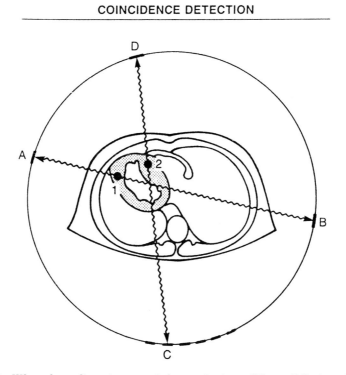

Figure 2-2. *When the radioactive atom 1 decays, it gives off 2 annihilation photons that strike detectors A and B simultaneously. The PET camera can then determine that the radioactive atom must lie somewhere on the line between A and B.*

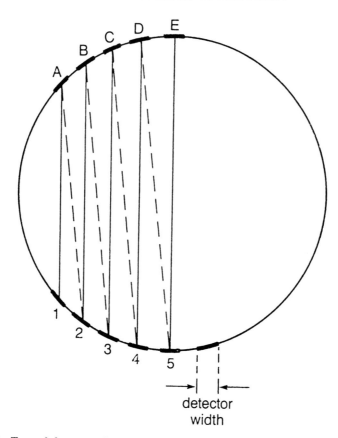

Figure 2-3. *Two of the many "views" or "projections" seen by a PET scanner. Coincidences between detector pairs A-1, B-2, C-3, etc., form one view, as shown by the solid lines. Coincidences A-2, B-3, C-4, etc., form another view, at a slightly different angle, as shown by the dashed lines.*

Coincidence detection serves the same purpose as the lens of the eye or the collimator of the gamma camera—it defines the angle at which the gamma rays have struck the two detectors. For example, as shown in Figure 2-3, if a coincidence event is observed by detectors A and 1, it can be assumed that the positron annihilated somewhere along the line connecting the 2 detectors. Similarly, coincidences between B and 2, C and 3, D and 4, etc., are produced by positrons annihilating along lines connecting each pair of detectors (solid lines in Figure 2-3). Together, the pairs provide a "view" of the object at a given angle. Coincidences between A-2, B-3, C-4, etc. (dashed lines on Figure 2-3), provide another view of the object, at a slightly different angle. The PET camera has electronic circuits that can distinguish coincidences from every possible pair of detectors in the field of view of the camera.

In Figure 2-3, the solid lines comprising one "view" or projection are spaced rather far apart. To allow the PET scanner to distinguish small objects from one another, it is desirable that these lines be as close together as possible.

This is accomplished by making the width of each detector small and placing the detectors as close together as possible. This decreases the spacing between lines and increases the number of possible angles (and therefore the number of views). Of course, increasing the total number of possible coincidences in this way increases the number of crystals, coincidence circuits, and other electronic components required, making the PET scanner more costly.

A factor that limits the number of crystals employed in a PET scanner is the number of photomultiplier tubes required. When a detector "detects" a gamma ray, it produces a small flash of light that is converted to an electronic pulse by a photomultiplier tube. Ideally each crystal would be attached to one photomultiplier tube, but the tubes cannot be made arbitrarily small and are quite expensive. Thus, manufacturers have devised schemes to allow one photo-multiplier tube to share many crystals. Realistically, even by cramming as many detectors as possible into a gantry, one often can't get enough of them around a ring to produce an image with satisfactory resolution. To compensate for this, many PET machines "wobble." That is, the whole gantry is made to move from side to side and up and down, usually in a circular, wobbling motion over a centimeter or more to fill in the missing "gaps" between detectors and therefore allow the spacing between lines to be smaller. A single "wobble" might take anywhere from 0.5 to several seconds.

Most scanners for cardiac imaging use several rings of detectors, often separated by lead shielding called "septa," to acquire data for multiple slices. To increase the number of slices, coincidences are often recorded between one detector in one ring, and an opposing detector in an adjacent ring. Such a slice would be called a "cross" slice. With 3 rings of detectors (numbered I, II, and III) 5 slices could be produced. The first would consist of all coincident events from opposing pairs of detectors in ring I (a direct slice), the second would be a cross slice consisting of all coincident events between 1 detector in ring I and an opposing detector in ring II (or vice versa), the third would be formed from events only in ring II, and so on. Some PET scanners have completely separate rings of detectors. With this design, what constitutes a cross slice and what constitutes a direct slice is obvious. Other scanners have crystals so close to-gether in the Z axis that the concept of physically separate rings no longer applies. What is important in any case is the final spatial resolution obtained (in all 3 directions) and the number of, and spacing between, slices.

Cardiac PET scanners reconstruct transaxial slices. The number and spac-ing of the slices should ideally be such that at least an 8 to 10 cm (and preferably larger) axial distance is encompassed by the slices, a thickness large enough to include the entire left ventricle in most subjects. It is often desirable to include some of the left atrium in the image also (even though it is not usually visualized well) to allow arterial blood concentrations of tracer to be measured. Some scanners permit a slight rotation and tilt of the gantry, but no scanner presently available can be positioned to yield true cardiac short-axis slices directly.

It is important to understand the quantity being measured in the recon-structed image obtained from a PET scan. Each of the projections described previously measures simply the total number of coincidences seen by each detector pair at a given angle during a specific time period (the scan time). For example, in Figure 2-3, one projection is formed by the solid lines A-1, B-2, etc. The quantity measured by each detector pair in this projection is the number of coincidences per second seen along the line, for example that formed by A-1. This "line" is not an infinitesimally thin line, but has a width, because the detector pair A and 1 both have finite width. The number of coincidences seen by the pair A and 1 are those produced by the radioactive material lying between them. The units of the measurement are therefore "coincidences per second per volume." These projection data are reconstructed to determine the number of coincidences arising from each point in the final reconstructed image. Since each point in the image also represents a small piece of volume in the object being imaged, the units are again coincidences per second per volume. Finally, it is assumed that the number of coincidences per second measured in a volume is directly proportional to the amount of radioactive material (usually measured in μCi or mCi) in that same volume. Providing all the corrections described below are made, this assumption is correct. The units of the PET scan can therefore be any of the following: coincidences/sec/cc, μCi/cc, or grams of radiolabeled material/cc. Use of the last unit is possible because microcuries can be easily converted to number of atoms or grams.

Resolution

The term "resolution" has been used above to describe a PET scanner. It requires more careful definition. The spatial resolution of a PET scanner is a measure of how well the scanner can distinguish 2 small objects placed closely together. Certain standard measurements of resolution have been adopted. With one, a very small spot of radioactivity is placed in the scanner's field of view and is imaged. If the range of the positron is very small (e.g., that of a positron from an isotope such as ^{18}F), then comparison of the apparent size of the object in the image and the actual size of the object allows calculation of the scanner's resolution. However, very small point sources of radioactive material are hard to construct. Instead, a thin rod of radioactive material—for example, a long thin needle or capillary tube filled with ^{18}F, may be used. Steel prevents the positrons from leaving the needle. The needle or rod is placed in the center of the scanner, with its long axis perpendicular to the plane of the ring (Figure 2-4). Data are acquired and the image is reconstructed as shown in Figure 2-5. The top right of the Figure shows a plot of the number of coincident events as a function of distance across the image. Typically such a plot follows a bell-shaped, approximately Gaussian curve. By convention, the width of this curve at half its maximum height (full width at half maximum, or FWHM) is used as a measure of spatial resolution. Since the initial measurement is obtained within one slice, or plane, it is called the "in-plane" resolution of the scanner. The in-plane resolution will usually be somewhat larger (perhaps a millimeter or so, depending on the scanner) when the measurement is made at the edge of the field of view, rather than at the center. Because the free wall or apex of the myocardium may be 10 cm or more from the center of

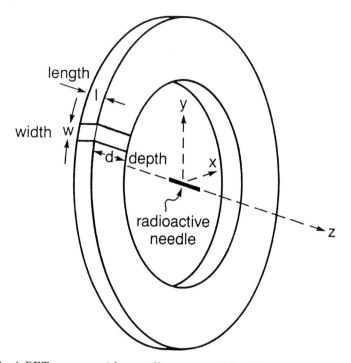

Figure 2-4. *A PET scanner with a needle source positioned to measure in-plane resolution. The dimensions of one typical crystal are also shown. The width W determines how closely spaced together the detectors are around the ring, and so influences the in-plane resolution. The length of the crystal, l, in the z direction similarly affects the axial resolution. The crystals have a depth, d.*

the field in a cardiac PET study, it is useful to know the PET scanner's resolution not just at the center, but also 10 or 15 cm from the center. In addition, at a given distance from the center of the scanner's field of view, the resolution in the anterior-posterior or Y direction may not be the same as that in the lateral, or X direction.

The scanner shown in Figure 2-3 is made up of crystals with a width W. The detectors of a real scanner, of course, would extend in and out of the plane of paper—that is, they would have a finite length, l, in the axial or Z direction, and would also have a depth, d, as shown in Figure 2-4. As pointed out previously the width, W, of the detectors influences the in-plane resolution. Similarly the length, l, of the detector in the Z direction determines, in part, the resolution of the scanner in the axial direction. To measure the resolution in this direction, a small "dot" of radioactive material, placed on the bed of the gantry, might be used. An image could be made of this dot of activity, the source could be moved through the gantry by 1 or 2 mm, and a second image made. Progressively moving the source of activity through the scanner in 1 or 2 mm steps, making an image at each location, would result in a series of images as a function of the Z axis position of the source. Plotting the number of coincident events in each image as a function of the Z axis position (clinically,

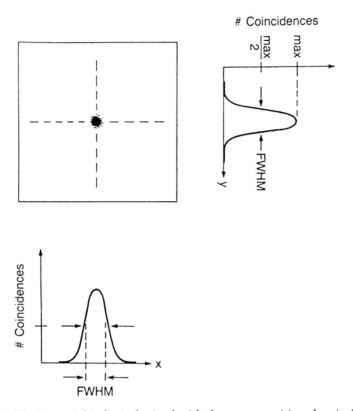

Figure 2-5. *The image (of 1 slice) obtained with the source positioned as in figure 2-4. The image is blurred because of the finite spatial resolution of the machine. The plot to the right shows the number of coincidences through the image in the vertical direction (the dotted line in the y direction). The lower plot shows the number of coincidences in the image along the horizontal (x direction) line. The FWHM of these plots defines the spatial resolution of the scanner.*

the bed position), would produce a plot similar to those in Figure 2-5. The FWHM resolution in the Z axis direction is often called the "slice thickness" because it is a measure of how far into the Z axis the slice extends. A PET scanner, then, has at least possibly two very different spatial resolutions: the in-plane resolution (made up of the resolution in the anterior-posterior direction and the lateral directions, which are usually about the same) and the Z axis, or axial resolution.

The axial resolution, or slice thickness, should not be confused with the separation between slices. The two are entirely independent of each other. Spacing between slices may be greater or less than the thickness of each slice. If the spacing between slices is less than the thickness of the slice (as measured by the FWHM), then the slices may be considered to partially overlap. Even if the spacing between slices is greater than the slice thickness, some overlap will be present because the "edges" of a slice are not sharp but exhibit a Gaussian distribution (Figure 2-5).

There are currently two schools of thought concerning optimal slice spacing and Z axis resolution for cardiac studies. According to one, the resolution in the Z direction should be the same as the in-plane resolution, theoretically making it easier to "re-slice" the data into short- and long-axis slices and to quantitate in 3 dimensions (an as yet unachieved goal). Proponents of this school of thought believe that detection of small abnormalities will be facilitated by good resolution along the Z axis, even if there are small gaps between slices. Others believe that it is acceptable (and even desirable) to have slightly thicker slices that overlap. They theorize that reslicing of thick or thin slices is equally accurate and since slices overlap, a defect could be found that would be missed if it were situated between the slices constructed by a machine that acquires thin, nonoverlapping slices. It is not yet clear which approach is the better one.

The resolution of a PET scanner is determined by:[17] the design of the machine (including crystal size and spacing, ring diameter, and wobbling radius among other factors); physical factors such as the finite range of positrons in tissue and the deviation of annihilation photons from exact collinearity; and processing, including smoothing (see below) performed on reconstructed images. The noncollinearity of the annihilation photons, which can be as much as several tenths of a degree, causes the FWHM to increase by a millimeter or so over its theoretical value. Positron range and image processing are to some extent controllable, as discussed below.

If the number of positrons detected is plotted as a function of distance in tissue from the source, the number decreases almost exponentially with distance.[2] However, some of the positrons travel relatively far, altering the resolution curve (Figure 2-5). The resolution curve produced by radioisotopes emitting very energetic positrons is a combination of the typical Gaussian curve illustrated in Figure 2-5 and the approximately exponential curve associated with positron penetration.[7] Therefore, the curve is roughly Gaussian in shape near the center, but exhibits a long, nearly exponential tail. The amount of degradation in resolution that would occur with use of a positron with a relatively long range in tissue, such as ^{82}Rb, can be estimated as follows:

$$\text{Final resolution} = (R^2 + 1.89*D^2)^{0.5} \qquad (1)$$

where R is the resolution of the scanner (including any smoothing) measured with a nearly zero-range positron source (e.g., when ^{18}F in a thin steel needle is used) and D is the average distance the positron travels, as shown in table 2-1.

For example, with a scanner with 7 mm useable resolution as measured with ^{18}F, the resolution expected with the use of ^{82}Rb is based on the average distance a ^{82}Rb positron travels (D), 2.3 mm. The resolution of ^{82}Rb scan can be calculated from the equation above to yield a final resolution of approximately 7.7 FWHM—about a 10% increase in FWHM resolution compared with that of a lower energy positron emitter. The factor of 1.89 is entered into equation 1 in consideration of the fact that the number of positrons decreases with distance in an exponential rather than a Gaussian manner. Because the resolution curve is not Gaussian with an isotope such as ^{82}Rb, specifying the FWHM does not tell the full story. Because the number of positrons decreases exponentially with distance from the source, many positrons will travel much farther than the average. Some ^{82}Rb positrons will travel more than a centimeter before annihilating. This produces an exponential tail on the resolution curve, in turn causing a small fraction of the counts in one part of an image to blur into other, distant parts of the image. To describe this effect, the full width at tenth maximum (FWTM) is measured in addition to FWHM. The FWTM for a ^{82}Rb image is approximately 19 mm compared with about 13 mm for ^{18}F.

To reduce the point-to-point random statistical fluctuations (called "noise") that are invariably present in a PET image, an image is often "smoothed" by averaging adjacent picture element (pixel) values together. Although this reduces image noise, it degrades resolution.

Various filters can be used at the time of reconstruction to facilitate smoothing. "Filtering" is the name given to the process of averaging neighboring pixels together[8] by replacing a pixel value with a weighted average of itself and its neighbors. For example, one commonly used filter replaces a pixel value with one-half times its own value plus one-eighth times each of its 4 nearest neighbor's values, so that the weighting factors for this filter would be $\frac{1}{2}$ and $\frac{1}{8}$. Such a filter will produce a less noisy image, but one with poorer spatial resolution. The filters most commonly used to smooth PET images are given names (e.g., the "Hanning" and "Butterworth" filters). Despite their specialized names, all filters do nothing more than average neighboring pixels together; they differ only in their weighting factors, which may be positive or negative.

In addition to filters that smooth but worsen resolution, filters exist that improve resolution and exaggerate noise. Unfortunately, it is a consequence of the basic laws of physics that it is impossible to simultaneously reduce noise and improve resolution, and because of statistical fluctuations caused by the limited numbers of coincident events, PET images almost always must be filtered with a smoothing, rather than a resolution-improving, filter. Available PET scanner software usually gives the investigator a choice of which smoothing filter to use at the time of image reconstruction. The term "filtered" in filtered back-projection does not, however, refer to these smoothing filters. Rather the "ramp" filter is a specialized filter (one that worsens noise) that is an intrinsic and fundamental part of the reconstruction process. For convenience, the smoothing and ramp filters are usually both applied at the same time.

Images reconstructed from detection of many photons (those, for example, acquired over a long interval or after injection of a large quantity of radioisotope), do not contain a great deal of noise. In such cases, it may be best to select a filter that does only a very minimal amount of smoothing to obtain the best spatial resolution possible. In contrast, under conditions in which imaging time is limited, or only a small amount of radioisotope can be administered, a filter that smooths the data more extensively may be necessary at the cost of resolution. Many different smoothing filters are available on commercial PET scanners. The best way to visualize their effects on image quality is to apply them to images of point or line sources in order to observe their effect on resolution, and to apply them to low count images, (e.g., a 20 cm uniform phantom imaged for only a short time) to observe their effect on noise.

It is important to clarify the difference between resolution and the distance between pixels. Imagine a PET scanner with 7 mm in-plane resolution (i.e., 7 mm FWHM) and a 41 cm field of view. The reconstructed image could be stored in an array (i.e., a digitized image) of 256 × 256 pixels. Each pixel would be 41 cm/256 or 1.6 mm apart. The 7 mm FWHM would therefore correspond to about 4.4 pixels. If instead the reconstructed image were stored in a 512 × 512 matrix, each pixel would comprise 41 cm/512 or 0.8 mm. The resolution would remain 7 mm FWHM which, with this matrix size, would be represented by 8.8 pixels. Resolution is a function of the scanner and any filtering that may be applied to the image; it cannot be improved by increasing the number of pixels in the image matrix. Below a certain number of pixels per centimeter, however, the image will no longer be able to reflect the resolution inherent in the scanner. In general, with PET images acquired in vivo, at least 3 pixels should be available for every FWHM.

Pixels are spaced a fixed distance apart in the x and y direction. With the use of a multislice machine, the data can be organized into pixels in the Z direction as well (e.g., if the transaxial slices are reorganized in coronal or sagittal views). A pixel, then, can be thought of as occupying a volume in space, in which case it is referred to as a voxel.

The Partial Volume Effect

Quantitative data are extracted from PET images with the aid of regions of interest drawn on the images. Analysis of the data contained in such regions yields either the total number of events per second occurring within the region that is proportional to the total activity in the region, or the mean number of events per second per pixel within the region that is proportional to the average concentration of activity in the region. The resolution of the PET scanner, the size and placement of the region of interest, and the true anatomic size of the structure imaged all influence the accuracy of such measurements. Collectively, such influences are referred to by the term partial volume effect.[9]

To better understand what the partial volume effect is, assume that a perfect PET scanner exists, and it is used to image a 2 cm diameter cylinder of radioactivity. Assume further that after imaging for 100 seconds, 100,000 coincident events would be detected (therefore 1000 events/sec) in a transaxial slice of the cylinder. The perfect scanner would produce an image like the one shown at the top left of Figure 2-6. All pixels within the cylinder would have the same value, and all pixels outside it would have the value zero. Placing a 2 cm diameter region of interest around the image of the cylindrical object would give the total number of coincidences per second coming from the object (i.e., 1000 coincidences/sec). All of the coincidences that were detected would occur within the region of interest.

If the same 2 cm diameter cylinder of radioactivity was imaged with an imperfect PET scanner (one with 7 mm FWHM resolution), the same 100,000

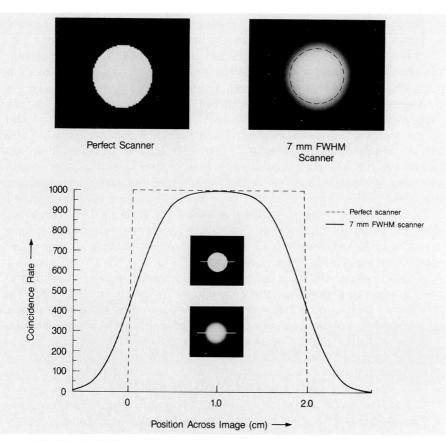

Figure 2-6. *(Top left) The image of a 2 cm diameter cylinder as produced with an "ideal" PET scanner. (Top right) The same 2 cm diameter cylinder imaged with a PET scanner with 7 mm FWHM resolution. (Bottom) Plot of counts across the 2 images. The ideal PET scanner gives a flat curve, with a value of 1000 events/sec everywhere inside the 2 cm region. The "actual" PET scanner gives only a small central region, which is flat. Note that many of the counts blur outside of the 2 cm borders (shown as dashed line) of the imaged object.*

coincidences (or 1000/sec) would be detected, but some of the coincidences would be blurred or spread out (Figure 2-6, top right). Some counts from pixels near the edge would be smeared into the region outside the true dimensions of the cylinder. Those from pixels near the center of the cylinder would not be affected as much because just as many counts would be blurred out as blurred into them from neighboring pixels. The same 2 cm diameter region of interest (shown as a dashed circle in the top right of Figure 2-6) would now produce a value of only 785 events/sec, the other 215 coincident events/sec being spread out over pixels outside of the region of interest. The percentage of the counts retained in the region of interest is termed the "recovery coefficient," 785 of 1000 or 78.5% in this case.

The term "partial volume effect" describes the resolution effect by which counts obtained from a region of interest applied to an image with finite resolution are fewer than those in the same region applied to an image from an "ideal" PET scanner. The poorer the resolution, the more blurred the data will be and the fraction of counts "recovered" within a given region of interest will be lower. As shown in Figure 2-6, a larger fraction of the total events can be recovered by enlarging the region of interest to more than the true 2 cm object size. Again referring to the example in Figure 2-6, if the region of interest were increased to 2.4 cm, 914 of the original total 1000 events/sec would be recovered. If the region were sufficiently large, all the original events would be recovered. Unfortunately, in patients, the size of the region drawn may be limited by the presence of substantial amounts of activity in structures close to the organ being imaged.

In the discussion so far, it has been tacitly assumed that the only quantity of interest is the total activity in the region, or the total number of events per second occurring in the "organ" (in this case, the cylinder). More commonly, the concentration of activity in a region being imaged is sought. For example, consider an image of myocardium obtained after intravenous administration of ^{18}F-fluorodeoxyglucose to a patient. Such an image is generally analyzed by dividing the image into small pieces (often by sector analysis or a circumferential profile method) and comparing selected anatomic regions to one another. The total activity in each piece will depend on the size (i.e., volume) of the piece chosen. Usually it is not useful or possible to analyze only pieces (regions) of the myocardium with exactly the same myocardial volume; instead, the size of pieces is varied to correspond to anatomic structure (free wall, apex, etc.) or territory supplied by a particular vessel. For this reason, the count rate obtained from each small piece is normalized by dividing by the number of pixels (i.e., the volume) in the region. This gives units of events per second per pixel. Since, as described previously, each pixel represents a small volume element, and events per second represent activity, the result is a measure of concentration of activity.

We must now reconsider what impact the partial volume effect will have on accuracy of measurements of concentrations of activity. Drawing "too large" a region in an effort to recover all the counts will actually have the opposite effect on activity concentration measurements. It will reduce the measured counts per second per pixel by increasing the total number of pixels. Again, consider the 2 cm diameter cylinder shown in Figure 2-6. The "ideal" PET scanner might, for example, yield 1000 events/sec total within the 2 cm diameter. If each pixel were 2 mm apart, this would correspond to about 0.75 counts per second per pixel. This value could be converted to a concentration of activity of perhaps 5 nCi/ml. The ideal PET scanner would, therefore, yield a value of 5 nCi/ml at every pixel within the 2 cm diameter, and zero outside. The mean value within any region of interest of 2.0 cm diameter or smaller would give the same value of 5 nCi/ml. If the region were enlarged to more than the true size of the object, however, the measured nanocuries per milliliter would fall because the region of interest would begin to include some pixels with 0 nCi/ml. For the 7 mm FWHM PET scanner producing the image in Figure 2-6 right, the 2.0 cm region of interest would yield too low a value for concentration of activity because events near the edge of the object would smear out to pixels outside the region. For the situation depicted in Figure 2-6, the drop would be from 5 to 3.9 nCi/ml, again with a recovery coefficient of 78.5%. If the region of interest were decreased in size, however, it would no longer include pixels near the edge and the concentration of activity would approximate the correct value of 5 nCi/ml. If the region of interest were 1.8 cm in diameter, the average counts per second per pixel would correspond to 4.3 nCi/ml (85% recovery), and if the region of interest were decreased still further to 1.6 cm, the value would be 4.5 nCi/ml (90% recovery). For measurements in nanocuries per milliliter or counts per second per pixel then, the smaller the region of interest in relation to the object size, the more accurate the value.

Unfortunately, as the region of interest gets smaller, so does the total number of events contained in it, causing statistical fluctuations (the standard deviation) to increase. Conversely, if the region of interest is too large (larger than the object being imaged), the mean "nCi/ml" value drops. A rule of thumb is that if the edge of the region of interest is more than 1 FWHM interior to the object's anatomic borders, the influence of the partial volume effect will be negligible. Unfortunately, myocardial walls are typically no thicker than 1 to 2 cm (except in certain disease states), whereas FWHMs are typically no less than 0.7 cm. It will often be impossible to draw a region that is 1 FWHM from both epi- and endocardial borders. Accordingly, myocardial PET images are significantly influenced by partial volume effects. In general, recovery coefficients are significantly less than 100%.

In summary: (1) To measure only the total activity within an organ, the region of interest should be drawn very generously (if there are no nearby structures containing activity) around the whole organ being imaged. Ideally, edges of the region of interest should be at least 1 FWHM larger than the true organ borders. This will lead to recovery of nearly all events that have "blurred out" of the organ. (2) To measure radioactive concentrations within an organ rather than simply activity: (a) the region must be smaller than the anatomic region of interest by 1 FWHM circumferentially; otherwise, recovery will be flawed, (b) for the same proportional size region of interest and the same PET resolution, thin myocardial walls will give lower recovery than thick walls, and (c) for a given myocardial wall thickness and a given PET spatial resolution, small regions will yield higher recovery values than large regions. Unfortunately, smaller regions will also give rise to greater statistical fluctuations because they contain fewer events. An important practical consequence of "b" above, is that, in general, activity concentrations measured from thin myocardial walls will be erroneously lower than those from thicker walls. This so-called partial volume effect may therefore significantly distort both the appearance of the image and the quantitative data derived from it.

It has been assumed that the activity concentration is uniform within the region of interest. If this is not the case, results should be suspect because the mean value within a region of interest will depend on the position of the region within the heterogeneous structure.

Another important factor that influences the accuracy of PET data is the effect of the finite resolution in the Z direction. Just as in-plane blurring causes counts to be smeared out within a slice, nonperfect resolution along the Z axis causes counts to be blurred out of the plane of a slice and may cause counts from objects outside the imaging plane to erroneously appear within it. If a set of transaxial slices is resliced into long- or short-axis pieces or into coronal or sagittal views, what was once Z axis blurring becomes part of in-plane blurring. This should be taken into account when drawing regions from the resliced data. If the Z axis resolution is different from that in the x and y resolutions, the data obtained after reslicing will have a spatial resolution that varies with direction, rendering assessment of the magnitude of the partial volume effect more complex.

It is possible to correct for the partial volume effect. If the true anatomic dimensions of the object being imaged and the resolution of the PET scanner producing the image are known, it is possible to calculate the recovery coefficients and use them to correct the data.[10] Unfortunately, the effects of cardiac wall motion also come into play. Sections of myocardium may move into and out of a region of interest as the ventricle contracts. In early generation scanners, the resolution was significantly greater than the magnitude of typical wall motion within a slice. In machines being used currently, this is no longer the case and wall motion may play a significant role in degrading quantitative data. By measurement of both the wall thickness and the wall thickening (for example, with a gated cardiac nuclear magnetic resonance system) the recovery coefficient at each myocardial segment can be defined and used to correct the image. To date, such a correction has not been reported.

Another method for correcting for partial volume effects will be discussed in chapter 5. It involves describing the clearance of radioactive tracer from the myocardium with the use of a mathematical model. The influence of the partial volume effects can sometimes be included in such models. When this is the case, data fits to the mathematical model can be used to calculate the recovery coefficient.[11]

Accidental Coincidences

The 2 gamma rays that cause a "coincidence" are assumed to strike their respective detectors simultaneously. However, the annihilation gamma rays do not always reach both detectors at exactly the same time. Because gamma rays travel at the speed of light, it takes them about $1.33 * 10^{-9}$ seconds (1.33 nsec) to travel the 40 cm or so from the center of the ring to one of the detectors. If an annihilation has taken place somewhere other than at the center, 1 of the 2 gamma rays will reach its detector earlier than the other. In addition, the detector/photomultiplier combination is usually not able to produce electronic pulses timed more accurately than within a few nanoseconds. For these reasons, "simultaneous" detection refers to detection within a so-called resolving time, τ, which is set electronically in the PET scanner. Typical resolving times for PET scanners are about 10 to 20 nsec. Any 2 photons that are detected within this resolving time are considered to have occurred in coincidence. Unfortunately, it is quite possible for 2 photons that did not come from the same

RANDOMS

- Two single, unrelated photons are <u>accidentally</u> detected at same time

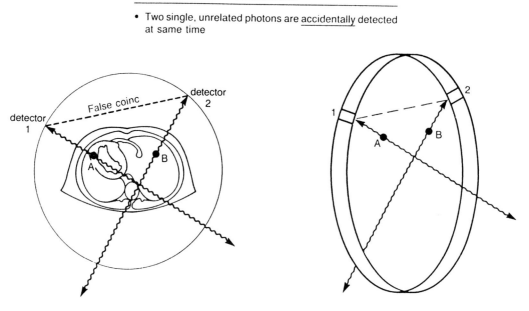

- # Randoms α (Activity)^2

Figure 2-7. *An "accidental" coincidence. Radioactive atom A decays at nearly the same instant as radioactive atom B. One of the photons emitted by A strikes detector 1. The other photon from A either misses its detector (as shown on the right) or passes through it without being detected. Similarly, one of the photons from atom B is detected by detector 2 while its opposing photon is not detected. Because detectors 1 and 2 both detect photons at nearly the same time, the PET camera falsely computes the location of the radioactive atom as lying on the line between the 2 detectors (the dashed line).*

annihilation event to be erroneously identified, quite by accident, as having occurred "simultaneously," or within the resolving time τ of the PET scanner. Figure 2-7 illustrates such a case. Only 1 of the photons from annihilation A has reached a detector; the other missed the ring. At nearly the same time atom B decayed. Only 1 of its photons was detected, the other also missing the ring. If these two separate events happen to occur at nearly the same time within the resolving time of the PET scanner, they will be considered to be in coincidence. The PET scanner then will falsely treat the detection of the 2 photons as if they reflected a single annihilation that took place along the line between the 2 detectors (the dashed line in Figure 2-7). Such false coincidence is called accidental, or random coincidence. It accounts for background activity in the reconstructed image that varies in magnitude at different positions over the image.

Accidental coincidences between unrelated photons must be distinguished from "true" coincidences between pairs of annihilation photons. The probability that an accidental coincidence will occur depends on the duration of the resolving time interval, τ: if it is very long, it becomes much more likely for 2 unrelated photons to be accidentally in coincidence. The resolving time of a PET scanner is therefore an important parameter defining how well the scanner will distinguish true coincidences from accidental ones.

A second factor influencing the number of accidental events recorded is the amount and location of activity detected by the PET scanner. If the activity within the patient is doubled, the number of true coincidences will of course double also. The number of accidental coincidences, however, will increase by a factor of 4, i.e., as the square of activity. This has important ramifications. At sufficiently high levels of activity, the number of accidental coincidences may equal or even exceed true coincidences. With administration of excessive amounts of tracer, the patient may, therefore, be exposed to a higher radiation risk without a comparable increase in the amount of useful information obtained. The amount of activity constituting an excess varies with the machine used; it may be only a few millicuries in the field of view or as much as 10 or more mCi.

The reason that accidental events increase as the square of activity can be discerned from consideration of Figure 2-7. Suppose that detector 1 measures S1 (S refers to singles) counts per second, independent of whether these counts were in coincidence with any other detector. The count rate observed by a single detector, as opposed to a coincident pair of detectors, is called the singles count rate of that detector. Suppose also that detector 2 measures a singles rate of S2 per second. Consider that 1 photon has just struck detector 1. If an unrelated photon were to hit detector 2 within the next τ seconds or has already hit detector 2 within the previous τ seconds, it will be in accidental coincidence with the event recognized by detector 1. Because there are S2 events detected by detector 2 each second, the number of these that will occur during the τ seconds before or the τ seconds after the event in S1 is S2 * 2τ. For every photon that strikes detector 1, there are therefore 2τ*S2 accidental coincidences per second. However, there are S1 photons striking detector 1 every second. Therefore the total number of accidental coincidences per second is:

$$\text{Accidental Coincidences/sec} = 2 * \tau * S1 * S2 \qquad (2)$$

If the activity in the patient is doubled, the singles rate for every detector is also doubled, so both S1 and S2 double, giving a factor of 4 increase in accidental coincidences.

Consideration of equation 2 suggests a way to correct for accidental coincidences. If the singles rate is measured at every detector, the number of accidental coincidences can be computed for every detector pair, and this number can be subtracted from the measured true events. Although measured singles rates include some counts from true coincidences, singles rates usually greatly exceed true coincidence rates. Thus, the error introduced by such a correction scheme is fairly small.

Another approach to correction for random coincidences is the delayed coincidence method. Consider a single pair of opposing detectors, one of which has a long wire connected to its output. This wire is passed through a special circuit (or even a long length of wire) that causes a prolongation of travel time for the signal, perhaps of several 100 nsec. This second wire is connected to the usual circuit, which determines whether the 2 pulses (from the delayed signal from the second wire of 1 detector, and the undelayed, first wire of the opposing detector) occurred within time τ of each other. If a true coincidence event occurs, the delayed signal traveling down the second wire will not register as a coincidence with the undelayed signal of the opposing detector. The signal traveling down the long wire would reach the coincidence electronics much later than the undelayed signal from the opposing detector. Any coincidences measured by this long wire would, therefore, only be accidental coincidences, and not true. They could, therefore, be subtracted from the total number of coincidences measured with the undelayed standard short wires of both detectors to yield the number of true coincidences. The delayed coincidence method is quite accurate. However, it is limited by low signal-to-noise ratios because the number of randoms measured by the second delayed wire is often quite small, which may introduce additional noise into the final corrected image (although a technique has been proposed to reduce such noise[12]). On the other hand, use of the singles method discussed previously adds little noise to the image because the number of singles recorded by each detector is so high. However, this method requires measurement of τ, which is possible but subject to inaccuracies.

Attenuation

If 511 keV annihilation gamma rays were made to travel through a substance with a very high atomic number, such as a lead brick, only a few of the photons would pass completely through the brick unaltered. Most of the photons would interact with the atoms of lead. Of those that interacted, some would do so by a process called the photoelectric effect, which involves both an atomic electron and the nucleus of the lead atom. In this process, the photon completely disappears. It is totally absorbed or "stopped" by the lead, its energy transferred to the nucleus and a fast-moving atomic electron. Other gamma rays passing through the lead brick would interact by a process called scattering (or more properly Compton scattering, after A.H. Compton, its discoverer). In this process, the photon strikes 1 of the atomic electrons surrounding the atom, the gamma ray is deflected from its original direction and continues in a new direction with reduced energy. The bigger the angle of deflection, the more energy the gamma ray will have lost. A photon undergoing such a collision is said to have scattered. In lead, the two processes—complete absorption or stopping, and scattering—are both likely. In soft tissue, complete absorption almost never occurs. Instead, essentially all interactions result in the photon scattering. Even in bone, 511 keV photons are absorbed only rarely. Instead they simply scatter.

In a small region of myocardium with an appreciable concentration of radiotracer many annihilation gamma ray pairs are emitted in all directions. Some small fraction of these photons will be headed in a direction such that both photons would strike a detector in the ring. As these photons travel toward the detector, they must pass through the tissue of the body. If either of the photons scatters, it will no longer be headed toward the detector. In all probability it will miss the ring entirely, or on those rare occasions that it does not, its energy will often be too reduced to be detected (what happens to those that still get detected after scattering will be considered subsequently). A coincident event that would have occurred in the absence of intervening tissue, now does not occur (Figure 2-8). The photons emanating from this small section of the myocardium are said to have been attenuated, and the loss of detected events due to interactions with atoms of the intervening tissue is termed attenuation. The number of photons that make it through unscathed decreases exponentially with the thickness (d) of interposed tissue

$$(\text{No. of photons reaching the detector}) =$$

$$(\text{No. of photons headed for detector}) * e^{-\mu d} \qquad (3)$$

The constant μ is the attenuation coefficient, and has a value 0.096 cm^{-1} for 511 keV photons in soft tissue. As seen from the equation, only half of the photons will make it through 7.2 cm of tissue. Lower energy photons, such as those emitted by ^{201}Tl (80 keV) are attenuated more easily, because μ is higher at lower energies. It takes only 4 cm of tissue to stop half the photons of ^{201}Tl from reaching their original destination. It would, therefore, seem that atten-

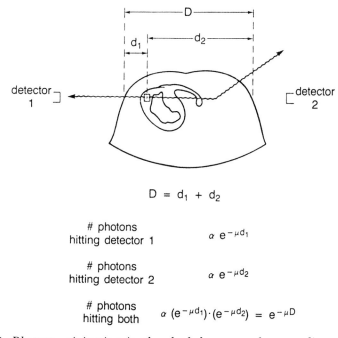

$$D = d_1 + d_2$$

# photons hitting detector 1	$\alpha\ e^{-\mu d_1}$
# photons hitting detector 2	$\alpha\ e^{-\mu d_2}$
# photons hitting both	$\alpha\ (e^{-\mu d_1})\cdot(e^{-\mu d_2}) = e^{-\mu D}$

Figure 2-8. *Photons originating in the shaded square of myocardium must travel through a distance d1 to reach detector 1 and a distance d2 to reach detector 2. The situation shown here illustrates that 1 of the 2 photons may be "attenuated" by being deflected from its path and never reach a detector (d2 in this case). The deflected photon will also be reduced in energy. The probability of both photons reaching their respective detectors is determined by the total attenuation, $e^{-\mu D}$.*

uation would be much more significant for thallium scans than for PET scans, because the low-energy Tl photons used for thallium scintigraphy are so much more easily attenuated. This presumption is incorrect, however. In a PET scan, both photons in a pair must reach their respective detectors. As illustrated in Figure 2-8, a photon P1, headed toward detector 1, must travel through a thickness of tissue d1 without interaction, and a photon P2 must travel through thickness d2 intact. The total attenuation is then

$$
\begin{aligned}
\text{No. of coincidences} &= (\text{No. headed in right direction}) * (\text{probability P1 gets} \\
&\quad \text{through}) * (\text{probability P2 gets through}) \\
&= (\text{No. headed in right direction}) * e^{-\mu(d1)} * e^{-\mu(d2)} \\
&= (\text{No. headed in right direction}) * e^{-\mu(d1+d2)} \text{ or} \\
\text{coincidences} &= (\text{No. headed in right direction}) * e^{-\mu*D}
\end{aligned}
\tag{4}
$$

where D is the total distance, d1 + d2, through the body. The attenuation occurring for a pair of photons in a PET scan can be calculated from equation 4 and measurements of d1 and d2 from an image as shown in Figure 2-8. Excluding the lungs (which attenuate about one-third as much as soft tissue), the distance through tissue might typically be about 23 cm. Equation 4 gives

$$
\text{No. of coincidences} = (\text{No. headed in right direction}) * (0.11)
\tag{5}
$$

Eighty-nine percent of the photons will be attenuated—only 11% will make it through the body in this direction. Photons traveling in other directions toward other detectors and those originating from other sections of the myocardium may be more extensively attenuated. In a 70 kg subject, attenuation by factors of 10 to 20 is common. Attenuation is even greater in obese subjects.

Obviously, attenuation has significant effects on the results of cardiac PET scans. Although this problem is serious with PET because both photons in a pair must survive intact (attenuation factor, $e^{-\mu(d1+d2)}$), accurate attenuation correction is possible. In contrast, with methods such as single-photon emission computed tomography (SPECT) in which only one photon is involved, such correction is not possible because the attenuation correction factor, $e^{-\mu d1}$, depends on measurement of the depth at which the isotope is located in tissue. This measurement cannot be made before imaging. The value necessary for attenuation correction of PET images, however, is (d1 + d2). This quantity is independent of how deep the isotope is located in the body and depends only upon the attenuation through the total body thickness, which can be measured accurately. The most common method for making this measurement involves performance of a "blank" scan and an "attenuation" scan (often called a transmission scan). Figure 2-9 illustrates this approach for one detector pair. Before the patient to be imaged is placed in the ring, a small positron-emitting source is placed at one side (as in Figure 2-9, top) and a scan, called the "blank," is

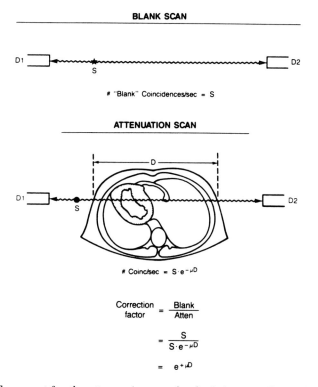

BLANK SCAN

D1 ⟵⟶ D2

S

\# "Blank" Coincidences/sec = S

ATTENUATION SCAN

D1 ⟵⟶ D2

S

\# Coinc/sec $= S \cdot e^{-\mu D}$

$$\frac{\text{Correction}}{\text{factor}} = \frac{\text{Blank}}{\text{Atten}}$$

$$= \frac{S}{S \cdot e^{-\mu D}}$$

$$= e^{+\mu D}$$

Figure 2-9. *To correct for the attenuation seen by the 2 detectors D1 and D2, the coincidences from a "blank" scan are measured by placing a source in the scanner without the patient (top), and then repeating the measurement with the patient in the gantry (bottom). The correction factor is the ratio of the 2 measurements.*

made. The position of the source is maintained, and the patient is positioned in the ring (before injection of the isotope). A second scan, the attenuation (or transmission) scan, is made (Figure 2-9, bottom). The difference in the counts detected in the blank and transmission scans results from attenuation through the patient. For example, if S coincident counts were recorded by the detector pair shown in Figure 2-9 in the blank scan, then $S*e^{-\mu*D}$ counts would be recorded by the same detector pair when the patient was interposed. The ratio of the blank scan counts to the transmission scan counts gives the factor $e^{+\mu*D}$, which is the factor needed to correct for attenuation for this detector pair. Making the same measurement for all detector pairs permits complete attenuation correction.

In practice, a cylindrical ring of activity is often used to obtain the blank and attenuation scans, so that all detector pairs can be measured simultaneously. Alternatively, a rod of activity can be used with its long dimension oriented along the Z axis (Figure 2-10). Such a rod is attached to a mechanism that rotates it at a fixed speed around the gantry. The rod source is far easier to handle and store (both ring and rod typically might contain a few mCi of activity), and more importantly, can produce better quality attenuation scans

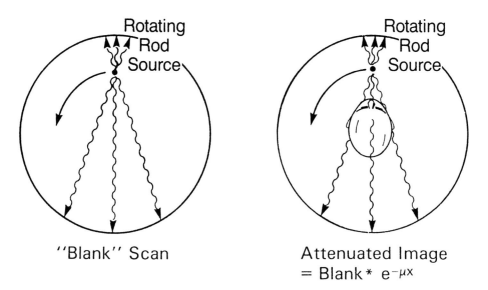

"Blank" Scan

Attenuated Image
= Blank * $e^{-\mu x}$

Figure 2-10. *To correct for the attenuation seen by all detectors, often a rod of activity is rotated about the gantry. The correction factor for each detector pair is computed from the ratio of the values obtained in the blank to the values obtained in the attenuation scan.*

than the ring. As the rod rotates, only those detectors that lie on the line formed by the detector, the rod, and the opposing detector can possibly be in coincidence. By turning on only the appropriate detectors as the rod rotates around the gantry, most accidental and scatter coincidences can be eliminated. The total count rate is, therefore, comprised primarily of true coincidence events. This yields a much higher quality scan in the same time that would be required if a ring were used because the ring gives a much larger fraction of random and scattered counts than the rod.

A typical scanning sequence is: (1) obtain a blank scan, (2) position the patient in the gantry and obtain a transmission scan, and (3) without moving the patient, inject the tracer and begin emission imaging. Unfortunately, tracers used for some scans (e.g., fluorodeoxyglucose) require up to a 30 minute delay after injection of the tracer before imaging. During this interval, the patient may move, in which case the attenuation correction factors computed from the blank and transmission scans will no longer apply. Very little information is available defining what the effects of patient motion might be in a given case, but they are likely to be appreciable. One approach to solving this problem has been to obtain the transmission scan after injection of the isotope[13,14] rather than before and to compensate for those photons emanating from the injected isotope. This minimizes the time delay between measurement of the attenuation correction factors and acquisition of the scan. The method has only been tested, however, for brain imaging. It is exceptionally sensitive to the values of certain of the correction factors discussed below and may be difficult to apply to thoracic imaging.

Scatter

When annihilation photons pass through tissue, they frequently collide with electrons. In these scattering collisions, the photon is deflected from its original direction and loses some fraction of its energy. The higher the angle of deflection, the greater the energy loss. The great majority of scattered photons never reach a detector, as illustrated in Figure 2-8. A small percentage of scattered photons, however, may still hit a detector in the ring and register coincidences, as shown in Figure 2-11. When this occurs, the PET camera erroneously computes the position of the radioactive atom (dotted line in Figure 2-11). Such mispositioning of events can cause false counts to appear in cold areas of an image when a hot region is nearby. In general, the phenomenon slightly blurs sources of radioactivity from one region into quite distant regions. This is of particular importance in cardiac imaging, since the observer is frequently trying to detect defects of uptake in segments of myocardium adjacent to normal regions.

Most PET scanners are designed to exclude errors resulting from detection of photons that have been scattered by quantifying photon energy and rejecting those photons with energy below a certain threshold value. Unfortunately, bismuth germinate (BGO) crystals (the most common crystals in use today) cannot measure the energy of the detected photons very accurately, but only to within about ± 150 keV. Thus, the best the threshold can be for this purpose

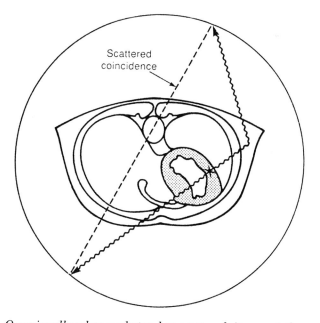

Figure 2-11. *Occasionally when a photon has scattered, it may strike another detector and be detected. This results in a false, "scattered" coincidence, as shown by the dotted line.*

is about 360 keV (511 minus 150). This energy threshold results in rejection of all photons that have been scattered by more than about 57°, but not those scattered less. Because photons are more likely to scatter at small angles, a large number of scattered photons will be detected. Attempts to raise the energy threshold to, for example, 400 keV, would result in the rejection of photons that had scattered by more than 44°, but a significant fraction of unscattered photons would be rejected as well, because of the failure of BGO crystals to quantify energy of individual photons accurately. Energy rejection can, therefore, be used to eliminate large-angle scattering, but can only eliminate smaller-angle scattering at the expense of eliminating unscattered photons as well. Accordingly, more empirical methods must be applied to correct for the remaining scatter.

The effect of scatter is to add an approximate exponential tail to the resolution curve. For example, if the resolution measurements that produced Figure 2-5 had been obtained in a scattering medium such as water (which simulates the properties of soft tissue), the resolution curves would not drop to zero quickly, but would fall off slowly (exponentially) with distance by exhibiting a long "tail." A similar phenomenon occurs when imaging is performed with a high-energy positron source except that the scattering tail declines much more slowly. One way to quantitate the effect of scattered photons in an imaging situation is to image a phantom consisting of a 5 cm diameter cylinder filled with water, which in turn is placed in a 20 cm diameter phantom filled with a mixture of water and a positron emitter. Ideally, no counts would be observed in the part of the image containing the 5 cm phantom. In practice, unless correction for scatter is employed, 10% to 30% (depending on the scanner's design) of the counts in the surrounding "hot" or radioactive areas will appear in the "cold" region (the one devoid of radioactivity). The fraction of events that appear in the cold cylinder is called the "scatter fraction." Such a measurement provides a standard for comparison of scatter in different scanners and yields a reasonable estimate of the amount of scatter to be expected in an imaging procedure for a static organ such as the brain. Cardiac studies, however, involve objects much larger than 20 cm. In addition, chests are elliptical, not cylindrical, in shape and contain lungs. For these reasons, the scatter fractions estimated from 20 cm phantoms may be lower than those actually seen in the neighborhood of the heart. When a 30 cm × 20 cm elliptical phantom with simulated lungs and a 5 cm cold cylinder at the approximate location of the heart is used, a scatter fraction of about 22% is observed (compared with about 16% obtained with the standard 20 cm phantom) with a particular scanner and at a particular energy threshold. While such results are dependent on the particulars of scanner design, they do demonstrate the geometry-dependent differences in scattering. Little data have been published to date concerning scatter fractions applied as correction factors for cardiac PET.

The major practical implication of scatter is that regions of myocardium devoid of radioactivity will appear to emit radioactivity because of scatter from neighboring regions containing radioactivity. Accordingly, defects in myocardium may appear to be significantly "hotter" than they should. Several schemes are available with commercial scanners for correcting for scatter,[15,16] most of which were initially developed for imaging the brain. They work reasonably well for the brain because of its relatively uniform activity and tissue homogeneity. The chest, on the other hand, is large and very inhomogeneous. The distribution of activity within it is nonuniform, especially with cardiac PET in which it is concentrated in the heart. The accuracy of scatter correction methods under such circumstances is not yet clear.

Deadtime

Quantitatively accurate PET studies require that the number of true coincidences be directly proportional to the concentration of radioactivity. In addition to physical phenomena such as scatter and accidental coincidences, a significant electronic effect in PET cameras can alter this relationship. Every time a photon produces a scintillation in a detector, a complex series of electronic events must occur: the light must be converted into an electronic pulse; the exact time of occurrence of the electronic pulse must be determined for use in timing coincidence; the magnitude of the pulse must be computed to allow rejection of scattered events; if one photomultiplier tube shares many detectors, the electronics must determine which detector produced the pulse; the electronic system must determine whether a coincidence occurred, i.e., if another pulse occurred or will occur during the previous or subsequent s seconds; and if a coincidence does occur, the electronic system must be able to screen out coincidences that are "impossible" (e.g., coincidences from adjacent detectors). All of this takes time. If a second photon should arrive before the processing of the previous pulse is complete, the second pulse may be lost. There is, therefore, a time interval after a photon has interacted with a crystal during which the PET scanner electronics may be unable to process further pulses. Pulses that occur during this interval, termed the "deadtime," are lost. The higher the count rate, the larger will be the fraction of lost pulses. Figure 2-12 illustrates the effect of lost pulses on a plot of true coincidences as a function of activity. The number of coincidences per second at first increases linearly with activity, but at high activities it deviates from linearity. Successive increases in activity produce successively smaller increases in coincidence rate. Manufacturers will frequently specify the activity concentration (nCi/cc in a 20 cm phantom) at which 50% of the counts will be lost due to deadtime.

The principal source of deadtime is often not the number of coincident events the machine must process per se, but rather the rate at which the system must process single, unpaired, photons. The singles rate recorded by a detector is often an order of magnitude or more, greater than the coincident rate. Usually, the deadtime loss of a detector can be predicted quite accurately as a function of the singles rate measured by the detector. This relationship is the basis for one effective method for correcting for deadtime. With this method the singles rates of individual detectors is measured as a function of time during the study. From the previously determined relationship between deadtime and singles rate, the fraction of time the machine is "dead" can be computed at each time point, and the coincidence data corrected appropriately. The corrections

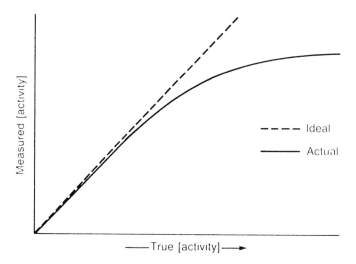

Figure 2-12. *Deadtime causes the activity concentration as measured by the scanner to deviate from the true concentration.*

are often quite large, especially with imaging techniques that require bolus injections of isotope. It is probably best to limit the amount of activity injected so that the required deadtime correction will be less than a factor of 2. Activity levels greater than this will result in increased radiation exposure to the patient without a comparable increase in true coincidences. In addition, the accuracy of larger correction factors is suspect.

Cardiac PET studies are especially susceptible to the effects of deadtime. This is particularly true with dynamic cardiac studies that attempt to measure the washin or washout of activity from the myocardium, or to measure arterial activity as a function of time by monitoring the activity in the atrial or ventricular cavities. During a bolus injection or even during a 1 minute infusion of isotope, the PET camera field of view may contain a large fraction of the entire injected dose. This is in marked contrast to the case in brain imaging studies in which only a small percentage of the injected dose is ever in the field of view. Quite frequently, the PET camera's deadtime characteristics (as well as random coincidences) limit the amount of activity that can be administered. Images that are already noisy because of a paucity of counts would be still further degraded because of failure of the PET camera's electronics system. Some of the older generation PET scanners have considerably better deadtime performance than newer scanners. New scanners often employ schemes by which many detectors share a single photomultiplier tube, especially for multislice machines. The result may be significantly greater deadtime.

PET Scanner Sensitivity and Calibration

Only a very small fraction of the annihilation photons produced in the field of view of a PET scanner are detected as coincidences. The sensitivity of a scanner is a quantitative measure of how big this fraction is. The undetected photons are wasted, increasing radiation dose to the patient, but producing no information. Sensitivity is an important characteristic of a PET scanner because nearly all types of PET imaging procedures are "count limited." That is, the total number of coincident photons detected is much smaller than one would like and results in an image that is noisy. The noise is caused by the statistical fluctuations always associated with radioactive decay and is amplified still further because of the mathematics of reconstruction (the filtered back-projection process). Having too few photons does not affect the spatial resolution of the scanner. It does, however, affect the ability to utilize this resolution, because it affects the observer's ability to distinguish real objects from noise. There are only 2 ways to compensate for an inadequate number of photons without degrading the image in any other way: increase the scan time or increase the amount of radioisotope administered (thereby increasing the radiation dose to the patient).

Why are so few emitted photons detected by PET scanners and why might one scanner have better sensitivity than another? The principal causes of photon loss are attenuation and geometry. Although attenuation is not a machine-dependent factor, geometry is. Of all the possible directions in which a pair of photons could travel, only a very small fraction of those directions (about 1 in 20 or fewer, depending on the ring dimensions) will result in the pair of photons striking the ring of detectors. The farther the detectors are away from the source, the lower the probability that photons emitted by a source at the center will be detected. Brain scanners need only a small diameter ring of detectors, typically 50 to 60 cm, whereas cardiac PET cameras require a larger patient aperture with a ring diameter of about 70 to 90 cm. Because sensitivity varies approximately as the reciprocal of ring diameter, all other things being equal, whole body scanners have a factor of 1.5 to 2 less sensitivity than brain scanners.

Sensitivity is dependent also on how efficiently the detectors are packed around the ring, which doesn't differ very much from one system to another. A second, nongeometrical factor affecting sensitivity results from photons passing through the detector without interacting to produce a flash of light of the required intensity. This is a function of the thickness of crystal through which the photon must travel (the "depth" of the crystal in Figure 2-4) and the material from which the crystal is made. Most PET cameras are made with BGO scintillation crystals. If a photon hits such a crystal head-on and the crystal is very deep (typically 30 mm), the probability is fairly high (50% to 80% or better) that the photon will interact with the crystal to produce a pulse above the energy threshold for detection. For coincidence, however, both photons must produce such a pulse. Thus, the probability that the coincident pair will produce a detectable pulse is the product of the individual detection probabilities, perhaps 25% to 64%. Some cameras, in particular "time of flight" cameras, use crystal materials (such as cesium or barium fluoride) that don't stop gamma rays as effectively as BGO, but instead, permit a shorter coincidence resolving time. PET cameras utilizing these faster detectors may have a lower sensitivity unless they also employ crystals of greater depth. Because sensitivity may vary from one PET scanner to another, the optimal imaging time and administered dose of isotope for a given study will be machine dependent.

To compare different scanners, standardized methods for measuring sensitivity have been devised. One is to scan a 20 cm hollow lucite cylinder filled with a mixture of ^{18}F and water and subsequently withdraw an aliquot for determination of the activity per milliliter in a calibrated scintillation counter. The image from the scanner is then reconstructed, correcting for random events and scatter, but not for attenuation. Sensitivity is defined as the total number of coincident events per second within the reconstructed image of the cylinder, divided by the activity per milliliter as determined from assay of the aliquot. The units of sensitivity are counts per second per activity concentration (or counts/sec/μCi/ml). Thus, sensitivity can be defined as the number of true, unscattered coincidences per second that the scanner detects from a 20 cm phantom filled with 1 μCi/ml of radioactive material. If an isotope such as gallium (Ga)-68 is used, a correction is required because of the fact that when ^{68}Ga decays it doesn't always emit a positron (11% of the time it emits something other than a positron). Fluorine-18, carbon-11, nitrogen-13, and oxygen-15 do not have this problem. To compare 2 scanners, it is important to make sure that the measurements were obtained in the same manner. If a measurement includes randoms and scatter, it overestimates sensitivity.

A measurement similar to the one used for sensitivity is necessary for calibration of a scanner. Typically, measurements of both the number of coincidences and the total activity or concentration of activity in an organ are desired. By reconstructing the data from a 20 cm cylindrical phantom, as described above but with attenuation correction, an image can be obtained with a uniform number of events at each pixel (apart from statistical fluctuations). The average number of events per second in each pixel within the cylinder divided by the measured activity concentration permits conversion from counts per second per pixel to microcuries per milliliter (events per second are proportional to activity, and a pixel is a volume element). This factor is the calibration factor for the scanner, and provides a means by which future measurements of coincidences per second per pixel can be converted into units of microcuries per milliliter. Using this calibration factor, the PET scanner can measure either activity concentrations (from events/sec/pixel) or total activity (from total events/sec in all pixels).

Conclusion

The driving force behind the initial commercial development of PET was the use of deoxyglucose for measuring glucose metabolism in the brain. When the method was first applied, it was already clear that quantitative measurements of glucose metabolism would require that PET instruments provide accurate measurements of activity concentrations in absolute terms. Much time and effort were expended in developing the many corrections necessary (those for attenuation, scatter, randoms, deadtime, and partial volume effects, etc., among others). PET emerged as one of the first truly quantitative approaches for determination of activity distributions in vivo. Applications for PET in cardiology quickly became apparent, and the corrections that had been so satisfactory for the brain were applied to cardiac imaging. It is not yet clear whether these corrections are adequate. The location of the heart, the large size of the chest, the inhomogeneity of surrounding tissue, and the fact that any intravenously injected material must pass through the chambers of the heart and the scanner field of view, make quantitative imaging of myocardium far more daunting than quantitative imaging of the brain.

The next few years are critical for cardiac PET imaging. There is a risk that undue haste to bring PET into clinical practice will result in inadequate attention being paid to the factors that can distort the data and the conclusions drawn from it. If, however, the technology is applied and interpreted with care, it will offer great promise. Never before has a nuclear medicine procedure been available with such great potential for accurate quantitative measurement of metabolism, perfusion, and cardiac cellular function.

References

1. Radionuclide Transformations: Energy and Intensity of Emissions. In: Sowby, FD, Ed. Annals of the ICRP Publication 38. New York: Permagon Press, 1983.
2. Evans RD. *The Atomic Nucleus*. New York:McGraw-Hill, 1955:pp 625–629.
3. Herman GT. *Image Reconstruction from Projections: The Fundamentals of Computerized Tomography*. New York:Academic Press, 1980.
4. Parker JA. *Image Reconstruction in Radiology*. Boca Raton: CRC Press, 1990.
5. Barrett HH, Swindell W. *Radiological Imaging: The Theory of Image Formation, Detection and Processing*. New York:Academic Press. 1981:II.
6. Budinger TF, Gullberg GT, Huesman, RH. Emission Computed Tomography. In: Herman GT, Ed. *Image Reconstruction from Projections: Implementation and Applications*. New York:Springer-Verlag, 1979; pp.147–242.
7. Phelps ME, Hoffman EJ, Huang SC, Ter-Pogossian MM. Effect of positron range on spatial resolution. J Nucl Med 1975; 16:649–652.
8. Collins SM, Skorton DJ. Fundamentals of Image Processing. In: Collins SM, Skorton DJ, eds. *Cardiac Imaging and Image Processing*, McGraw Hill, 1986.
9. Hoffman EJ, Huang SC, Phelps ME. Quantitation in positron emission computed tomography: 1. Effect of object size. J Comput Assist Tomogr 1979; 3:299–308.
10. Wisenberg G, Schelbert HR, Hoffman EJ, Phelps ME, Robinson GD Jr., Selin CE, Child J, Skorton D, Kuhl DE. In vivo quantitation of regional myocardial blood flow by positron-emission computed tomography. Circulation 1981; 63:1248–1258.
11. Iida H, Kanno I, Takahashi A, Miura S, Murakami M, Takahashi K, Ono Y, Shishido F, Inugami A, Tomura N, Higano S, Fujita H, Sasaki H, Nakamichi H, Mizusawa S, Kondo Y, Uemura K. Measurement of absolute myocardial blood flow with $H_2^{15}O$ and dynamic positron emission tomography: Strategy for quantification in relation to the partial-volume effect. Circulation 1988; 78:104–115.
12. Casey ME, Hoffman EJ. Quantitation in positron emission computed tomography: 7. A technique to reduce noise in accidental coincidence measurements and coincidence efficiency calibration. J Comput Assist Tomogr 1986; 10:845–850.
13. Carson RE, Daube-Witherspoon ME, Green MV. A method for postinjection PET transmission measurements with a rotating rod source. J Nucl Med 1988; 29:1558–1567.
14. Thompson CJ, Ranger NT, Evans AC. Simultaneous transmission and emission scans in PET. IEEE Trans Nucl Sci 1989; 36:1011–1016.

15. Bendriem B, Soussaline F, Campagnolo R, Verrey B, Wajnberg P, Syrota A. A technique for the correction of scattered radiation in a PET system using time of flight information. J Comput Assist Tomogr 1986; 10:287–295.
16. Bergstrom M, Ericksson L, Bohm C, Blomqvist G, Litton J. Correction for scattered radiation in a ring detector positron camera by integral transformation of the projection. J Comput Assist Tomogr 1983; 7:42–50.
17. Hoffman EJ, Phelps ME. Resolution limits for positron imaging devices. J Nucl Med 1978; 18:491–492.

Chapter 3

Myocardial Metabolism Pertinent to Cardiac Positron Tomography

Charles K. Stone, M.D. and A. James Liedtke, M.D.

Cardiac muscle is second only to brain in its obligate aerobic needs. It requires large amounts of high-energy phosphates to satisfy the demands of contractile performance. Autoregulation of coronary flow and a coronary reserve of approximately fivefold permits increases in oxygen delivery at high workloads. Substrates, including fatty acids, carbohydrates, ketones, and amino acids serve as fuel for myocyte production of adenosine triphosphate (ATP) and phosphotocreatine. Investigations spanning more than a century have characterized the metabolic pathways involved, their regulation, and dysfunctions secondary to myocardial ischemia and reperfusion.[1-4]

This chapter focuses on metabolic phenomena with particular relevance to cardiac positron emission tomography (PET) and is designed to aid physicians in identifying appropriate diagnostic indications for use of this modality.

Historical Considerations

Opie[5] divided the development of investigation of cardiac metabolism into five eras: classical cardiac physiology, sampling techniques in the coronary sinus allowing for the measurement of arteriovenous differences of metabolites across myocardial perfusion beds of interest, isolated heart preparations with controlled coronary perfusion and perfusate containing trace-labeled metabolites, suborganelle preparations permitting the monitoring of local biochemical events and membrane/enzyme kinetics, and the current multidisciplinary approach featuring an increasing number of new measuring techniques, instruments, and preparations directed toward an understanding of phenomena at

This work was supported in part by PHS Grants HL32350 and HL41914, AHA Grant 88951, The Rennebohm Foundation of Wisconsin, and the Oscar Mayer Cardiovascular Research Fund.

From *Positron Emission Tomography of the Heart* edited by Steven R. Bergmann, MD, PhD and Burton E. Sobel, MD © 1992, Futura Publishing Inc., Mount Kisco, NY.

the molecular level. Taegtmeyer has reviewed these historical milestones,[6] summarized here and quotes Bing[7] who cited the initial reference to myocardial metabolism as that in the 1878 lecture of Hugo Kronecker, a Berlin physiologist, on the nutritional supplies of frog hearts. Dr. Kronecker correctly observed that continued performance of heart muscle was dependent on blood rather than saline in the coronary perfusate, but erroneously deduced that oxygen had no influence on cardiac activity. This was soon rectified when Yeo[8] reported not only that oxygen delivery was important to cardiac function, but also that oxygen consumption varied directly with heart rate. In 1904, glucose was identified as an essential exogenous substrate for the heart.[9] For several decades, glucose and other carbohydrates were viewed as the only important myocardial carbon fuels. The concept of alternate competing substrates was slow to gain acceptance, although fatty acids were identified as one possibility as early as 1933.[10] Bing et al. recognized considerable extraction of fatty acids in the postabsorption state in both patients and dogs.[11] Opie and co-workers,[12] using an isolated perfused rat heart preparation and isotopic techniques, identified a hierarchical preference of substrates in mammalian hearts. They concluded that fatty acids were the preferred substrate of myocardial metabolism and that fatty acids inhibited glycolysis.

Cellular Metabolism

Four major classes of substrates are available for metabolism by cardiac myocytes. In addition to the carbohydrates and fatty acids, amino acids and ketone bodies contribute under certain circumstances. Specific substrates exhibit specific cellular transmembrane transport properties, cytosolic metabolism, and mitochondrial membrane transport and metabolism. Utilization is dependent upon the abundance of the substrate in the cell and perfusate, the availability of competing substrates, and the metabolic state of the cell.

Cellular metabolism comprises cytosolic and mitochondrial components including the citric acid cycle, respiratory chain, and oxidative phosphorylation. The citric acid cycle (Figure 3-1) utilizes 8 enzyme systems adherent to the inner mitochondrial membrane or the mitochondrial matrix. The site of entry into the cycle for most metabolic fuels is acetyl-CoA that, with oxaloacetate, forms citrate by the enzyme citrate synthase. The entire cycle entails catabolism of acetyl residues to reducing equivalents in the form of 3 pyridine nucleotide (NADH) molecules, 1 flavoprotein ($FADH_2$) molecule, and 1 high-energy phosphate guanosine triphosphate (GTP). Oxaloacetate is regenerated with each turn of the cycle such that it acts as a catalytic unit.

The reducing equivalents are converted to high-energy phosphate bonds through oxidative phosphorylation by the respiratory chain (Figure 3-2). The inner mitochondrial membrane contains the enzyme complexes of the respiratory chain that are in close proximity to those of the citric acid cycle. Coupled reactions of oxidation and reduction occur down the chain with increasing redox potential. The last cytochrome in the chain, cytochrome oxidase, is responsible for the reduction of molecular oxygen to water. Phosphorylation of ADP to ATP occurs through ATP synthase.

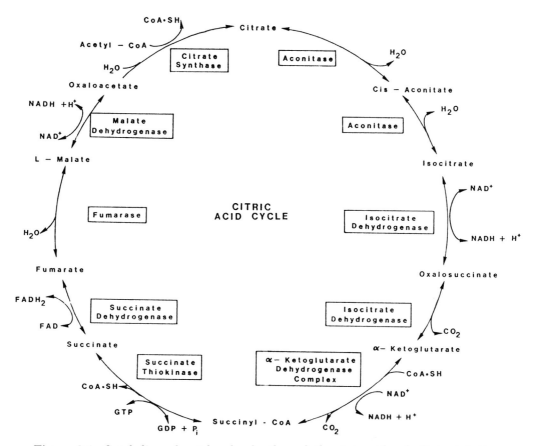

Figure 3-1. *Catabolism of acetyl molecules through the citric acid cycle. Entry into the cycle starts with the formation of citrate from oxaloacetate and acetyl-CoA. In one turn of the cycle, 3 molecules of reduced nicotinamide adenine dinucleotide (NADH), 1 molecule of reduced flavin adenine dinucleotide (FADH₂), and 1 molecule of the high-energy phosphate guanosine triphosphate (GTP) are produced from 1 molecule of acetyl-CoA with regeneration of the intermediary compound oxaloacetate. Enzymes of the cycle are shown in boxes. All of the enzymes are in the mitochondrial matrix or along the inner membrane. (Adapted from Murray RK, Granner DK, Mayes PA, Rodwell VW: Harper's Biochemistry. Appleton & Lange, 1988, with permission of the publisher.)*

Several hypotheses have been proposed to explain the coupling of oxidation and phosphorylation. The most widely held theory, that of chemiosmosis, envisions coupling through an electrochemical potential with the passage of hydrogen ions outside of a coupling membrane by the respiratory chain complexes.[13] Passage of these ions back across the coupling membrane drives the ATP synthase-regulated phosphorylation of ADP to ATP. The oxidation of NADH to NAD^+ yields 3 ADP molecules to ATP whereas that of $FADH_2$ to FAD^{++} yields only 2 ATP molecules since the entry of hydrogen ions in the respiratory chain occurs farther down the chain at the ubiquinone site (coenzyme Q). Thus, each turn of the citric acid cycle ultimately produces 12 high-energy phosphate

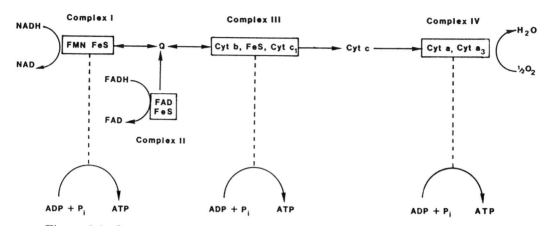

Figure 3-2. *Components of the respiratory chain. Final common pathway of substrate metabolism is the phosphorylation of ADP to ATP by the oxidation of NADH and FADH$_2$. Protons pass through the cytochrome complexes of the respiratory chain with reduction of molecular oxygen to water as the final step. Cytochrome complexes of the respiratory chain are complex I, NADH/ubiquinone oxidoreductase; complex II, succinate/ubiquinone oxidoreductase; complex III, ubiquinol/ferricytochrome c oxidoreductase; complex IV, ferrocyochrome c/oxygen oxidoreductase. (Abbreviations) Q, ubiquinone; P$_i$, inorganic phosphate. Other abbreviations as in Figure 3-1). (Adapted from Murray RK, Granner DK, Mayes PA, Rodwell VW:* Harper's Biochemistry. *Appleton & Lange, 1988, with permission of the publisher.)*

bonds (11 ATP molecules from the oxidation of the 3 NADH molecules and 1 FADH$_2$ and 1 GTP molecule from the cleavage of CoA from succinyl-CoA at the substrate level).

Metabolism of Glucose in Aerobic Myocardium

Although glucose alone is inadequate to support high rates of oxidative phosphorylation in aerobic hearts, its fate is relevant to the understanding of uptake of ^{18}F-2-deoxy-2-fluoro-D-glucose (FDG) used in PET. ^{18}FDG detects only transport and the initial phosphorylation step of glycolysis because the tracer is undirectionally trapped as the phosphate derivative. These two proximal steps may not parallel overall rates of glucose metabolism. Glucose utilization is controlled at key steps outside the mitochondria, including glucose transport and reactions regulated by hexokinase, glycogen synthetase, glycogen phosphorylase, phosphofructokinase, and pyruvate kinase and dehydrogenase[1,3](Figure 3-3). Factors influencing flux through specific reactions are listed in Table 3-1.[4]

Energy from glucose utilization is derived from anaerobic glycolysis (the Embden-Meyerhof pathway), the citric acid cycle, and the respiratory chain. However, anaerobic glycolysis provides only trivial fractions of ATP comprising myocardial energy requirements. Glycolysis is limited by the rates of disposal of glycolytically produced NADH in cytosol and by the activity of glyceral-

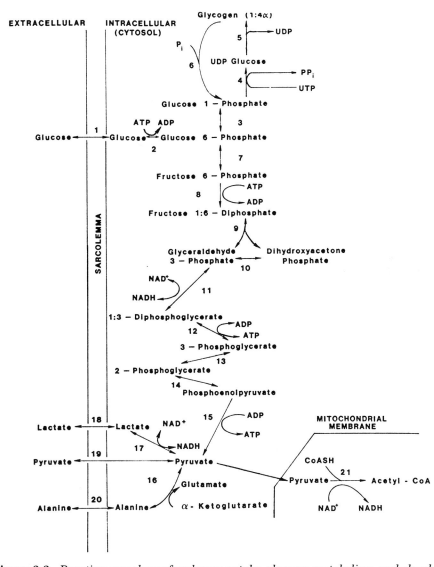

Figure 3-3. *Reactions are shown for glucose uptake, glycogen metabolism, and glycolysis in heart muscle. Numbers represent regulating steps or enzymes within this pathway and include: 1, glucose transport; 2, hexokinase; 3, phosphoglucomutase; 4, UDPG pyrophosphorylase; 5, glycogen synthetase; 6, phosphorylase; 7, phosphoglucose isomerase; 8, phosphofructokinase; 9, aldolase; 10, triosephosphate isomerase; 11, glyceraldehyde-3-phosphate dehydrogenase; 12, 3–phosphoglycerate kinase; 13, phosphoglyceromutase; 14, enolase; 15, pyruvate kinase; 16, alanine aminotransferase; 17, lactate dehydrogenase; 18, 19, lactate and pyruvate transport (not proved); 20, alanine transport; and 21, pyruvate dehydrogenase. (Adapted from Randle and Tubbs,[3] with permission of the American Physiological Society.)*

Table 3-1
Glycolysis and Glycogen Synthesis and Breakdown

Major Rate-Regulating Steps	Substrates(s)	Product(s)	Chief Regulating Mechanism*	Changes in Flux With	
				Anoxia†	Ischemia†
Glucose transport	Glucose	Glucose	Hormonal, chiefly insulin	Increased	Increased
Hexokinase	Glucose; ATP	Glucose-6-P; ADP	Product inhibition	Increased	Increased
Phosphofructokinase	Fructose-6-P; ATP	Fructose-1,6-P; ADP	Allosteric control	Increased	Increased
Glyceraldehyde-3-P dehydrogenase	Glyceraldehyde-3-P; NAD^+	1,3-diphosphoglycerate; NADH	Product inhibition	Increased	Decreased
Pyruvate dehydrogenase	Pyruvate, coenzyme-A, NAD^+	Acetyl-CoA, CO_2, NADH	Allosteric and product inhibition; covalent modification	Decreased	Decreased
Glycogen synthetase	Uridine-diP-glucose	Glycogen	Allosteric and product inhibition; covalent modification	Unknown	Unknown
Glycogen phosphorylase	Glycogen, Pi	Glycose-1-P	Allosteric and product inhibition; covalent modification	Increased	Increased

* Under aerobic physiologic conditions.
† Complies with definitions described in text, i.e., anoxia indicates normal-to-high coronary perfusion with deoxygenated perfusate, ischemia indicates low flow with oxygenated perfusate.
Reprinted from Liedtke,[4] by permission of the W. B. Saunders Company.

dehyde-3-phosphate dehydrogenase (especially at high flux rates).[14] Glucose as a sole substrate in experiments in rat hearts fixes the availability of acetyl-CoA and the citric acid cycle behaves in a "run-down" manner, as reflected by reduced levels of acetyl-CoA, citrate, and isocitrate; decreased mitochondrial NADH/NAD$^+$ ratios; and increased oxaloacetate levels. Oxidative phosphorylation is constrained by the availability of NADH.

Glucose transport is stereospecific, but relatively unselective since it inwardly channels a number of metabolized and nonmetabolized sugars, including glucose, mannose, 2-deoxyglucose and [18]FDG, 3-O-methyl glucose, D-xylose, and L-arabinose.[3] This nonenergy-dependent entry process is termed carrier-mediated transport or facilitated diffusion.[1] Sugars are transferred bidirectionally across the lipid membrane. A number of nutritional and other factors influence sugar uptake. Transport is obviously very sensitive to insulin levels in the perfusate, but can operate in its absence. Increasing plasma glucose concentrations, presence of NADH in anoxia, high cardiac work, growth hormone, epinephrine, and uncouplers of oxidative phosphorylation all stimulate transport. Conversely, availability of competing substrates and oxidation of fatty acids, ketones, and pyruvate all inhibit transport. Glucose-6-phosphate (and its analogous compounds deoxyglucose phosphate and [18]FDG phosphate) at concentrations that inhibit the hexokinase reaction do not inhibit transport. With respect to the overall rate of glucose utilization, glucose transport under the experimental conditions of no insulin and low workloads becomes rate limiting.

A second step in glucose and [18]FDG transport is hexokinase-mediated phosphorylation, rate limiting at high transport rates.[1,3,4,] Although accelerated by increasing intracellular glucose, its rate is strongly inhibited by glucose-6-phosphate as well as ATP, ADP, AMP, inorganic phosphate (P_i), oxidation of fatty acids and ketones, starvation, and diabetes. The reaction is essentially irreversible in heart muscle and governed predominantly by 2 hexokinase isoenzymes bound to mitochondria.[3]

Neely and Morgan[15] considered glucose metabolism (utilization) a five-step process: glucose uptake (transport and the hexokinase reaction), glycogen metabolism (reactions between the formation of glucose-6-phosphate and glycogen), glycolysis (glucose-6-phosphate to pyruvate), pyruvate metabolism (pyruvate to either lactate, acetyl-CoA, or alanine), and the citric acid cycle. In brain in the absence of glycogen formation, flux rates of glucose uptake are tightly linked to those of glycolysis, and [18]FDG uptake is a valid marker of glycolytic flux. Such is not the case in myocardium, in which glycogen formation exists in competition with glycolysis. Most of the glucose extracted by heart muscle is synthesized to glycogen in fasting and fed states. In normal volunteers in the postabsorption state, arterial levels of fatty acids determine glucose uptake. Of glucose extracted, 20% is oxidized, 13% is metabolized to lactate and released, and 60% to 70% is stored as glycogen. In hyperglycemic subjects, the percentage of glucose oxidized increases modestly. Most is still stored as glycogen.[16,17] Thus, [18]FDG uptake does not necessarily parallel the rate of glycolysis or of anaerobic energy production in aerobic or in ischemic myocardium.

A final point that complicates the use of PET for estimation of glucose metabolism is the dependency of myocardial glucose metabolism on substrate competition. Most information regarding myocardial substrate preference has been acquired in isolated perfused hearts. Thus, results may not be directly applicable to intact hearts perfused with whole blood perfusate containing multiple substrates in concentrations that vary with nutritional state. In hearts of fasting patients, [18]FDG uptake is unpredictable, making reliable clinical diagnoses difficult and requiring regional analysis. Marshall et al.[18] have used a protocol in which a carbohydrate-containing meal is followed by additional oral glucose loading (40 to 50 g) 60 to 90 minutes before injection of [18]FDG. This stimulates an increase in circulating insulin, which has been shown experimentally to directly and indirectly enhance glucose uptake and decrease peripheral lipolysis, arterial levels of free fatty acids, and myocardial uptake of fatty acids.[19] Empirically, by use of this approach, the quality of the PET scintigrams was much improved, and the feeding protocol has become part of the standard diagnostic format.

Lactate at sufficiently high arterial concentrations (4.5 mmol/l) (such as those induced by exercise[20]) is utilized preferentially over both glucose and fatty acids.[21] Pyruvate is another potentially highly competitive substrate. Pyruvate dehydrogenase is the key enzyme regulating its metabolism and is stimulated by pyruvate and inhibited by fatty acylcarnitine derivatives and ketones.[22] At high intramitochondrial concentrations of pyruvate, this substrate can diminish palmitoylcarnitine oxidation by 40%.[23] Thus, findings with PET and [18]FDG are dependent on the nutritional state of the patient and the availability and concentrations of several competing substrates in whole blood.

Fatty Acid Metabolism in Aerobic Myocardium

Fatty acid utilization is illustrated in Figure 3-4. Major rate-regulatory steps and mechanisms are listed in Table 3-2. Regulation occurs with transfer of free fatty acids (FFA), bound to either albumin or glycerol, from plasma to cardiomyocytes with intracellular activation to stored triacylglycerols, or further steps to oxidation including transfer as the acyl ester across the mitochondrial membrane via carnitine-dependent reactions, and with beta- and acetyl-CoA oxidation within mitochondria.[1,3–5] At low workloads in aerobic hearts, flux rates in the citric acid cycle determine rates of acetyl-CoA oxidation.[24] At high workloads, rates of acyl translocation across the inner mitochondrial membrane limit oxidation. Fatty acids exhibit a high first-pass extraction ratio in myocardium, although the capillary endothelium represents a major barrier to entry. Uptake is dependent on arterial concentrations of FFA in coronary perfusate, which can vary from 0.1 to 2.0 mM under various physiologic conditions, albumin/FFA molar ratio in perfusate, chain length and degree of unsaturation of the fatty acid, energy requirements of the cell, and size of existing endogenous fatty acid and lipid pools.[3,4] Entry occurs through selective channels by either passive diffusion or nonenergy-dependent saturable binding between proteins. After entry and activation, fatty acids are distributed among several carbon pools. A small fraction is not metabolized and

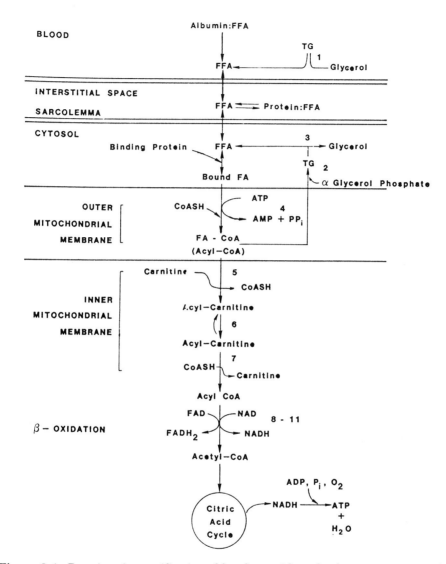

Figure 3-4. *Reactions in esterification of free fatty acids and subsequent transport into, and β-oxidation and respiratory oxidation within mitochondria. Numbers represent regulating enzymes and include 1, endothelial lipoprotein lipase; 2, enzymes of triacylglycerol (TG) esterification; 3, enzymes of lipolysis; 4, acyl-CoA synthetases; 5, carnitine palmitoyltransferase I; 6, carnitine-acylcarnitine translocase; 7, carnitine palmitoyltransferase II; 8–11, enzymes of β-oxidation including acyl-CoA dehydrogenase, enoyl-CoA hydrase, 3–hydroxyacyl-CoA dehydrogenase, and 3-oxoacyl-CoA thiolase. (Adapted from Corr et al.,[5] with permission of the American Heart Association, Inc.)*

Table 3-2
Long-Chain Fatty Acid Oxidation*

Major Rate-Regulating Steps	Substrates	Products	Chief Regulating Mechanism†	Changes in Flux With Oxygen Deficiency‡
Cellular uptake by plasma membrane binding sites and anatomic channels	FFA, triacylglycerols	FFA	Plasma FFA concentrations; FFA:albumin molar ratio; FA properties; metabolic activity of cell; hormones	Decreased
Cytosolic activation by acyl-CoA synthetases	FFA, coenzyme-A, ATP	Acyl-CoA, AMP, Pi	Product inhibition; coenzyme-A availability	Decreased
Cytosol-Mitochondrial transfer by carnitine acyl transferase-translocase	Acyl-CoA, coenzyme-A; acyl-carnitine; carnitine	Acyl-CoA; coenzyme-A; acyl-carnitine; carnitine	Ratio of substrates to products	Decreased
β-oxidation	Acyl-CoA, FAD^+, NAD^+	Remaining acyl-CoA(-2 carbons); acetyl-CoA, $FADH_2$, NADH	Metabolic activity of cell; oxygen availability; flux through citric acid cycle	Profoundly decreased chief inhibited step

* Exclusive of nonoxidative pathways to neutral and polar lipids.

† Under aerobic physiologic conditions.

‡ Includes both anoxia and ischemia. FFAs are free long-chain fatty acids bound in albumin or intracellular proteins.

Reprinted from Liedtke,[4] by permission of the W. B. Saunders Company.

undergoes backdiffusion, and a small but critically important fraction proceeds directly to acetyl-CoA oxidation. The remainder is distributed into a relatively stable phospholipid and a dynamic triacylglycerol pool with the potential for rapid turnover and variable transit times. Esterification of acyl-CoA to mono–, di–, and triacylglycerols exceeds hydrolysis of triacylglycerols with increased availability of FFA, anoxia, and ischemia. The reverse is true when FFA is depleted, work is increased, or when the heart is exposed to catecholamines.

PET with carbon-11 (^{11}C)-palmitate has been used to estimate fatty acid metabolism. This tracer, unlike ^{18}FDG, has potential for interrogation of the entire pathway of utilization from substrate entry to complete oxidation. Unfortunately, the half-life of the tracer may introduce sampling errors. As shown in Figure 3-4, fatty acid utilization is complex, with the possibility of diversion of tracer at membrane transfer and of dispersal and temporary storage of same in lipid carbon pools. In studies with carbon-14 (^{14}C)-palmitate equilibrium infusion labeling, we have shown that $^{14}CO_2$ production does not reach steady-state levels for at least 20 to 30 minutes in aerobically perfused myocardium.[25–27] More recently, we have observed (unpublished data) that a storage lipid pool, presumably triacylglycerols, continues to contribute additional carbons to fatty acid oxidation for at least 40 minutes in aerobically perfused myocardium. These carbons may eventually provide a large portion of the fuel for oxidative metabolism and would be incompletely labeled by a positron-emitting isotope of short-lived radioactivity. This bias toward undercharacterizing events distal in the pathway of fatty acid metabolism and the complicated kinetics of tracer compartmentalization within the pathway, both argue for caution in interpreting PET studies with fatty acids. Nevertheless, decreased FFA metabolism is a hallmark of irreversibly injured myocardium, as discussed in Chapter 6.

Metabolism of Glucose in Ischemic Myocardium

A myriad of untoward consequences of restricted oxygen delivery have been reported with assessments of substrate metabolism in cardiac tissue.[1,3,4,28] Not only is oxygen supply threatened in this aerobic organ, but critical washout of inhibitory intermediate products is curtailed, impairing overall flux within metabolic pathways. Key steps within glucose utilization and glycolytic pathway are regulated in disparate fashions (Table 3-1), with increases occurring in glucose transport and the hexokinase, phosphofructokinase, and glycogen phosphorylase reactions and decreases in the glyceraldehyde-3-phosphate dehydrogenase and pyruvate dehydrogenase reactions. Overall rates of glycolysis are determined by the absolute restrictions on coronary flow. Glyceraldehyde-3-phosphate dehydrogenase, because of its inhibition by rising intracellular concentrations of NADH, hydrogen ion, and lactate with ischemia, is considered the chief rate-limiting enzyme in glycolysis. Its continued activity is dependent on the washout of these metabolites, as demon-

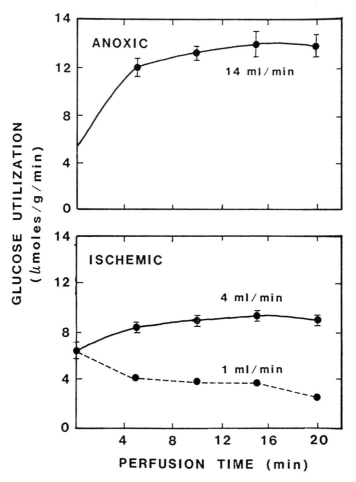

Figure 3-5. *Effects of restricted oxygen delivery by the imposition of anoxia (top) or ischemia (bottom) on glucose utilization (glycolytic flux) estimated by release of ³H₂O from 2-³H-glucose or 5-³H-glucose in isolated working rat hearts. In anoxic hearts, coronary flow of blood-free perfusate was maintained at about 14 ml/min. In ischemic hearts, coronary flow was either maintained at 4 ml/min (solid line) or allowed to decline to 1.0 ml/min (broken line). Each value represents the mean ± SEM for 6 determinations. (Adapted from Rovetto et al.,[29] with permission of the American Heart Association, Inc.)*

strated by Rovetto et al.[29](Figure 3-5). With isolated, working rat hearts perfused with Krebs-Henseleit bicarbonate buffer containing 11 mM glucose as substrate, glycolytic flux was measured under conditions of oxygen deprivation induced either by equilibrating the perfusate with 95% N_2-5% CO_2 with flow maintained at 14 ml/min (Figure 3-5, top), or by decreasing flow to either 4 or 1 ml/min with the perfusate equilibrated with 95% O_2-5% CO_2 (Figure 3-5, bottom). With reduced oxygen delivery but preserved flow, hypoxia, and, to a lesser extent, ischemia (at 4 ml/min of flow) were associated with accelerated glucose utilization. When washout was critically reduced, however, such that inhibitory intermediates could no longer be removed from ischemic myocardium (1 ml/min flow), glycolytic flux was impaired.

These data indicate that ischemic damage occurs in a graduated fashion, with at least initial partial preservation of metabolic function. With respect to oxidative metabolism, ischemia is not an "all or none" phenomenon. Fatty acids remain the preferred substrate in the presence of mild-to-moderate flow reductions, suggesting some maintenance of mitochondrial performance in reversibly injured tissue. Only with more advanced forms of ischemic injury does glucose become the main carbon source. Even in dense zones of ischemia/infarction residual oxidative metabolism persists, with more than 90% of ATP production being derived oxidatively.[30]

Traditionally, [18]FDG has not been used in the evaluation of *acute* ischemia. Nearly all of the experimental and clinical data to date have characterized myocardium, some time (hours to months) after a coronary event, such as myocardial infarction.[18,31,32] Hence, the flow/[18]FDG metabolic mismatch that has most popularized this tracer and its use in predicting myocardial viability is a reflection of *chronic* reperfusion rather than acute hypoperfusion. Whether a mismatch reflects consequences at some level of chronic ischemia is open to debate because [18]FDG only tracks glucose uptake and not glycogen synthesis/degradation or glycolysis in heart muscle.

The overall rates of glycolysis and glucose uptake may diverge with myocardial ischemia (Table 3-1), and estimation of glycolysis based on monitoring glucose uptake is subject to error. This still leaves open the question of cell viability. The argument is persuasive that [18]FDG uptake, even if used only for qualitative assessment of glucose transport and initial phosphorylation, is a valid tool for clinical evaluation of the presence of jeopardized myocardium under conditions of coronary hypoperfusion. Integrity and preservation of an element of metabolic performance a priori should mean integrity and viability of some cells. Perhaps such is the case under conditions of chronic reperfusion after a coronary event, but not necessarily in settings of acute hypoperfusion with actual tissue injury. Sebree et al.[33] recently reported that in rabbit hearts subjected to coronary occlusion, myocardium destined for unequivocal histologic necrosis accumulated ^{14}C-deoxyglucose to only a slightly to moderately reduced extent compared with nonischemic regions. This maintenance of metabolic activity was unexplained and could have reflected uptake of ^{14}C-deoxyglucose in inflammatory cells that migrated into the infarct zone. The authors concluded that use of radiolabeled deoxyglucose, and by analogy [18]FDG, was inadequate for detecting myocardial viability in areas surrounding recently infarcted cardiac muscle.

Fatty Acid Metabolism in Ischemic Myocardium

Every step in the fatty acid utilization pathway is inhibited by reductions in coronary flow, and oxidative metabolism is critically curtailed[1,3,4](Table 3-2). The level of physiologic compromise is determined by the magnitude of reduction in coronary flow and attributable to deleterious effects of metabolic derangements rather than due to limitation of overall substrate delivery.[34] The chief rate-limiting step is β-oxidation due to the build-up of NADH and FADH$_2$, which in the absence of adequate oxygen delivery, cannot be processed through the electron transport chain. ATP production is commensurately decreased and, with it, mechanical performance declines and intermediate products accumulate. Certain of these latter products, including long-chain acyl CoA and carnitine and lysophosphoglycerides, further impair cellular functions secondarily during ischemia.[1,3–5,35,36] Fatty acid esters at monomer to micellar concentrations can: 1) alter the gel-fluid interface of biolipid membranes, and in so doing, influence protein and ionic channels within membranes, and 2) form nonspecific detergents that act to threaten membrane integrity. Examples of this influence on several enzymatic activities are listed in Table 3-3. Lysophosphoglyceride, a breakdown product of phospholipids that are cleaved during ischemia by the increased activity of phospholipase A$_2$ under the influence of calcium ion, has been strongly implicated in the propagation of life-threatening arrhythmias.[5,37] To a greater or lesser extent, triacylglycerols also increase during ischemia, and in areas of dense ischemia or peri-infarction border zones deposits of micro- and/or macro-lipid droplets are seen.[38]

[11]C-palmitate was used in early PET applications to characterize myocardial ischemia in experimental preparations. One of its potential strengths is that unlike [18]FDG, metabolism of ^{11}C-palmitate conforms directly to the pathway of physiologic utilization of fatty acid substrate. Thus, the altered metabolism of fatty acids that occurs with ischemia will affect the fate of the radiolabeled substrate similarly. Weiss et al.,[39] in isovolumically beating rabbit hearts

Table 3-3
Enzymatic Activities Affected by Amphiphiles

Activity	Amphiphile	Effect
Sarcolemmal Ca^{++} ATPase	Fatty acid acyl carnitine	Inhibits
Sarcolemmal (Na, K) ATPase	Fatty acid acyl carnitine	Inhibits
Plasma membrane (Na, K) ATPase (kidney)	Acyl CoA	Stimulates
Mitochondrial NADH dehydrogenase	Fatty acid	Inhibits
Mitochondrial F component of the ATP synthetase	Fatty acid	Uncouples or dissipates proton conductance
Mitochondrial adenine nucleotide translocase	Acyl CoA	Inhibits
Cytosolic triglyceride lipase	Fatty acids Acyl CoA Acyl carnitine	Inhibits

Adapted from Liedtke and Shrago,[36] by permission of Kluwer Academic publishers.

that were rendered ischemic, observed diminished myocardial uptake and tissue avidity for ^{11}C-octanoate and ^{11}C-palmitate and a decreased extraction fraction for both isotopes after reductions in coronary flow. Lerch et al.[40] confirmed these findings and reported a decrease in rate of tracer clearance and a change from homogeneous to heterogeneous clearance in dogs with coronary stenoses of > 70%. Schelbert and colleagues[41] confirmed that the time-activity curve for ^{11}C-palmitate comprises two phases: an early, rapid-turnover and a later, slow-turnover pool. The first phase primarily represents fatty acid oxidation with generation of [11]CO_2. The second primarily reflects incorporation of the tracer into lipids being synthesized and their slower turnover. Ischemia decreased the net extraction fraction and relative magnitude of the early component and prolonged the half-time of clearance of tracer attributable to it. A disproportionally greater fraction of tracer entered the slow-turnover pool but its clearance half-time was unchanged. More recently, Fox et al.[42] noted, with both ischemia and hypoxia, that a considerable amount (40.6% and 48.7%, respectively) of the ^{11}C-palmitate extracted by myocardium effluxed back out into the coronary effluent in a nonmetabolized form. This was further characterized by Rosamond and coworkers,[43] who described the biochemical fate and tissue distributions of 1-^{11}C and 1-^{14}C palmitate in aerobic and ischemic myocardium (Figure 3-6). Both tracers were administered as intracoronary bolus injections. 1-^{11}C palmitate was used to estimate [11]CO_2 and labeled fatty acids in blood and to acquire myocardial residue time-activity curves by external detection. 1-^{14}C palmitate was used to define the intracellular distribution of radiolabeled tracer, cocalibrated to be expressed as ^{11}C residual activity, in left ventricular biopsy samples. Although sampling bias of nonequilibrium pool labeling with the use of a short-lived ^{11}C isotope (20.4 minutes half-time) could have influenced the data (see section on Fatty Acid Metabolism in Aerobic Hearts), the results are nevertheless instructive. In aerobic hearts 10.3% of initially extracted tracer was retained in complex lipid pools (2.9% in triacylglycerols, 3.5% in phospholipids, and 3.9% in other lipid and aqueous fractions), 73.7% was oxidized, and 16.1% was backdiffused as nonmetabolized substrate. In ischemic hearts both expected and unanticipated shifts within lipid species were observed. Of initially extracted tracer, 28.1% was retained in complex lipids (18% in triacylglycerols, 6.0% in phospholipids, and 4.1% in other lipid and aqueous fractions), 27.2% was oxidized, and 44.4% was backdiffused. The authors concluded that surveillance of fatty acids by external detection with PET does not reliably define the metabolic behavior of the tracer used and that the large shift in backdiffusion of nonmetabolized substrate in ischemia essentially precludes quantitative estimation of rates of substrate oxidation with the use of a single tracer of fatty acid metabolism under conditions of reduced flow.

The problems encountered with ^{11}C-palmitate for this purpose are both methodologic and metabolic. In addition to possible errors in equilibrium labeling, sampling bias, and quantitation, limitations are attributable to lack of biochemical specificity. The PET-generated time-activity curve for ^{11}C-palmitate after bolus administration is an integral of several substrate utilization events occurring simultaneously. A specific portion of the time-activity curve

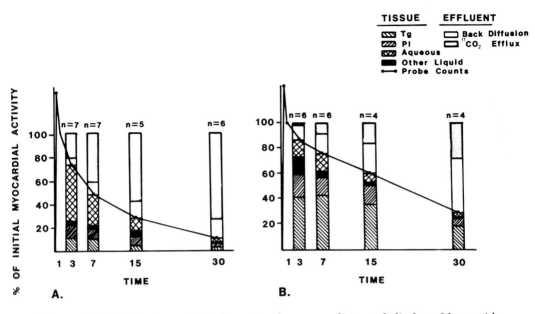

Figure 3-6. *Distributions of initially retained tracer predict metabolic fate of fatty acids in myocardium. 1-^{11}C palmitate was used to follow $^{11}CO_2$ production and backdiffusion of nonmetabolized substrate in coronary venous effluent and to develop a time-activity curve of tracer residue by external detection with a beta probe. 1-^{14}C palmitate was used to detect tracer distributions into various tissue lipid pools, including triacylglycerols (Tg), phospholipids (Pl), and other lipid and aqueous fractions. The quantitative analysis of the metabolic fate of radiolabeled palmitate in myocardial tissue and venous effluent during aerobic (A) and ischemic (B) perfusion is shown. The mean residue time-activity curve is plotted on a linear scale. Histograms below the time-activity curve indicate the mean percentage of initially extracted tracer activity at each biopsy time point within aqueous and lipid extractable tissue pools. Histograms above the mean residue time-activity curve indicate the mean cumulative contribution of $^{11}CO_2$ and 1-^{11}C palmitate (i.e., coronary venous efflux) to clearance of tracer from the myocardium in the venous effluent expressed as a percentage of 1 minute residue activity. Time on the abscissa is in minutes of post-tracer injection. (Reproduced from Rosamond et al.,[43] with permission of the Society of Nuclear Medicine.)*

does not track any specific element of the utilization pathway, which includes myocyte incorporation of fatty acids, fatty acid activation, lipid storage, mitochondrial transfer of fatty acid esters, β-oxidation, and entry into the citric acid cycle. PET imaging with ^{11}C-palmitate is useful as a qualitative tool with which to estimate overall fatty acid utilization in heart muscle, and to identify overall diminished metabolic function in ischemia. However, it cannot differentiate ischemic from irreversibly injured myocardium with static imaging at only one interval.

Metabolism of Glucose in Reperfused Myocardium

After reversible ischemic injury, heart muscle becomes mechanically and metabolically inefficient. Myocardial stunning or a failure to rapidly recover mechanical function despite reperfusion is a well-known consequence of reflow and has been explained by several hypotheses. Defects in energy metabolism may contribute to stunning.[44] Other proposed mechanisms include loss of intracellular calcium homeostasis and injury resulting from free-radical formation.[45] Mitochondria are ultrastructurally damaged in reversibly injured heart muscle with compromise of function.[46] In reperfused pig hearts, we have shown a clear reduction in the production of ATP in vitro, respiratory dysfunction compatible with partial uncoupling, and decreases in the activity of the critical transport enzyme adenine nucleotide translocase. Neubauer et al.[47] described oxygen wasting in reperfused mitochondria and a lower than expected P/O ratio, indicative of impaired oxidative phosphorylation, in glucose-perfused hearts.

The question of whether the damaged mitochondria can perform adequately with regard to intermediary and substrate utilization needed to sustain energy production during reflow has not yet been resolved. Much of the early information relevant to this issue was acquired by PET in attempts to define metabolic performance in response to reflow after induction of severe ischemia in dogs[48] or after infarction in patients. This work led to the recognition of a flow/metabolic mismatch with [18]FDG, which many regard as a clinical marker of myocardial viability in previously injured heart muscle. However, results of several recent studies are pertinent to interpretation.

Myears et al.[49] conducted studies in reperfused dog hearts after 1 hour of coronary occlusion. Coronary perfusate was whole blood, and ^{3}H-glucose and ^{14}C-palmitate were administered to follow substrate metabolism. Extraction fraction of labeled glucose and glycolysis were both increased during 1 hour of early reflow, whereas lactate utilization was nil. Most glycolysis was anaerobic, as judged from the observation that only 25% of exogenous glucose was oxidized. Schwaiger et al.[50] studied metabolic behavior 24 hours after a more severe ischemic stress (3 hours of coronary occlusion) in reperfused dog hearts with the use of D-6-^{14}C glucose and L-U-^{13}C lactate. They noted enhanced glucose uptake and glycolysis that was again largely anaerobic and accompanied by a large outpouring of lactate, over 90% of which came from exogenous glucose. Under less stringent ischemic conditions (60% hypoperfusion for 45 minutes) in blood-perfused porcine hearts in early reflow, we also observed only a modest use of glucose in oxidative metabolism, and this was accompanied by similar declines in pyruvate and lactate oxidation.[51,52] We explained this suppression of carbohydrate utilization by the preferred use of fatty acids available in the coronary perfusate and resulting allosteric inhibition (Figure 3-7). Approximately 80% to 90% of ATP produced with reflow was derived from fatty acid oxidation in these studies.[51–53]

How do these data bear on the flow/metabolic mismatch? The findings support the view that increased glycolysis, initiated during ischemia, persists during *early* reflow. This pattern of activity is largely nonoxidative. Comparatively little glucose enters oxidative metabolism. Thus, the amount of resulting ATP production is trivial. Whether this pattern persists in more chronic states of reperfusion (days to months) unsupported by other substrate utilization or oxidation, as suggested by clinical [18]FDG data, is conjectural. It seems unlikely

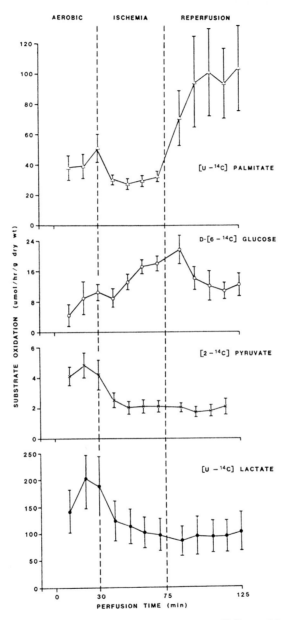

Figure 3-7. *A composite of data reported by Renstrom,[51,52] Liedtke,[56] and their colleagues in intact, working, extracorporeally perfused pig hearts. Regional $^{14}CO_2$ production curves from labeled palmitate (A), glucose (B), pyruvate (C), and lactate (D) are shown for whole-blood perfused hearts containing excess fatty acids. Aerobic perfusion was from 0 to 30 minutes, ischemic hypoperfusion from 30 to 75 minutes, and reperfusion from 75 to 125 minutes. Fatty acid oxidation, which rebounded above aerobic values in reflow, was associated with decreased oxidation of glucose, pyruvate, and lactate. (Adapted with permission of the American Heart Association, Inc.)*

that anaerobic glycolysis alone could sustain energy needs over long periods in viable, respiring myocardium, even if it were mechanically stunned or "hibernating."

A second problem concerns hypoperfusion. Although during acute ischemia some capacity for residual oxidative metabolism is maintained early, ultimately, oxygen delivery must be restored or the tissue will die. In heart muscle this threshold is thought to occur in 20 to 40 minutes. Unlike the case with mechanical stunning, no data support the notion that heart muscle somehow subsists on dramatically reduced energy demands in a "metabolically suspended" but viable state over long intervals of ischemia. It is unlikely that myocardium could remain viable for weeks to months if perfusion were less than 50% of aerobic levels. The American Heart Association Advanced Cardiac Imaging and Technology Committee on Nuclear Magnetic Resonance, PET, and Computed Tomography recently released an advisory on cardiac PET.[54] In it they stated that "two areas of potential clinical application (for PET) have emerged: detection and characterization of coronary artery disease and identification of ischemically injured but viable myocardium." It is our opinion that before such recommendations are widely implemented, fundamental issues regarding energy supply derived solely from glycolysis and the absolute magnitude of flow reduction must be resolved more fully.

Metabolism of Fatty Acid in Reperfused Myocardium

[11]C-palmitate time-activity curves generally are not used to estimate oxidative metabolism in clinical studies of reperfusion. In animal studies, such curves acquired in canine hearts showed delayed clearance of ^{11}C-palmitate activity over 90 minutes of reflow after a 20 minute coronary occlusion[55] and for up to 1 week after a 3 hour coronary occlusion.[48] Such curves represent integrations of several simultaneous biochemical events in the fatty acid utilization pathway. Results are not tightly coupled with fatty acid oxidation, at least early after reperfusion. Myears and coworkers[49] described a 52% decline in fatty acid uptake during early reflow. Nevertheless, oxidation of this substrate accounted for 63% of total oxygen consumption. The authors concluded that fatty acids continued to comprise the primary substrate for oxidative metabolism. Both Lopaschuk et al. and our group[53,56] noted full recovery of palmitate oxidation rates in reperfused hearts with early reflow. In our studies, a rebound occurred above aerobic values. This may have reflected a partial uncoupling of electron transport as observed in impaired mitochondria[46] or a mass-action effect in the proximal portion of the utilization pathway pushing the reaction toward oxidation.[57] However, these phenomena may not be observed with longer periods of reperfusion.

Amino Acid Metabolism in Aerobic Myocardium

Although amino acids are the major precursors in protein synthesis, their role in aerobic energy metabolism is less substantial. They do not represent a major source of carbon groups for ATP synthesis. Cellular availability of amino acids is dependent, at least in part, on 1) entry from the extracellular perfusate, 2) exit from the intracellular compartment, 3) incorporation and release by protein synthesis and degradation, and 4) intracellular synthesis and degradation by transamination and oxidation. Membrane transport of amino acids occurs over 4 membrane systems: system A for short, polar side chains; system ASC for alanine, serine, and cysteine; system L for amino acids with side chain rings; and system Ly$^+$ for cationic amino acids. Passage of amino acids across these systems is known to be bidirectional, with the net flux dependent on the amino acid gradient, the particular transport system involved, and the cell type. The rate of transport is affected also by inhibitory and stimulatory feedback controls of intracellular concentrations of amino acids and stimulation by hormones such as insulin.[58,59] The relative rates of protein synthesis and degradation are major determinants of intracellular amino acid concentration and are influenced by several factors, including the contractile state of the myocardium, the specific energy substrate of the tissue, degree of hormonal stimulation, availability of free amino acids, and oxygen availability. Synthesis and oxidation of individual amino acids have an impact on intracellular amino acid concentrations. The major pathway of synthesis of amino acids is transamination of citric acid cycle intermediates (see below). Amino acid levels may be decreased as a result of oxidative deamination with glutamate dehydrogenase in which ammonia is released from glutamate to enter the urea nitrogen cycle.

With regard to energy metabolism in aerobic hearts, the two major metabolic functions of amino acids, excluding tyrosine and phenylalanine, are to provide intermediates for the citric acid cycle and to serve as a shuttle system for the transfer of reducing equivalents into the mitochondria. The catabolism of amino acids to compounds within the citric acid cycle is by diverse pathways, depending on the particular amino acid. The most common catabolic step for all amino acids is the removal of the amino group by transamination (Figure 3-8). The principal transaminases, alanine and aspartate transaminases, catalyze the transfer of the amino group to pyruvate, to form alanine, and to α-ketoglutarate to form glutamate, converting the amino acid to the α-keto acid. In some cases, transamination is sufficient to obtain the citric acid cycle intermediate from the amino acid; for instance, aspartate is directly converted to oxaloacetate, and glutamate is degraded to α-ketoglutarate. With other amino acids, several steps are required to convert the amino acid to the citric cycle intermediate: histidine requires four steps before conversion to glutamate. Other amino acids form an intermediate before entering the citric acid cycle (e.g., the conversion of alanine or glycine to pyruvate). Transamination is an equilibrium reaction that allows for the formation of amino acids from citric acid cycle intermediates when amino acid concentrations decrease.

The second major metabolic function of aspartate and glutamate is participation in the malate-aspartate shuttle for transmitochondrial membrane transport of reducing equivalents (Figure 3-9). The passage of reducing equivalents (NADH) from the cytosol into the mitochondria occurs under 2 constraints: 1) the much higher NADH/NAD$^+$ ratio in the mitochondrial than in

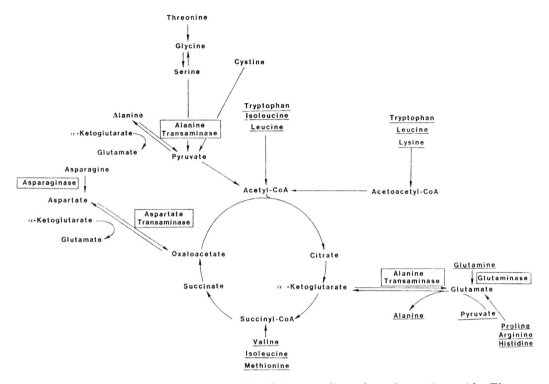

Figure 3-8. *Formation of citric acid cycle intermediates from free amino acids. The catabolism of some amino acids to the cycle compounds is relatively simple, requiring only transamination, while other amino acids require extensive catabolic steps before entry into the citric acid cycle. Major points of entry for amino acids is through glutamate to α-ketoglutarate; aspartate to oxaloacetate; alanine to pyruvate; leucine, lysine, and tryptophan to acetoacetyl-CoA; and isoleucine, methionine, and valine to succinyl-CoA. (Adapted from Taegtmeyer,[6] by permission of Raven Press, and from Murray RK, Granner DK, Mayes PA, Rodwell VW:* Harper's Biochemistry. *Appleton & Lange, 1988, with permission of the publisher).*

the cytosolic compartment, which prevents simple diffusion of NADH into the mitochondria,[60] and 2) the impermeability of the mitochondrial membrane to oxaloacetate. The transfer of reducing equivalents is facilitated by the oxidation of NADH and reduction of oxaloacetate to malate in the cytosol. Malate is then transported across the mitochondrial membrane by a specific membrane carrier. In the mitochondria, NADH is reformed with the oxidation of malate to oxaloacetate. Cytosolic levels of oxaloacetate are maintained at least in part by 1) the mitochondrial transamination of oxaloacetate and glutamate to aspartate and α-ketoglutarate, 2) transport of glutamate and aspartate to the cytosol across the mitochondrial membrane by the aspartate-glutamate antiport system, and 3) the regeneration of oxaloacetate by transamination of α-ketoglutarate and aspartate to oxaloacetate and glutamate.

A challenge in measuring rates of turnover of proteins and amino acids in myocardium is accounting for the diverse sources of amino acid synthesis and

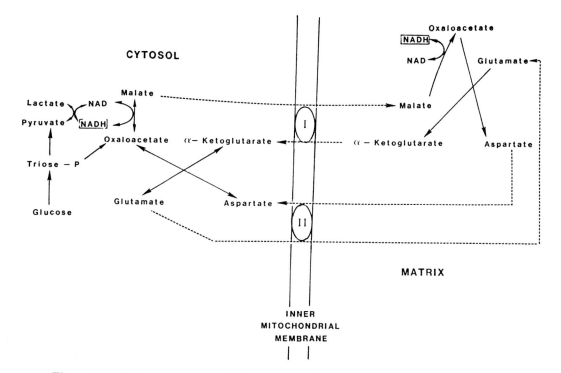

Figure 3-9. *Malate-aspartate cycle for transport of reducing equivalents from the cytosol to the mitochondrial matrix. Passage of reducing equivalents against a mitochondrial/ cytosol gradient occurs with the reduction of oxaloacetate to malate in the cytosol and exchange of malate for mitochondrial α-ketoglutarate by the malate-α-ketoglutarate exchange carrier (I). Cytosolic concentrations of oxaloacetate are maintained with exchange of cytosolic glutamate and mitochondrial aspartate by the mitochondrial membrane aspartate-glutamate antiport system (II). (Triose-P includes glyceraldehyde-3-P and α-glycerophosphate). (Adapted from Safer,[78] with permission of the American Heart Association, Inc.)*

depletion. Two amino acids, tyrosine and phenylalanine, are neither synthesized nor degraded by the heart, making them suitable for labeling studies to measure protein turnover.[61] PET imaging with ^{13}N-labeled compounds has reflected the complexities of measuring amino acid flux (see Chapter 8). In one study, transamination of 30% of the labeled amino group of glutamate to aspartate and alanine was observed within 6 minutes after uptake of tracer in isolated rabbit hearts.[62]

Amino Acid Metabolism in Ischemic Myocardium

The role of free amino acids in anaerobic metabolism was first identified by Hochachka and associates in studies of diving vertebrates.[63] Subsequent work with anoxic or hypoxic isolated papillary muscles, isolated hearts, or regionally ischemic myocardium has supported their observations. Specifically, two alterations in amino acid flux occur in the settings of low oxygen tension: alanine synthesis increases, and glutamate is converted to succinate in the citric acid cycle. In hypoxia or anoxia, net alanine synthesis has been demonstrated in a number of skeletal and cardiac muscle preparations.[64] The stimulus for this increase may be an increase in levels of pyruvate, which cannot enter aerobic metabolism. The rise in alanine production is accompanied by a decrease in concentrations of glutamate attributable to transamination.[64](Figure 3-10). Taegtmeyer and coworkers, using an isolated, right ventricular, papillary muscle preparation, demonstrated inhibition of alanine synthesis by blocking pyruvate production with the glycolytic inhibitors 2-deoxyglucose and iodoacetate.[64] Furthermore, synthesis of alanine by transamination was demonstrated by its suppression with the aminotransferase inhibitors L-cycloserine and aminooxyacetic acid. Although addition of glutamate further stimulated alanine synthesis, infusion of aspartate was without effect. This is in contrast to the findings of Peuhkurinen et al., who demonstrated reciprocal changes in alanine and aspartate concentrations in the isolated rat heart.[65] Concentrations of glutamate were unchanged, consistent with regeneration of α-ketoglutarate by aspartate transaminase (Figure 3-10).

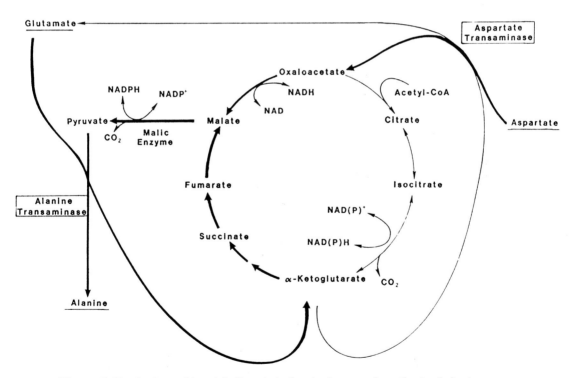

Figure 3-10. *Amino acid metabolism in ischemia. Increased synthesis of alanine occurs with transamination of glutamate and pyruvate by alanine transaminase. Isolated rat heart studies have demonstrated the utilization of aspartate, which has not been verified in isolated rabbit papillary muscle experiments. Increased synthesis of succinate from the transamination of glutamate to α-ketoglutarate also occurs in ischemia. (Adapted from Peuhkurinen et al.,[65] with permission of the American Physiological Society.)*

From a teleologic viewpoint, the importance of alanine synthesis during anaerobic metabolism is twofold. Alanine is a major substrate for hepatic gluconeogenesis. Its release from muscle during anaerobic metabolism allows for hepatic production of glucose for a continued supply of organic carbons for peripheral glycolysis. Second, the conversion of pyruvate to alanine decreases the cellular accumulation of lactate, a potent inhibitor of glycolysis at high concentrations.[64] The role of alanine in gluconeogenesis and suppression of lactate formation during anaerobiosis underlies the rationale for the use of glutamate in perfusion solutions to ameliorate ischemic episodes.

The second major role of amino acids at low oxygen contents is the conversion of glutamate and aspartate to succinate. Taegtmeyer,[66] using ^{14}C-labeled glutamate and aspartate, demonstrated a marked increase in succinate during anoxia. Concomitant increases in fumarate synthesis suggested that the conversion of aspartate to succinate occurs through fumarate. Under conditions of low oxygen availability, succinate formation via amino acid metabolism results in the generation of reducing equivalents and high-energy phosphates by the oxidation of α-ketoglutarate to succinate. However, the role of residual oxidation of α-ketoglutarate at low oxygen tension is controversial, and its occurrence has not been reproducibly observed under all experimental conditions. Furthermore, data from anoxic, isolated rat heart cells have suggested that the increase in ATP generation noted with infusion of malate, fumarate, and α-ketoglutarate may be attributable to the elimination of glycolytic inhibition by increased NADH. This increase in ATP generation was out of proportion to that in succinate.[67] NADH may be depleted as an alternate electron acceptor with the reduction of malate to succinate.

In recent studies in open-chest canine preparations of regional ischemia, changes in amino acid flux with hypoxia or anoxia similar to those previously observed in smaller mammals have been documented.[68] These reports confirm an increase in alanine efflux and succinate levels. Aspartate utilization was not increased during regional ischemia, consistent with the results of rabbit papillary muscle experiments in vitro.[66]

Changes in amino acid metabolism during ischemia have been evaluated, both in normal subjects and in patients with coronary artery disease (CAD), by measurement of arteriovenous differences in metabolites across the myocardium at rest and during cardiac pacing.[69] Increased alanine release was demonstrated in resting patients with CAD as compared with normal subjects (22 ± 3 vs 5 ± 4 nmol/ml, $p < 0.001$). With pacing to 140 beats/min, significant release of alanine occurred in the normal subjects (10 ± 4 nmol/ml), but it was still less than that in the patient group (23 ± 3 nmol/ml, $p < 0.05$). Glutamate uptake was seen in both groups, although again, it was significantly greater in the patient group. With pacing, net glutamate uptake decreased essentially to zero in the control group, but was still evident in the patient group. The findings indicate that net alanine synthesis is greater in patients with CAD under both resting and stressed conditions, as predicted from animal studies. These results have been confirmed by others. Enhanced extraction of glutamate during ischemia has been demonstrated with ^{13}N-glutamate PET imaging. In these studies, increased uptake of the tracer occurred in zones of reversible stress thallium defects and was correlated with percent ^{201}Tl redistribution.[70]

Amino Acid in Reperfused Myocardium

Data relevant to the flux of amino acids in reperfused hearts are scanty. In working isolated guinea pig hearts, reperfusion decreased the total glutamate and aspartate concentrations and increased the alanine synthesis.[71] Although a causal link with functional recovery was not tested, the results suggest a possible contribution of the amino acids to mechanical performance in vitro with reperfusion. Some clinical studies have suggested a possible benefit of glutamine infusions on postischemic contraction as well.[72]

Uptake and Kinetics of Ketone Bodies and Acetate

With the exception of PET data with ^{11}C-acetate (Chapters 9 and 11), relatively little information is available concerning acetate and ketone body metabolism with ischemia and reperfusion in human hearts. The principal ketone bodies are acetoacetate and D-3-hydroxybutyrate, produced by the liver. Acetate is present in only negligible quantities under physiologic conditions. In human subjects in the fed state, circulating levels of ketone bodies are quite low (0.1 mM),[73] but with starvation, pregnancy, hypoglycemia, or untreated diabetes, marked increases can occur. Peripheral metabolism of ketone bodies is relatively uniform compared with that of other substrates. Both 3-hydroxybutyrate and acetoacetate are readily taken up into the cytosolic compartment of most cells, with uptake limited principally by their availability in blood. Oxidation is through the citric acid cycle, with the mitochondrial membrane being permeable to both substrates (Figure 3-11). Ketones participate in cytosolic lipogenesis through conversion to butyryl-CoA or acetyl-CoA in some cells. Acetate enters the citric acid cycle after rapid conversion to acetyl-CoA by acetate thiokinase, present in the mitochondria. The rapid entry of this ketone with direct access to mitochondrial respiration, unencumbered by complicated transport or transfer mechanisms, is the chief rationale for its use as ^{11}C-acetate in estimating rates of cellular oxidation.[74]

Ketone Body Metabolism in Ischemic Myocardium

Because the circulating levels of ketones are low under physiologic conditions, data defining changes in their metabolism with ischemia and reperfusion are sparse. In the heart, ketones inhibit glucose uptake by inhibiting phosphofructokinase through increased levels of citrate (Figure 3-12). The increase in fructose 6-phosphate concentration inhibits hexokinase activity and thereby decreases glucose uptake.[75] Cardiac performance may be impaired, perhaps because of inhibition by ketonemia of α-ketoglutarate dehydrogenase.[76] An increase in the NADH/NAD$^+$ ratio may account for the inhibition. Nevertheless, infusion of 3-hydroxybutyrate compared with saline after coronary occlu-

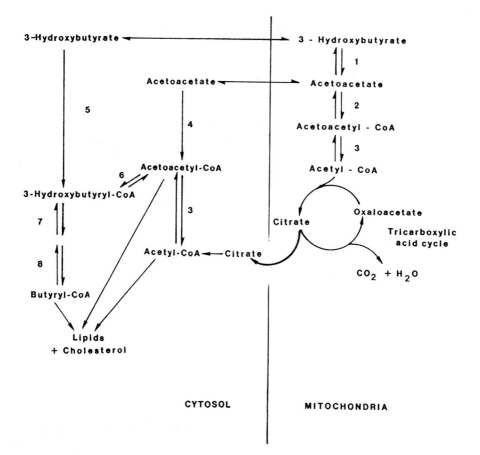

Figure 3-11. *Peripheral cellular catabolism of ketone bodies. Primary fate of ketone bodies is oxidation in the citric acid cycle or lipogenesis. Lipogenesis is of minor importance in the cardiomyocyte. Enzymes: 1, 3-hydroxybutyrate dehydrogenase; 2, 3-oxoacid-CoA transferase; 3, acetoacetyl-CoA thiolase; 4, acetoacetyl-CoA synthetase; 5, 3-hydroxybutyryl-CoA synthetase; 6, acetoacetyl-CoA reductase; 7, enoyl-CoA hydratase; 8, enoyl-CoA reductase. (Reprinted from Robinson and Williamson,[73] with permission from the American Physiological Society.)*

sion in open-chest dogs can provide partial protection against mechanical dysfunction.[77]

Summary

    In conclusion, an overview of myocardial metabolism indicates that substrate utilization for oxidation in normal, ischemic, and reperfused myocardium depends on the circulating and cellular concentrations of specific substrates and the oxygen tension of the myocardium. Complexities of fatty acid metabolism, glucose uptake, and phosphorylation underscore some of the chal-

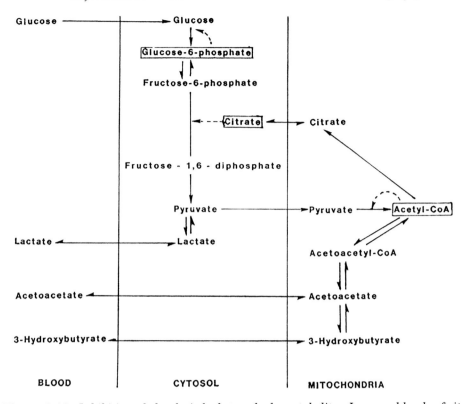

Figure 3-12. *Inhibition of glycolysis by ketone body metabolites. Increased levels of citrate in the cytosol with metabolism of acetoacetate inhibit phosphofructokinase activity. Increase in glucose 6-phosphate with the increase in fructose 6–phosphate inhibits hexokinase activity, thereby decreasing glucose uptake. The second and probably less important site of inhibition in the heart is pyruvate dehydrogenase. It is thought that increased levels of acetyl-CoA activate pyruvate dehydrogenase kinase and stimulate phosphorylation of pyruvate dehydrogenase. Dashed arrows indicate sites of inhibition. (Reprinted from Robinson and Williamson,[73] with permission of the American Physiological Society.)*

lenges in using labeled forms of these substrates (^{11}C-palmitate and ^{18}F-FDG) to quantitate myocardial metabolism by PET. PET imaging with analysis of washout of ^{11}C-acetate activity may provide more consistent quantitation of myocardial oxidative phosphorylation rates. However, because rates of anaerobic glycolysis are not measured, ^{11}C-acetate imaging at a single interval may not differentiate ischemic or "viable" myocardium from infarction. The diversity of myocardial metabolism allows the heart to continue to function in a variety of metabolic milieus. The same diversity poses a challenge for noninvasive assessment of myocardial metabolic rates and argues for the use of more than one tracer for determination of myocardial metabolism by PET.

Acknowledgments: The art work of Donna Hotz, Kathleen Carroll, Larry Whitesell, Brita Renstrom, and Catherine Kidd and the secretarial assistance of Shelley Kroncke and Candyce Carlson are greatly appreciated.

References*

1. Neely JR, Rovetto MJ, Oram JF. Myocardial utilization of carbohydrate and lipids. Prog Cardiovasc Dis 1972; 15:289–329.
2. Randle PJ, Tubbs PK. Carbohydrate and fatty acid metabolism. In: *Handbook of Physiology. The Cardiovascular System I*. Steiner DF and Freinkel N (Eds). American Physiological Society, Washington, D.C., 1979; 805–844.
3. Liedtke AJ. Alterations of carbohydrate and lipid metabolism in the acutely ischemic heart. Prog Cardiovasc Dis 1981; 23:321–336.
4. Corr PB, Gross RW, Sobel BE. Amphipathic metabolites and membrane dysfunction in ischemic myocardium. Circ Res 1984; 55:135–154.
5. Opie LH. Substrate utilization and glycolysis in the heart. Cardiology 1971/1972; 56:2–21.
6. Taegtmeyer H. Myocardial metabolism. In: Phelps M, Mazziotta J and Shelbert H, Eds. *Positron Emission Tomography and Autoradiography: Principles and Applications for the Brain and Heart*. New York: Raven Press, 1986; 149–195.
7. Bing RJ. The course of science and cardiac metabolism. Circ Res 1976; 38 (suppl I):I-15—I-155.
8. Yeo GF. An attempt to estimate the gaseous interchange of the frog's heart by means of the spectroscope. J Physiol (London) 1885; 6:93–121.
9. Locke FS, Rosenheim O. The disappearance of dextrose when perfused through the isolated mammalian heart. J Physiol (London) 1904; 31:14–15.
10. Cruickshank EWH, Startup CW. The respiratory quotient, oxygen consumption and glycogen content of the mammalian heart in aglycaemia. J Physiol (London) 1933; 80:179–192.
11. Bing RJ, Siegel A, Ungar I, Gilbert M. Metabolism of the human heart. 2. Studies on fat, ketone and amino acid metabolism. Am J Med 1954; 16:540–545.
12. Opie LH, Evans JR, Shipp JC. Effect of fasting on glucose and palmitate metabolism of perfused rat heart. Am J Physiol 1963; 205:1203–1208.
13. Mitchell P, Keilin's respiratory chain concept and its chemiosmotic consequences. Science 1979; 206:1148.
14. Gobayashi K, Neely JR. Control of maximum rates of glycolysis in rat cardiac muscle. Circ Res 1979; 44:166–175.
15. Neely JR, Morgan HE. Relationship between carbohydrate and lipid metabolism and the energy balance of heart muscle. Annu Rev Physiol 1974; 36:413–459.
16. Wisneski JA, Stanley WC, Neese RA, Gertz EW. Effects of acute hyperglycemia on myocardial glycolytic activity in humans. J Clin Invest 1990; 85:1648–1656.
17. Wisneski JA, Gertz EW, Neese RA, Mayr M. Myocardial metabolism of free fatty acids: Studies ^{14}C-labeled substrates in humans. J Clin Invest 1987; 79:359–366.
18. Marshall RC, Tillisch JH, Phelps ME, Huang S-C, Carson R, Henze E, Schelbert HR. Identification and differentiation of resting myocardial ischemia and infarction in man with positron computed tomography, ^{18}F-labeled fluorodeoxyglucose and N-13 ammonia. Circulation 1983; 67:766–778.
19. Barrett BJ, Schwartz RG, Francis CK, Zaret BL. Regulation by insulin of myocardial glucose and fatty acid metabolism in the conscious dog. J Clin Invest 1984; 74:1073–1079.
20. Gertz EW, Wisneski JA, Stanley WC, Neese RA. Myocardial substrate utilization during exercise in humans: Dual carbon-labeled carbohydrate isotope experiments. J Clin Invest 1988; 82:2017–2025.
21. Drake AJ, Haines JR, Noble MIM. Preferential uptake of lactate by the normal myocardium in dogs. Cardiovasc Res 1980; 14:65–72.
22. Dennis SC, Padma A, DeBuysere MS, Olson MS. Studies on the regulation of pyru-

---

* A complete citation list is available from the author.

vate dehydrogenase in the isolated perfused rat heart. J Biol Chem 1979; 254:1252–1258.

23. Brosnan JT, Reid K. Inhibition of palmitoylcarnitine oxidation by pyruvate in rat heart mitochondria. Metabolism 1985; 34:588–593.

24. Oram JF, Bennetch SL, Neely JR. Regulation of fatty acid utilization in isolated perfused rat hearts. J Biol Chem 1973; 248:5299–5309.

25. Liedtke AJ, Nellis SH. Effects of carnitine isomers on fatty acid metabolism in ischemic hearts. Circ Res 48:859–866, 1981.

26. Liedtke AJ, Nellis SH, Mjos OD. Effects of reducing fatty acid metabolism on mechanical function in regionally ischemic hearts. Am J Physiol 1984; 247 (Heart Circ Physiol 16):H387–H394.

27. Miller WP, Liedtke AJ, Nellis SH. Effects of 2–tetradecylglycidic acid on myocardial function in swine hearts. Am J Physiol 1986; 251 51 (Heart Circ Physiol 20):H547-H553.

28. Liedtke AJ, Demaison L, Eggleston AM, Cohen LM, Nellis SH. Changes in substrate metabolism and effects of excessive fatty acids in reperfused myocardium. Circ Res 1988; 62:535–542.

29. Rovetto MJ, Lamberton WF, Neely JR. Mechanisms of glycolytic inhibition in ischemic rat hearts. Circ Res 1975; 37:742–751.

30. Opie LE. Effects of regional ischemia on metabolism of glucose and fatty acids: Relative rates of aerobic and anaerobic energy production from myocardial infarction and comparison with effects of anoxia. Circ 1976; Res 38 (suppl I):I-52-I-74.

31. Schwaiger M, Brunken R, Grover-McKay M, Krivokapich J, Child J, Tillisch JH, Phelps ME, Schelbert HR. Regional myocardial metabolism in patients with acute myocardial infarction assessed by positron emission tomography. J Am Coll Cardiol 1986; 8:800–808.

32. Tillisch J, Brunken R, Marshall R, Schwaiger M, Mandelkern M, Phelps M, Schelbert H. Reversibility of cardiac wall-motion abnormalities predicted by positron tomography. N Engl J Med 1986; 314:884–888.

33. Sebree L, Bianco JA, Subramanian R, Wilson MA, Swanson D, Hegge J, Tschudy J, Pyzalski R. Discordance between accumulation of C-14 deoxyglucose and Tl-201 in reperfused myocardium. J Mol Cell Cardiol 1991; 23:603–616.

34. Fox KAA, Nomura H, Sobel BE, Bergmann SR. Consistent substrate utilization despite reduced flow in hearts with maintained work. Am J Physiol 1983; 244 (Heart Circ Physiol 13):H799-H806.

35. Liedtke AJ. Lipid burden in ischemic myocardium. J Mol Cell Cardiol 1988; 20 (suppl II):65–74.

36. Liedtke AJ, Shrago E. Detrimental effects of fatty acids and their derivatives in ischemic and reperfused myocardium. In: *Pathophysiology of Severe Ischemic Myocardial Injury.* Piper,HM, (Ed.) Kluwer Academic Publishers, Dordrecht/Boston/London, 1990; 149–166.

37. Corr PB, Gross RW, Sobel BE. Arrhythmogenic amphiphilic lipids in the myocardial cell membrane. J Mol Cell Cardiol 1982; 14:619–626.

38. Bilheimer DW, Buja LM, Parkey RW, Bonte FJ, Willerson JT. Fatty acid accumulation and abnormal lipid deposition in peripheral and border zones of experimental myocardial infarcts. J Nucl Med 1978; 19:276–283.

39. Weiss ES, Hoffman EJ, Phelps ME, Welch MJ, Henry PD, Ter-Pogossian MM, Sobel BE. External detection and visualization of myocardial ischemia ^{11}C-substrates in vitro and in vivo. Circ Res 1976; 39:24–32.

40. Lerch RA, Ambos HD, Bergmann SR, Welch MJ, Ter-Pogossian MM, Sobel BE. Localization of viable, ischemic myocardium by positron-emission tomography with ^{11}C-palmitate. Circulation 1981; 64:689–699.

41. Schelbert HR, Henze E, Keen R, Schone HR, Hansen H, Selin C, Huang S-C, Barrio JR, Phelps ME. C-11 palmitate for the noninvasive evaluation of regional myocardial fatty acid metabolism with positron-computed tomography. IV. In vivo evaluation of acute demand-induced ischemia in dogs. Am Heart J 1983; 106:736–750.

42. Fox KAA, Abendschein DR, Ambos HD, Sobel BE, Bergmann SR. Efflux of metabolized and nonmetabolized fatty acid from canine myocardium: Implications for quantifying myocardial metabolism tomographically. Circ Res 1985; 57:232–243.
43. Rosamond TL, Abendschein DR, Sobel BE, Bergmann SR, Fox KAA. Metabolic fate of radiolabeled palmitate in ischemic canine myocardium: Implications for positron-emission tomography. J Nucl Med 1987; 28:1322–1329.
44. Neely JR, Grotyohann LW. Role of glycolytic products in damage to ischemic myocardium: Dissociation of adenosine triphosphate levels and recovery of function of reperfused ischemic hearts. Circ Res 1984; 55:816–824.
45. Jolly SR, Kane WJ, Bailie MB, Abrams GD, Lucchesi BR. Canine myocardial reperfusion injury. Its reduction by the combined administration of superoxide dismutase and catalase. Circ Res 1984; 54:277–285.
46. Huang XQ, Liedtke AJ. Alterations in fatty acid oxidation in ischemic and reperfused myocardium. Mol Cell Biochem 1989; 88:145–153.
47. Neubauer S, Hamman BL, Perry SB, Bittl JA, Ingwall JS. Velocity of the creatine kinase reaction decreases in postischemic myocardium: A ^{31}P-NMR magnetization transfer study of the isolated ferret heart. Circ Res 1988; 63:1–15.
48. Schwaiger M, Schelbert HR, Ellison D, Hansen H, Yeagman L, Vinten-Johansen J, Selin C, Barrio J, Phelps ME. Sustained regional abnormalities in cardiac metabolism after transient ischemia in the chronic dog model. J Am Coll Cardiol 1985; 6:336–347.
49. Myears DW, Sobel BE, Bergmann SR. Substrate use in ischemic and reperfused canine myocardium: Quantitative considerations. Am J Physiol 1987; 253 (Heart Circ Physiol 22):H107-H114.
50. Schwaiger M, Neese RA, Araujo L, Wyns W, Wisneski JA, Sochor H, Swank S, Kulber D, Selin C, Phelps M, Schelbert HR, Fishbein MC, Gertz EW. Sustained nonoxidative glucose utilization and depletion of glycogen in reperfused canine myocardium. J Am Coll Cardiol 1989; 13:745–754.
51. Renstrom B, Nellis SH, Liedtke AJ. Metabolic oxidation of glucose during early myocardial reperfusion. Circ Res 1989; 65:1094–1101.
52. Renstrom B, Nellis SH, Liedtke AJ. Metabolic oxidation of pyruvate and lactate during early myocardial reperfusion. Circ Res 1990; 66:282–288.
53. Lopaschuk GD, Spafford MA, Davies NJ, Wall SR. Glucose and palmitate oxidation in isolated working rat hearts reperfused after a period of transient global ischemia. Circ Res 1990; 65:546–553.
54. Statement from the advanced cardiac imaging and technology committee on NMR, PET, and CT. Council on Clinical Cardiology Newsletter. Ed: GM Pohost. Winter 1990, 15.
55. Schwaiger M, Schelbert HR, Keen R, Vinten-Johansen J, Hansen H, Selin C, Barrio J, Huang S-C, Phelps ME. Retention and clearance of C-11 palmitic acid in ischemic and reperfused canine J Am Coll Cardiol 1985; 6:311–320.
56. Liedtke AJ, DeMaison L, Eggleston AM, Cohen LM, Nellis SH. Changes in substrate metabolism and effects of excessive fatty acids in reperfused myocardium. Circ Res 1988; 62:535–542.
57. Renstrom B, Liedtke AJ, Nellis SH. Mechanisms of substrate preference for oxidative metabolism during early myocardial reperfusion. Am J Physiol 1990; 259:H317-H323.
58. Schwartz RG, Barrett EJ, Francis CK, Jacob R, Zaret BL. Regulation of myocardial amino acid balance in the conscious dog. J Clin Invest 1985; 75:1204–1211.
59. Schimke RT. Regulation of protein degradation in mammalian tissues. Mammalian Protein Metab 1970; 4:177–228.
60. Williamson JR, Browning ET, Scholz R. Control mechanisms of gluconeogenesis and ketogenesis: I. Effects of oleate on gluconeogenesis in perfused rat liver. J Biol Chem 1969; 244:4607–4616.
61. Morgan HE, Earl DCN, Broadus A, Wolpert EB, Giger KE, Jefferson LS. Regulation of protein synthesis in heart muscle. I. Effect of amino acid levels on protein synthesis. J Biol Chem 1971; 246:2152–2162.

62. Krivokapich J, Keen RE, Phelps ME, Shine KI, Barrio JR. Effects of anoxia on kinetics of ^{13}Nglutamate and ^{13}NH$_3$ metabolism in rabbit myocardium. Circ Res 1987; 60:505–516.

63. Hochachka PW, Storey KB. Metabolic consequences of diving in animals and man. Science 1975; 187:613–621.

64. Taegtmeyer H, Peterson MB, Ragavan VR, Ferguson AG, Lesch M. *De novo* alanine synthesis in isolated oxygen deprived rabbit myocardium. J Biol Chem 1977; 252:5010–5018.

65. Peuhkurinen KJ, Takala TES, Nuutinen EM, Hassinen IE. Tricarboxylic acid cycle metabolites during ischemia in isolated perfused rat heart. Am J Physiol 1983; 244:H281-H288.

66. Taegtmeyer H. Metabolic responses to cardiac hypoxia. Increased production of succinate by rabbit papillary muscles. Circ Res 1978; 43:808–815.

67. Wiesner RJ, Rosen P, Grieshaber MK. Pathways of succinate formation and their contribution to improvement of cardiac function in the hypoxic rat heart. Biochem Med Metab Biol 1988; 40:19–34.

68. Wiesner RJ, Deussen A, Borst M, Schrader J, Grieshaber MK. Glutamate degradation in the ischemic dog heart: Contribution to anaerobic energy production. J Mol Cell Cardiol 1989; 21:49–59.

69. Mudge GH Jr, Mills RM Jr, Taegtmeyer H, Gorlin R, Lesch M. Alterations of myocardial amino acid metabolism in chronic ischemic heart disease. J Clin Invest 1976; 58:1185–1192.

70. Zimmermann R, Tillmanns H, Knapp WH, Helus F, Georgi P, Rauch B, Neumann F-J, Girgensohn S, Maier-Borst W, Kubler W. Regional myocardial nitrogen-13 glutamate uptake in patient with coronary artery disease: Inverse post-stress relation to thallium-201 uptake in ischemia. J Am Coll Cardiol 1988; 11:549–556.

71. Pisarenko OI, Oleynikov OD, Shulzhendo VS, Studneva IM, Ryff IM, Kapelko VI. Association of myocardial glutamate and aspartate pool and functional recovery of postischemic heart. Biochem Med Metab Biol 1989; 42:105–117.

72. Lazar HL, Backberg GD, Manganero AJ, Becker H, Maloney JV Jr. Reversal of ischemic change with amino acid substrate enhancement during reperfusion. Surgery 1980; 88:702–709.

73. Robinson AM, Williamson DH. Physiological roles of ketone bodies as substrates and signals in mammalian tissues. Physiol Rev 1980; 60:143–187.

74. Walsh MN, Geltman EM, Brown MA, Henes CG, Weinheimer CJ, Sobel BE, Bergmann SR. Noninvasive estimation of regional myocardial oxygen consumption by positron emission tomography with carbon-11 acetate in patients with myocardial infarction. J Nucl Med 1989; 30:1798–1808.

75. Randle PJ, England PJ, Denton RM. Control of the tricarboxylate cycle and its interactions with glycolysis during acetate utilization in rat heart. Biochem J 1970; 117:677–695.

76. Taegtmeyer H. On the inability of ketone bodies to serve as the only energy providing substrate for rat heart at physiological work load. Basic Res Cardiol 1983; 78:435–450.

77. Lammerant J, Huynh-Thu T, Kolanowski J. Stabilization of left ventricular function with D-(-)-3-hydroxybutyrate after coronary occlusion in the intact dog. J Mol Cell Cardiol 1988; 20:579–583.

78. Safer B. The metabolic significance of the malate-aspartate cycle in heart. Circ Res 1975; 37:527–533.

Chapter 4

Radiopharmaceuticals for Cardiac Positron Emission Tomography

Michael J. Welch, Ph.D. and Arooj M. Shaikh M.D.

Production of Isotopes

Many radiopharmaceuticals have been developed for studies of myocardial perfusion and metabolism with positron emission tomography (PET). Most require the incorporation of positron-emitting radionuclides into the tracer of interest using novel, rapid, synthetic schemes.

Positron-emitting radionuclides can be produced in one of two ways, either with an on-site accelerator or with a generator. Use of an on-site cyclotron can support production of oxygen-15 (^{15}O, half-life 2.04 minutes), nitrogen-13 (^{13}N, half-life 10 minutes), carbon-11 (^{11}C, half-life 20.4 minutes), and fluorine-18 (^{18}F, half-life 110 minutes). Because of these short physical half-lives, with the possible exception of radiopharmaceuticals labeled with ^{18}F, production of tracers with these radionuclides at a remote site is not practical. Because labeling of compounds of particular physiologic and pharmacologic importance is facilitated with these positron-emitting radionuclides, a dedicated, on-site cyclotron is advantageous.

At present, approximately 50 PET centers perform cardiologic studies: those centers with a major research interest and that utilize a wide variety of radiopharmaceuticals; and those centers that utilize a limited number of radiopharmaceuticals (i.e., only a flow and/or a metabolism tracer) for clinical assessment of perfusion or myocardial viability.

Three types of cyclotrons are currently available: 30 MeV machines that accelerate protons, deuterons, helium-3, and alpha particles with a proton energy of 30 MeV; dual-particle, 8 MeV deuteron, 16 MeV proton accelerators; and 11 MeV proton-only accelerators. A center with a major research commitment would necessarily select 1 of the first 2 accelerators. A center with more

From *Positron Emission Tomography of the Heart* edited by Steven R. Bergmann, MD, PhD and Burton E. Sobel, MD © 1992, Futura Publishing Inc., Mount Kisco, NY.

limited requirements could obtain radioisotopes with a smaller accelerator. Alternatively, if only 1 or 2 radiopharmaceuticals are required, an additional option is to obtain ^{18}F from a regional delivery center and a flow tracer from either a radionuclide generator or from a compact ^{15}O-production system.

At present, large cyclotrons are available from at least 3 manufacturers: Japan Steel Works (Japan), Scanditronix (Sweden), and Ion Beam Applications (IBA, Belgium); medium-energy, dual-particle machines are available from Japan Steel Works, Scanditronix, and IBA; and proton-only machines from Siemens/CTI and Oxford Instruments. Scanditronix has recently announced a design of a proton-only cyclotron.

Development of ultracompact, simple-to-use accelerators is likely to impact favorably on the future of PET centers. Table 4-1 lists some new accelerators that have become commercially available or been described in the literature recently. They can provide a number of radiopharmaceuticals inexpensively and simply. With the exception of the Cyclone-3, all of these units are linear accelerators that are lightweight, require less power than cyclotrons, and are simpler to operate. If such accelerators can be used to produce all of the radionuclides required, operation of cardiac PET facilities will be simpler and less expensive than is currently the case.

Production of positron-emitting radionuclides with generators, whereby a short-lived daughter radionuclide is rapidly separated from a longer-lived parent, can be advantageous in that the parent radionuclide can be produced at a remote site and less expensively than cyclotron-produced radiopharmaceuticals. To date, generator-produced radiopharmaceuticals suitable for cardiac studies are limited to agents used to image the blood pool or estimate perfusion.

Table 4-1
Recently Developed Accelerators Available for Production of Positron-Emitting Radionuclides

Company	Type of Accelerator	Particle(s)	Comment
Ion Beam Applications Belgium	Cyclone (Cyclone-3)	3 MeV deuterons	^{15}O-only accelerator; Size of a soda vending machine
Science Applications Int'l Corp. San Diego, CA	Radio-frequency quadruple accelerator	8 MeV ^{3}He	With shielding 1/9 weight of cyclotron; ^{15}O and ^{11}C produced carrier added
ACCSYS Technology Pleasanton, CA	Ion linac	Several designs; 3 MeV deuterons 11 MeV protons	Lightweight high current machine
Science Research Lab, Inc. Somerville, MA	Electrostatic accelerator (TCA)	3.7 MeV protons and deuterons	Very high current accelerator; high yield production of ^{18}F and ^{15}O has been demonstrated

Table 4-2
Parent-Daughter Generator Systems by which Flow Tracers Have Been
Developed

Parent Decay Isotope	Parent Half-Life	Daughter Isotope	Daughter Half-Life	Daughter Positron Yield (%)	Daughter Positron Energy (MeV)	Daughter Product (Stable)
^{68}Ge	288 days	^{68}Ga	68.1 min	90	1.899	^{68}Zn
^{82}Sr	25.0 days	^{82}Rb	75 sec	96	3.15	^{82}Kr
^{62}Zn	9.2 hour	^{62}Cu	9.74 min	98	2.93	^{62}Ni

Generators used for cardiac applications are listed in Table 4-2. Unlike the radionuclides that can be produced with a cyclotron, these nuclides are not normal chemical constituents of molecules of biological interest. The costs of generators are not negligible. For example, an infusion system for a strontium/rubidium generator costs over $50,000 and the strontium column, which needs to be replaced monthly, costs approximately $25,000. Because the inexpensive accelerators described in Table 4-1 are anticipated to cost under $1,000,000, such relatively inexpensive accelerators may be cost effective compared with many generators.

Staffing and Quality Control

Centers producing positron-emitting isotopes require both high-level and low-level radiochemistry laboratories in addition to a cyclotron room and a control room. Cyclotron operators, radiochemists, and radiopharmacists are required. Several controls are necessary pertinent to administration of radio-pharmaceuticals produced on-site including: 1) pharmaceutical quality control, 2) chemical quality control, and 3) radionuclidic and radiochemical quality control. Rigorous testing is needed to ensure sterility and lack of pyrogenicity. Most tracers are also passed through a 0.22 μm filter just prior to administration. Because of the short half-life of positron-emitting radionuclides, some tests cannot be performed on every batch—but representative batches (e.g., every tenth) should be tested. Chemical quality control involves measurement of the amounts of chemical impurities present with exclusion of chemical impurities that may arise from synthetic precursors and/or chemicals used in the purification of the final compound. Chemical quality control usually involves high-performance liquid chromatography (HPLC). In some circumstances, such as those requiring compounds that label receptors, the presence of unlabeled impurities that bind to the receptor can inhibit uptake of the tracer at the site of interest.

Radionuclidic quality control can be performed simply by measuring the decay pattern and half-life of the nuclide. In the case of the positron-emitting radionuclides discussed in this chapter, it is unlikely that radionuclides, other than positron-emitting species, will contaminate the final preparation. Periodic checks of half-life are usually sufficient to exclude them. Determination of radiochemical impurity is more difficult, however. For example, with 2-fluoro-2-deoxyglucose, possible impurities include free fluoride ion and the isometric ^{18}F-2-fluoro-2-deoxymannose. Thus, sophisticated HPLC separations are needed to define the amount of 2-fluoro-2-deoxymannose in the final preparation.

Tracers Used to Quantify Perfusion

Myocardial perfusion can be measured with PET using the diffusible tracers ^{15}O-labeled water or ^{11}C- or ^{15}O-labeled butanol, or with extractable tracers such as ^{13}N-labeled ammonia, rubidium-82 (^{82}Rb), copper-62 (^{62}Cu) pyruvaldehyde bis(N^4-methylthiosemicarbazone)(PTSM), and complexes of gallium-68 (^{68}Ga). Schemes of the synthesis will be described only in brief, general terms. Details for some novel syntheses under development are provided in the Appendix.

^{15}O-labeled Water

^{15}O is generally produced by the ^{14}N [d,n]^{15}O reaction.[1] If a cyclotron with only a proton beam is used, ^{15}O can be produced with the ^{15}N[d,n]^{15}O reaction and an enriched ^{15}N target, but at a higher cost. With the use of a nitrogen gas target containing a trace of oxygen, ^{15}O is formed as $O^{15}O$ gas.[2] The labeled oxygen can be incorporated into labeled water by two processes: it can be mixed with hydrogen and passed over a catalyst or combusted to form $H_2{}^{15}O$,[3] or it can be converted to carbon dioxide and water when $CO^{15}O$ is dissolved in aqueous solution:[3]

$$CO^{15}O + H_2O \rightleftharpoons H_2CO_2{}^{15}O \rightleftharpoons H_2{}^{15}O + CO_2$$

Bubbling of $CO^{15}O$ through normal saline produces ^{15}O-labeled water in a form suitable for intravenous injection. An alternative route of administration is the inhalation of $CO^{15}O$ after inhalation of gaseous $CO^{15}O$ that is converted to ^{15}O-water in the lungs and blood. Production (which takes about 5 minutes) can be completely automated with routine synthesis of > 200 to 400 mCi per run and a purity of > 99%. A total of 20 to 70 mCi are usually needed for cardiac studies.

^{11}C- and ^{15}O-butanol

Butanol labeled with either ^{11}C or ^{15}O has been proposed as an alternative diffusible tracer for assessment of perfusion. Although ^{11}C-butanol has been used for estimates of myocardial perfusion, the labeled alcohol has not been used extensively. An automated production scheme for ^{15}O-butanol has recently been described.[4]

^{13}N-ammonia

^{13}N is best produced with a biomedical cyclotron via the ^{16}O [p,α]^{13}N nuclear reaction with the use of a water target to yield the radionuclide as a mixture of nitrate, nitrite, and ammonium ions that can be converted readily to ^{13}N-ammonia by reduction with the use of titanium [III] chloride or other reducing agents.[5] Production takes 20 to 30 minutes and results in up to 200 to 300 mCi/run with a specific activity of 200 to 400 mCi/μmol and a purity of > 99%. Ten to 20 mCi is typically administered.

Rubidium-82 (^{82}Rb)

^{82}Rb flow tracers have been synthesized with generator production systems (Table 4-2). The strontium-82 (^{82}Sr)/^{82}Rb generator system, which has been approved by the U.S. Food and Drug Administration,[6] consists of a tin dioxide absorbent from which ^{82}Rb can be eluted selectively in normal saline. The parent ^{82}Sr is produced by bombardment of a molybdenum target with high-energy protons and contamination with ^{85}Sr in at least a 1:1 ratio. The rubidium produced can be injected directly into the patient as a solution of Rb$^+$ ions. Use of a computer-controlled infusion system permits adjustment of the dose of ^{82}Rb, the total volume of solution, and infusion rate to predetermined values. The tracer can be eluted in NaCl from the generator every 5 to 10 minutes. Thirty to 60 mCi are typically eluted with minimal ^{82}Sr breakthrough and administered directly. Because the half-life of the ^{82}Sr parent is 25 days, a single generator can be used for approximately 4 weeks.

^{62}Cu-PTSM

Green and colleagues have described the production and evaluation of ^{62}Cu-labeled copper-II pyruvaldehyde bis (N^4-methylthiosemicarbazone) (PTSM).[7–9] ^{62}Cu has a 9.74 minute half-life, suitable for (PET) and measurement of myocardial blood flow.[10–12] A zinc-62/^{62}Cu generator has been developed that is capable of yielding 100 to 400 mCi of ^{62}Cu, which, in turn, can yield ^{62}Cu-PTSM in approximately 6 to 8 minutes after elution of the generator.[13] Despite the need for replacement of the generator almost daily, Cu-PTSM is a promising alternative to ^{82}Rb as a generator-produced flow tracer.

Gallium-68 (^{68}Ga)

Gallium-68–1,1,1-tris(5-methoxysalicylaldiminomethyl) ethane was the first generator-produced gallium agent developed to measure myocardial blood flow,[14] but its clearance from the myocardium was too rapid and its use required a blood pool subtraction technique. Two alternative ligands, tetrakis(2-hydroxy-3,5-dimethylbenzyl)ethylene diamine[15] and ^{68}Ga-BAT-TECH, may be superior.[16] However, all ^{68}Ga imaging agents developed to date clear rapidly from myocardium so that the quality of perfusion images is suboptimal[17] compared with that obtainable with other flow tracers.

Blood Pool Tracers

A number of tracers of the vasculature have been developed. These are often used to delineate the vasculature (for reference in identification of myocardial structures) as well as to assess myocardial blood volume, cardiac chamber motion, and correctional factors required in algorithms pertinent to the vascular pool.

Carbon Monoxide

The tracer most commonly used to visualize the blood pool is carbon monoxide labeled with ^{11}C or [15]O. ^{11}C-carbon monoxide can be formed by passing ^{11}C-carbon dioxide produced in a cyclotron target chamber over zinc metal heated to approximately 450°C.[1,2] One hundred to 500 mCi of ^{15}O-labeled carbon monoxide can be formed from ^{15}O-oxygen produced in a nitrogen target by passage over charcoal heated to > 900°C.[1,2] Thirty to 50 mCi of C[15]O are administered by inhalation. In both schemes, only a minute amount of carrier carbon monoxide is produced.

[68]Ga and [62]Cu Proteins and Red Cells

Both the germanium/gallium and zinc/copper generators have been used to produce labeled proteins and red cells for blood pool evaluations. In the most common germanium/gallium generator, gallium is eluted as a chloride in 1M HCl. Neutralization with citrate buffer forms a gallium citrate that, on injection, leads to the formation in vivo of gallium transferrin[18] as a result of the large stability constant of the complex.[19] ^{68}Ga-labeled red cells can be produced by a technique similar to that used for labeling blood components with indium-111 (^{111}In). When ^{68}Ga-8-hydroxyquinoline is incubated with separated red cells, high labeling yields are obtained.[20] Labeling of albumin and other proteins for use as blood pool tracers with either ^{68}Ga or with [62]Cu can be accomplished by functionalizing the protein with a strong chelate.[21,22]

Tracers of Metabolism

[18]F-fluorodeoxyglucose

Fluorodeoxyglucose is an analog of glucose widely used for assessment of myocardial viability. ^{18}F-fluorodeoxyglucose can be produced in a biomedical cyclotron via either the $^{20}Ne(d,\alpha)^{18}F$ or the $^{18}O(p,n)^{18}F$ nuclear reactions. A neon target containing 0.1% to 1% fluorine gas is used for labeling. Bombardment of enriched $H_2{}^{18}O$ produces an aqueous fluoride ion that can be converted into reactive fluoride. 2-Fluorodeoxyglucose was initially produced by the use of labeled fluorine gas (Appendix),[23] but most centers producing this compound now use fluoride ion and a procedure initially developed by Hamacher et al.[24] (Appendix). Synthesis time is typically 1 hour with a yield of 20 to 30 mCi with a specific activity of ~1.2 Ci/mmol. Radiochemical purity is ~95%. Five to 10 mCi are needed for administration. Automated production systems have been developed.

Labeling of Fatty Acids with ^{11}C

Because fatty acids are the primary physiologic substrate for oxidative metabolism in normal myocardium, radiolabeled fatty acids are attractive agents for the elucidation of regional metabolism. The first ^{11}C-fatty acid synthesized for this purpose, via the reaction of the corresponding Grignard compound with $^{11}CO_2$, was 1-^{11}C-palmitic acid. $^{11}CO_2$ can be produced by use of a nitrogen gas target via the $^{14}N(p\,\alpha)^{11}C$ reaction, although an alternate boron oxide target can be used to produce ^{11}C via the $^{11}B(p,n)^{11}C$ or $^{10}B(d,n)^{11}C$ reactions.[25] Details are provided in the Appendix:

$$R\text{-}MgX\ +\ {}^{11}CO_2 \longrightarrow [R^{11}CO_2MgX] \xrightarrow{\text{hydrolysis}} R^{11}CO_2H$$
$$\quad\text{I} \qquad\qquad\qquad\qquad\quad \text{II} \qquad\qquad\qquad \text{III}$$

^{11}C-labeled Acetate

As pointed out in chapter 9, assessment of myocardial oxidative metabolism is readily accomplished with radiolabeled acetate. The synthesis of ^{11}C-acetate developed by Pike et al.[26] utilizes the following reactions:

$$^{11}CO_2\ +\ CH_3MgBr \xrightarrow[\text{(Et)}_2O]{} CH_3{}^{11}COOMgBr \xrightarrow{\text{6N HCl}}$$

$$CH_3{}^{11}COOH \xrightarrow{\text{NaHCO}_3} CH_3{}^{11}COO^-_{\text{aq}}$$

The reaction scheme starts with dry bromomethane and involves preparation of methylmagnesium bromide in diethyl ether under nitrogen and its carbonation with $^{11}CO_2$. The 1-^{11}C-acetate is obtained by acid hydrolysis, and sodium bicarbonate solution is added to facilitate efficient extraction of the aqueous layer containing the 1-^{11}C-acetate from the ethereal phase. It is necessary to heat the solution at 60°C for 5 minutes under nitrogen to remove dissolved ether before the final 0.22 μm filtration is performed to prepare a sterile solution suitable for intravenous injection. The method has been adapted for use by others with routine production of 100 to 200 mCi with a synthesis time of 30 minutes, a specific activity of > 1 Ci/mmol and radiochemical purity $>$ 98%. Fifteen to 30 mCi are used for administration.[27]

^{11}C-labeled Pyruvic Acid

Overall flux through the pyruvate dehydrogenase pathway has been assessed with ^{11}C-labeled pyruvic acid. Several procedures have been developed for its synthesis, as outlined in the Appendix.

Fatty Acids Labeled with ^{18}F

Because of the central role of fatty acid in myocardial metabolism, a number of centers without on-site cyclotrons have been interested in the labeling of fatty acids with the longer-lived ^{18}F isotope.

The development of radiopharmaceuticals labeled with the positron-emitter ^{18}F has progressed rapidly over the last 10 years with the evolution of several new procedures. Thus, ^{18}F-labeled tracers can be transported to sites distant from the site of production. Details for their production are provided in the Appendix.

^{18}F-fluoromisonidazole

Fluoromisonidazole is a member of the class of compounds referred to as "hypoxic sensitizers" which accumulate in hypoxic but viable cells. The synthesis of ^{18}F-fluoromisonidazole has been recently described.[28] The synthesis consists of adding ^{18}F to K_2CO_3 and Kryptofix 222, heating under N_2 and drying with CH_3CN. The residue is taken up in anhydrous CH_3CN transferred to a vial containing (2R) (-)glycidyl tosylate and heating. The resultant ^{18}F-epifluorhydrin is isolated by passing the reaction mixture through a short silica column and eluted with CH_3CN. The epifluorhydrin solution is mixed with nitroimidazole, $NaHCO_3$ and water, heated with stirring, and the product purified by preparative HPLC on a silica column. Overall synthesis time is 2 hours with a radiochemical purity of $> 99\%$ in specific activity of > 400 Ci/mmol. The tracer is dissolved in saline and is radiochemically stable for at least 4 hours at room temperature. Five to 15 mCi are used for administration.

Labeling of Sympathetic Nervous System Receptor Ligands with Positron Emitters

The characterization of receptors with PET in vivo is a significant challenge. Although neuro- and tumor receptors have been studied extensively, myocardial receptors were among the first to be characterized in animals.[29,30] Early work on the development of agents for imaging the adrenergic system of the heart focused on labeling β-adrenergic antagonists such as practolol and pindolol.[31] More recent work has concentrated on newer tracers such as ^{11}C-labeled hydroxyephedrine and metaraminol. Their uses are outlined in chapter 10. Pertinent syntheses are shown in the Appendix.

Practical Present and Future Considerations

The number of radiopharmaceuticals labeled with positron-emitting radionuclides is limited only by the imagination of radiochemists and the development of novel schemes to incorporate these relatively short-lived nuclides into compounds of interest. To date, only blood flow agents have been labeled with generator-produced radionuclides. Although a greater variety of compounds can be synthesized with an on-site cyclotron, such an installation involves a major commitment of space, personnel, and funds. Advances in accelerator technology are likely to reduce the cost and complexity of the production of positron-emitting radionuclides and will likely revolutionize the application of positron emission tomography in cardiac centers.

APPENDIX

A comprehensive compendium of the synthetic schemes of all radiopharmaceuticals used for cardiac studies is impossible. Listed below are some typical schemes used for synthesis of common radiopharmaceuticals and schemes for those requiring novel radiochemical procedures.

Synthesis of 2-FDG with Fluorine Gas or Fluoride Ion

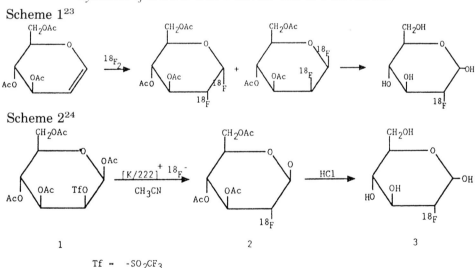

Scheme 1[23]

Scheme 2[24]

1   2   3

$Tf = -SO_2CF_3$

Synthesis of ^{11}C-fatty Acids and Fatty Acid Analogs

In general, ^{11}C-fatty acids are synthesized from a Grignard reagent prepared with a reaction vessel containing approximately 100 mg of dry magnesium and a small iodine crystal. After the reaction vessel is purged of air with an inert gas such as argon, a solution containing alkyl halide (about 1 g in 1 ml) dissolved in dry tetrahydrafuran (THF) is added to the apparatus. The vessel is slowly warmed until the iodine loses its color, with reflux maintained by gentle addition of the remaining alkyl bromide solution. After 90 to 180 minutes of reaction, the mixture is cooled to room temperature and the solution containing the reagent is ready for carboxylation with $^{11}CO_2$. After the preparation and acid decomposition of the intermediate, the palmitic acid is extracted into an organic solvent that is removed before the dissolution of the product in an injectable solution.

Many approaches to synthesis designed to reduce radiation exposure to the chemist have been tested, including several remote-controlled synthetic methods[32–35] and recently, a completely automated system for the production of 1-^{11}C-fatty acids.[36] Automating the extraction procedure is the most difficult step in such a system, but with the use of a specially designed "isobaric separator" (isobaric Sepaltor, made by Kokubo Seiki Co. Ltd. of Japan), this problem has been solved. Complete separation of the organic layer from the aqueous layer is accomplished by passing the nonpolar solvent hexane from the water-hexane mixture through a round porous membrane made of Teflon™. The totally automated system consists of a synthesis unit in a shielded box and an operation console made up of a microcomputer, printer, and cathode ray tube. Via a series of interfaces, the system controls the solenoid valves by a time-sequence program, and receives signals from optical liquid level sensors. Pressurized helium gas is used for transferring and agitating the reaction mix.

A novel method of synthesizing 1-^{11}C-fatty acids from H-^{11}CN has been described.[37,38] Its advantages are accommodation of relatively small amounts of substrate starting material and the lack of a need for absolutely anhydrous solvents. ^{11}C-hydrogen cyanide is synthesized from $^{11}CO_2$ according to the following reaction scheme by use of an automated synthesis system:

$$^{11}CO_2 \xrightarrow[\text{Ni}(400°C)]{\text{H}_2} \; ^{11}CH_4 \xrightarrow[\text{Pt }(920°C)]{\text{NH}_3} \; \text{H-}^{11}CN$$

The reaction starts with 1-bromo-alkane and the −Br is replaced by −CN, followed by hydrolysis to the 1-^{11}C-fatty acid:

$$CH_3(CH_2)_{14}CH_2Br \; + \; \text{H-}^{11}CN \xrightarrow[\text{DMSO}]{\text{KOH}} \xrightarrow[\text{DMSO}]{\text{6N NaOH}} CH_3(CH_2)_{14}CH_2 \, ^{11}COOH$$

To emulsify the labeled fatty acid, 1 ml of an ethanolic solution of Tween 20 is added to the fatty acid solution, and the ethanol is completely evaporated under vacuum. To the residue, 1 ml of an aqueous solution of human albumin (2 g/100 ml) is added while shaking at 50°C. The solution is then filtered through a 0.22 μm sterile filter to make it suitable for intravenous injection.

The above method makes it possible to synthesize labeled fatty acids by the use of only a few milligrams of alkyl bromides, although the overall radiochemical yield after synthesis is lower than that of the Grignard synthesis.

1-^{11}C-beta-methyl-heptadecanoic acid [1-^{11}C-BMHDA] has been synthesized recently.[39] The β-methyl group appears to inhibit β-oxidation of the labeled fatty acid analog.[40] Thus, radioactivity is trapped within the myocardium. This tracer may accumulate in myocardial cells as a fatty acid analog,[41] but trapping is not complete[42] with consequent backdiffusion.

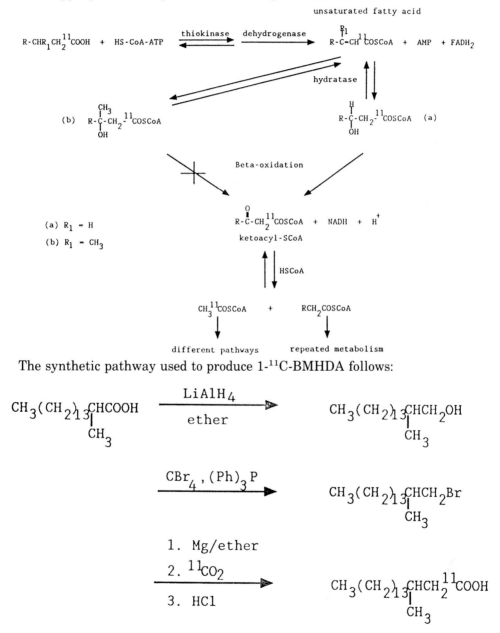

The synthetic pathway used to produce 1-^{11}C-BMHDA follows:

The products of this reaction are more than 99% radiochemically pure after HPLC.

Procedures for Labeling Fatty Acids with [18]F

Fluorine has striking nucleophilic character—the strongest among the halogens. One procedure of labeling fatty acids with ^{18}F consists of 2 steps, an exchange reaction involving fluorine substitution for another halogen (e.g., bromine) in the halogenated methylester derivative of the fatty acid and saponification of the ester via hydrolysis.[43,44] The methylester group serves to protect the omega end of the compound from fluorination:

$$Br-CH_2(CH_2)_{14}CH_2\overset{\overset{O}{\|}}{C}OCH_3 \xrightarrow{\;^{18}F^-\;} \;^{18}F-CH_2(CH_2)_{14}CH_2\overset{\overset{O}{\|}}{C}OCH_3$$

$$\xrightarrow{\;OH^-\;} \;^{18}F-CH_2(CH_2)_{14}CH_2COOH$$

The ^{18}F-fatty acid is extracted from the hydrolysis mixture by use of an organic solvent such as n-heptane and can be purified further by HPLC. Reaction time is approximately 1 hour. The radiochemical yield is approximately 30% for 17-^{18}F-heptadecanoic acid.

The position of the fluorine label within the fatty acid moiety has interesting effects on the biochemical distribution of the tracer. It has been shown that the distribution of α-fluoro fatty acids in the heart is poor, and that ω-fluoro fatty acids in the heart are not confined to the heart long enough for optimal imaging. Accordingly, synthesis of ^{18}F-labeled 6– and 7-fluoropalmitic acids has been developed.[45]

The approach consists of fluoride replacement of the reactive group methanesulfonate, which is introduced in the central portion of the molecule, and hydrolysis of the benzyl-group to form the fatty acid:

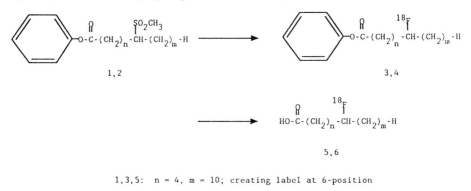

1,3,5: n = 4, m = 10; creating label at 6-position

2,4,6: n = 5, m = 9; creating label at 7-position

The total time for the preparation is 105 minutes, with the labeling step requiring 30 minutes. The yield is 20%.

In view of the relatively low yields obtained by typical fluorine exchange reactions, the nucleophilic activity of the fluorine anion has been enhanced. Nucleophilic substitution reactions are optimal in dipolar, aprotic (without H^+) solvent, such as acetonitrile. The use of neutral-phase transfer catalysts, in combination with positively charged alkali carrier in acetonitrile, is one way this can be accomplished.

The carrier, usually potassium bicarbonate, accompanies the catalyst, which is optimally a bicyclic polyether such as aminopolyether 2.2.2. (APE).[46] Together they are added to water containing the ^{18}F in a glass carbon vessel, and a solution of APE-potassium fluoride/carbonate is produced. The K^+ cation is encapsulated by the polyether, and reduces its interactions with the F^- anion. Thus the fluoride anion appears more "naked" because it is not solvated to any appreciable extent, and it more readily participates in nucleophilic reactions.

This procedure, with a typical radiochemical yield of 82%, is shown below:

$$^{18}F^-_{aqueous} + K_2CO_3 + APE \text{ (Kryptofix 222)} \xrightarrow{CH_3CN} [K/222]^+ \ ^{18}F^-$$

$$Br\text{-}CH_2(CH_2)_{14}CH_2COCH_3 \xrightarrow{[K/222]^+ \ ^{18}F^-} \xrightarrow{KOH} \ ^{18}F\text{-}CH_2(CH_2)_{14}CH_2COOH$$

The use of APE allows the labeling reaction to proceed under mild conditions that do not lead to decomposition of the final product. This method is not as sensitive to traces of water as the homologous reaction in plain acetonitrile and is promising as a high-yield technique of fluorinating temperature-sensitive aliphatic compounds.

The synthesis of ^{18}F-fatty acids that exhibit efficient myocardial uptake despite structural features that inhibit subsequent metabolism and egress of the label is likely to be particularly useful. Recently the synthesis of 17-^{18}F-3-methyl-heptadecanoic acid has been described.[47] By varying the length of the omega methoxyalkylacylchloride substrate, a series of 3-methyl-fatty acids can be prepared:

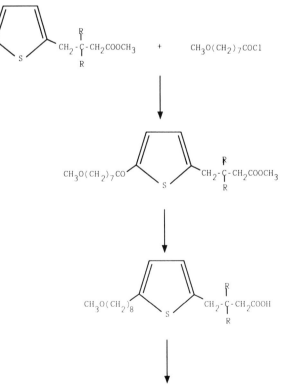

The reaction solution is passed through a cation-exchange column and the 3-^{11}C-pyruvate is eluted with water. After the addition of phosphate buffer and adjustment of pH with NaOH, the solution is sterilized by 0.22 μm filtration into a sterile vial.

The total synthesis time is approximately 35 minutes, and the product is more than 99% pure after HPLC, with a decay-corrected radiochemical yield of approximately 73%. The combination of the 2 enzymes is a novel approach to the use of the enantiomeric mix of D and L alanine.

β-Receptor Ligands

A simple method of producing labeled β-adrenergic receptor ligands is N-alkylation with ^{11}C, as has been developed by Antoni et al.[51] It employs the N-alkylating agent 2-^{11}C-isopropyl iodide. The alkylating agent is synthesized in polar aprotic solvent for a yield of 40% by the following scheme.

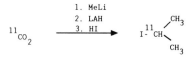

The alkylation reactions are carried out in polar aprotic solvent (dimethylformamide [DMF] or dimethylsulfoxide [DMSO]) for 10 minutes:

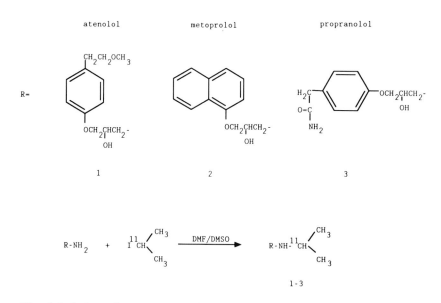

The labeled products are purified by HPLC, evaporated, and filtered appropriately for biological application. The radiochemical yield ranges from

5% to 30% with a reaction time of 40 to 50 minutes beginning with exposure to $^{11}CO_2$.

The false neurotransmitter metaraminol has been labeled with ^{18}F and found to accurately map the neuronal distribution of the heart.[52] The structures of the in vivo neurotransmitter norepinephrine (NE) and the false agent are shown below:

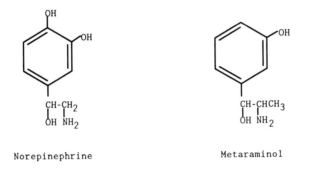

Norepinephrine   Metaraminol

Metaraminol is actively accumulated by the ends of adrenergic nerves and displaces NE from intraneuronal storage vessels. It is released on transmission of a nerve impulse, but is much less potent in exciting postsynaptic adrenergic receptors, making it a potentially excellent tracer, not only of tissue content of NE, but also of active neural activity.

One labeling scheme used is as follows:

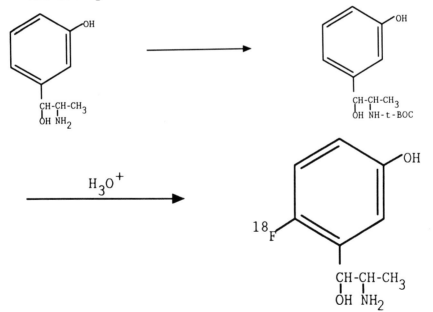

Another agent that appears to have high sympathetic neuroselectivity in myocardium is ^{11}C-metahydroxyephedrine (HED), which is synthesized by direct N-methylation of metaraminol with ^{11}C-methyl iodide.[53]

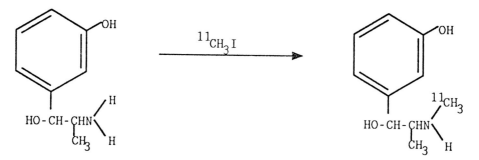

HED is purified by purification of metaraminol by HPLC. Total synthesis time is 25 minutes; the yield is 30% to 40% product that is more than 98% chemically pure.

References

1. Clark JC, Buckingham PD. *Short-lived radioactive gases for clinical use.* London: Butterworths, 1975:pp.150–157.
2. Welch MJ, Ter-Pogossian MM. Preparation of short half-lived gases for medical studies. Radiat Res 1968; 36:580–587.
3. Welch MJ, Lifton JF, Ter-Pogossian MM. Preparation of millicurie quantities of ^{15}O-labeled water. J Label Compounds 1969; 5:168–174.
4. Berridge MS, Cassidy EH, Terris AH. A routine, automated synthesis of oxygen-15-labeled butanol for positron tomography. J Nucl Med 1990; 30:1727–1731.
5. Tilbury RS, Dahl JR, Monahan WG, Laughlin, JS. Production of nitrogen-13 labeled ammonia for medical use. Radiochem Radioanal Lett 1971; 8:317–323.
6. Gennaro GP, Neirinckx RD, Bergner B, Muller WR, Waranis A, Haney TA, Barker SL, Loberg MD, Yarnais A. A Radionuclide Generator and Infusion System for Pharmaceutical Quality Rb-82. In: Knapp FF Jr, Butler TA, eds. *Radionuclide Generators*, Washington, D.C.: American Chemical Society, 1984.
7. Green MA, Klippenstein DL, Tennison JR. Copper(II) bis(thiosemicarbazone) complexes as potential tracers for evaluation of cerebral and myocardial blood flow with PET. J Nucl Med 1988; 29:1549–1557.
8. John EK, Green MA. Structure-activity relationships for metal-labeled blood flow tracers: comparison of ketoaldehyde bis(thiosemicarbazonato) copper(II) derivatives. J Med Chem 1990; 33:1764–1770.
9. Green MA. A potential copper radiopharmaceutical for imaging the heart and brain. Nucl Med Biol 1987; 14:59–61.
10. Shelton ME, Green MA, Mathias CJ, Welch MJ, Bergmann SR. Kinetics of copper-PTSM in isolated hearts: a novel tracer for measuring blood flow with positron emission tomography. J Nucl Med 1989; 30:1843–1847.
11. Shelton ME, Green MA, Mathias CJ, Welch MJ, Bergmann SR. Assessment of regional myocardial and renal blood flow using copper-PTSM and positron emission tomography. Circulation 1990; 82:990–997.
12. Green MA, Mathias CJ, Welch MJ, McGuire AH, Perry D, Fernandez-Rubio F, Perlmutter JS, Raichle ME, Bergmann, SR. ^{62}Cu-labeled pyruvaldehyde bis(N^4-methylthiosemicarbazonato)copper (II): synthesis and evaluation as a positron emission tomography tracer for cerebral and myocardial perfusion. J Nucl Med 1990; 31:1989–1996.
13. Mathias CJ, Margenau WH, Brodack JW, Welch MJ, Green MA. A remote system

for the synthesis of copper-62 labeled Cu(PTSM). Int J Appl Rad Isotopes 1991; 42:317–320.

14. Green MA, Mathias CJ, Welch MJ. 1,1,1-tris (5-methoxysalicylaldimino-methyl) ethane: a chelating agent for the preparation of lipophilic gallium and indium radiopharmaceuticals. J Labeled Compound Radiopharm 1984; 21:1001–1002.

15. Madsen SL, Welch MJ, Weisman RA, Motekaitis RJ, Martell AE. Synthesis and investigation of N,N,N,N-tetrakis(2-hydroxy-3,5-dimethylbenzyl) ethylene-diamine: a potential generator produced tracer for PET imaging. J Nucl Med 1990; 31:768.

16. Kung HF, Liu BL, Mankoff D, Kung MP, Billings JJ, Francesconi L, Alavi A. A new myocardial imaging agent: synthesis, characterization, and biodistribution of [^{68}Ga]BAT-TECH. J Nucl Med 1990; 31:1635–1641.

17. Green MA. The potential for generator-based PET perfusion tracers. J Nucl Med 1990; 31:1641–1645.

18. Mintun MA, Dennis DR, Welch MJ, Mathias CJ, Schuster DP. Measurements of pulmonary vascular permeability with PET and gallium-68 transferrin. J Nucl Med 1987; 28:1704–1716.

19. Harris WR, Pecoraro VI. Thermodynamic binding constants for gallium transferrin. Biochemistry 1983; 22:292–299.

20. Welch MJ, Thakur ML, Coleman RE, Patel M, Siegel BA, Ter-Pogossian MM. Gallium-68 labeled red cells and platelets. New agents for positron tomography. J Nucl Med 1977; 18:558–562.

21. Wagner SJ, Welch MR. Gallium-68 labeling of albumin and albumin microspheres. J Nucl Med 1979; 20:428–433.

22. Mathias CJ, Welch MJ, Green MA, Diril H, Meares CF, Gropler RJ, Bergmann SR. In vivo comparison of copper blood pool agents: potential radiopharmaceuticals for use with copper-62. J Nucl Med 1991; 32:475–480.

23. Ido T, Wan C-N, Fowler JS, Wolf AP. Fluorination with F_2. A convenient synthesis of 2-deoxy-2-fluoro D-glucose. J Org Chem 1977; 42:2341–2342.

24. Hamacher K, Coenen HH, Stocklin G. Efficient stereospecific synthesis of no-carrier-added 2-[^{18}F]-fluoro-2-deoxy-D-glucose using amino-polyether supported nucleophilic substitution. J Nucl Med 1986; 27:235.

25. Fowler JS, Wolf AP. The synthesis of carbon-11, fluorine-18, and nitrogen-13 labeled radiotracers for biomedical applications. Nuclear Medicine Series NAS-NS-3201, Technical Information Center, U.S. Department of Energy.

26. Pike VW, Eakins MN, Allan RM, Selwyn AP. Preparation of (1-^{11}C)acetate-an agent for the study of myocardial metabolism by positron emission tomography. Int J Appl Radiat Isot 1982; 33:505–512.

27. Brown M, Marshall DR, Sobel BE, Bergmann SR. Delineation of myocardial O_2 utilization with C-11(acetate). Circulation 1987; 76:687–696.

28. Hwang D-R, Dence CS, Bonasera TA, Welch MJ. No-carrier-added-synthesis of 3-[^{18}F]fluoro-1-(2-nitro-1-imidazolyl)-2-propanol. J Label Compounds Radiopharm 1989; 40:117–126.

29. Francis B, Eckelman WC, Grissom MP, Gibson RE, Reba RC. The use of tritium labeled compounds to develop gamma-emitting receptor-binding radiotracers. Int J Nucl Med Biol 1982; 9:173–179.

30. Eckelman WC, Alter III WA, Grissom MP, Vieras F, Phillips J, Eng R,Gibson RE, Reba RC. Comparison of myocardial uptake and distribution of thallium-201 and two prototype receptor-binding radiopharmaceuticals in the normal and ischemic canine heart. Int J Nucl Med Biol 1984; 11:287–290.

31. Prenanat C, Sastre J, Crouzel C, Syrota A. Synthesis of (C-11)pindolol. J Labeled Compounds Radiopharm 1987; 24:227–232.

32. Welch MJ, Wittmer SL, Dence CS. Radiopharmaceuticals labeled with 11-C and 18-F: considerations related to the preparation of (11-C)palmitate. In: Root J and Krohn K, eds.,*Short-lived Radionuclides in Chemistry and Biology,* Washington, D.C.: ACS Advances in Chemistry Series Monograph, American Chemical Society.

33. Welch MJ, Dence CS, Marshall DR, Kilbourn MR. Remote system for production of carbon-11 labeled palmitic acid. J Label Compounds Radiopharm 1983; 20:1087–1095.

34. Padgett HC, Robinson GD, Barrio JR. (1-^{11}C)Palmitic acid: improved radiopharmaceutical preparation. Int J Appl Radiat Isot 1982; 33:1471.

35. Pike VW, Eakins MM, Allan RM, Selwyn AP. Preparation of carbon-11 labeled acetate and palmitic acid for the study of myocardial metabolism by emission-computerized axial tomography. J Radioanal Chem 1981; 64:291.

36. Takahashi T, Ido T, Iwata R, Hatano K, Nakanaishi H, Shinohara M, Ilda S. Automated synthesis system with computer control for the production of (1-^{11}C)fatty acids. Int J Radiat Appl Instrument (Part A) 1988; 39:659–665.

37. Iwata R, Ido T, Takahashi T, Nakanishi H, Ilda S. Optimization of (C)HCN production and no-carrier-added (1-^{11}C)amino acid synthesis. Int J Rad Appl Instrument (Part A) 1987; 38:97–102.

38. Takahashi T, Ido T, Kentaro H, Iwata R, Nakanishi H. Synthesis of 1-C- labeled fatty acid from (^{11}C)HCN. Int J Radiat Appl Instrument (Part A) 1990; 41:649–654.

39. Livni E, Elmaleh DR, Levy S, Brownell GL, Strauss WH. Beta-methyl(1-^{11}C)heptadecanoic acid: a new myocardial metabolic tracer for positron emission tomography. J Nucl Med 1982; 23:169–175.

40. van der Waal EE. Myocardial imaging with radiolabeled free fatty acids: applications and limitations. Eur J Nucl Med 1986; 12:S11-S15.

41. Elmaleh DR, Alpert NM, Buxton RB, Strauss HW, Livni E. In vivo measurement of myocardial fatty acid metabolism with 1-beta-methyl(^{11}C)heptadecanoic acid. J Nucl Med 1989; 30:797–780.

42. Abendschein DR, Fox KAA, Ambos HD, Sobel BE, Bergmann SR. Metabolism of beta-methyl(1-^{11}C)heptadecanoic acid in canine myocardium. Int J Rad Appl Instrument (Part B) 1987; 14:579–585.

43. Knust EJ, Kupfernagel CH, Stocklin G. Long-chain (F-18)fatty acids for the study of regional metabolism in heart and liver; odd-even effects of metabolism in mice. J Nucl Med 1979; 20:1170–1175.

44. Knust EJ, Schuller M, Stocklin G. Synthesis and quality control of long-chain (F-18)fatty acids. J Labeled Compound Radiopharm 1980; 17:353–363.

45. Berridge MS, Tewson TJ, Welch MJ. Synthesis of (F-18) labeled 6- and 7-fluoropalmitic acids. Int J Appl Rad Isotopes 1983; 34:727–730.

46. Coenen HH, Klatte B, Knochel A, Schuller M, Stocklin G. Preparation of N.C.A. 17-(F-18)fluoroheptadecanoic acid in high yields via aminopolyether supported, nucleophilic fluorination. J Label Compounds Radiopharm 1986; 23:455–466.

47. Goodman MM, Knapp FF. Radiochemical synthesis of (F-18)-3-methyl-branched omega fluorofatty acids. J Label Compounds Radiopharm 1989; 26:233–235.

48. Pochapsky SS, VanBrocklin HF, Welch MJ, Katzenellenbogen JA. Synthesis and tissue distribution of fluorine-18 labeled trifluorohexadecanoic acids. Considerations in the development of metabolically blocked myocardial imaging agents. Bioconjug Chem 1990; 1:231–244.

49. Kilbourn MR, Welch MJ. No-carrier-added synthesis of (1-^{11}C)pyruvic acid. Int J Appl Radiat Isot 1982;33:359–361.

50. Bjurling P, Watanabe Y, Langstrom B. The synthesis of (3-^{11}C), a useful synthon, via an enzymatic route. Int J Appl Rad Isotopes (Part A) 1988; 39:627–630.

51. Antoni G, Malmborg P, Ulin J, Langstrom B. Synthesis of the N-(2-C11-isopropyl)-labeled β-adrenergic ligands atenolol, metoprolol, and propanolol. J Label Compounds Radiopharm 1989; 26:208–210.

52. Mislankar SG, Gildersleeve DL, Wieland DM, Massin CC, Mulholland K, Toorongian SA. 6-(F-18)fluorometaraminol: a radiotracer for in vivo mapping of adrenergic nerves of the heart. J Med Chem 1988; 31:362–366.

53. Haka MS, Rosenspire KC, Gildersleeve DL, VanDort ME, Sherman PS, Wieland DM. Synthesis of (C-11)-m-hydroxyephedrine (HED) for neuronal cardiac imaging. J Nucl Med 1989; 30:783.

Chapter 5

Quantification of Myocardial Perfusion with Positron Emission Tomography

Steven R. Bergmann, M.D., Ph.D.

Assessment of myocardial perfusion is crucial for determination of the physiologic significance of coronary artery disease and for evaluation of its severity. In addition, it is needed for definitive evaluation of the efficacy of pharmacologic, mechanical, or surgical interventions designed to augment nutritive perfusion.

The severity of stenosis, generally determined visually from angiograms, does not accurately predict maximal flow in response to a physiologic or pharmacologic stimulus.[1] Even though quantitative arteriography has improved the accuracy and reproducibility of assessments of macrovascular coronary artery disease, such measurements cannot define nutritive perfusion per se. Coronary artery Doppler flow velocity measurements have recently been introduced as a means to more accurately assess the vasodilatory capacity of particular coronary artery beds.[1] Assessment of the physiologic response to a vasodilator appears to predict the necessity for further mechanical or surgical interventions.[2] Nonetheless, coronary artery Doppler flow velocity measurements at rest and after pharmacologic vasodilation reflect only bulk conductance flow in limited vascular territories. Unless velocity measurements are coupled with assessment of diameter, flow itself cannot be evaluated. Furthermore, nutritive perfusion may not parallel macrovascular flow.

Nuclear medicine procedures such as planar or single-photon emission computed tomography with perfusion agents such as thallium-201 (^{201}Tl), technetium-99m (^{99m}Tc) isonitriles, or boronic acid technetium oximes have played a significant role in the assessment of regional myocardial perfusion. Despite their convenience, methods using single-photon-emitting radiotracers are of limited sensitivity because of inadequate correction for depth-dependent attenuation of photons and for the complex behavior of nonphysiologic tracers within

From *Positron Emission Tomography of the Heart* edited by Steven R. Bergmann, MD, PhD and Burton E. Sobel, MD © 1992, Futura Publishing Inc., Mount Kisco, NY.

myocardium. Accordingly, estimates of regional perfusion with such tracers cannot quantify myocardial perfusion in absolute terms (i.e., ml/min/g).[3]

Positron emission tomography (PET) has emerged as the most accurate approach for quantification of regional myocardial perfusion. It provides for sensitive and specific identification of patients with coronary artery disease. Delineation of perfusion defects is straightforward in patients with single-vessel coronary artery disease, in whom a region of the heart supplied by a relatively normal coronary artery can be used for qualitative, comparative measures of net uptake and clearance. Heterogeneity of accumulation and clearance of tracers indicative of disparities in regional perfusion can be observed in subjects at rest or after hyperemic stress induced with intravenous dipyridamole or adenosine. All the tracers used for estimation of myocardial perfusion with PET have permitted identification of coronary artery disease in patients with stenoses of greater than approximately 40%.[4–11]

Quantitative estimates of perfusion in absolute terms are crucial for the evaluation of patients in whom uptake and clearance of flow tracers is homogeneous (i.e., without regional disparities), such as those with chest pain and angiographically normal coronary arteries, cardiac allografts, or cardiomyopathy. In addition, quantitative estimates of myocardial perfusion and perfusion reserve may be important in patients with balanced or multivessel coronary artery disease, in whom regional disparities may not be obvious. When mathematically and physiologically appropriate models are used to describe the biological behavior of the administered radiotracers in blood and in myocardial tissue over time, quantitative estimates of regional myocardial perfusion can be obtained.

Accurate tomographic measurement of perfusion requires satisfaction of assumptions inherent in the models of tracer kinetics on which interpretations are based. Quantification of myocardial perfusion in absolute terms typically requires dynamic scanning with which the time-activity history of tracer in blood and in myocardium can be followed. Because limitations of spatial resolution in the current generation of PET tomographs leads to underestimation of the true content of radioactivity in regions less than approximately two times the full-width at half-maximum resolution of the scanner, and because of volume averaging imposed by cardiac and respiratory motion, time-activity curves from blood and myocardium must be corrected for partial volume and spillover effects (see Chapter 2). Corrections can be performed with independent measurements of the dimensions of structures with modalities such as echocardiography, computed tomography, or magnetic resonance imaging. However, the technical limitations of dual-modality scanning are considerable. In addition, such measurements cannot be readily corrected for the tomographic slice interrogated, and measurements may be altered with changing loading or physiologic conditions.

Effects of cardiac motion are particularly problematic. Motion results in spatial averaging. Although gating can partially overcome motion effects and has been successfully implemented, it greatly reduces the amount of data obtained because of diminution of the duration of the acquisition interval. The loss of data becomes critical when rapid kinetic data are being acquired. Ac-

Table 5-1
Positron-emitting Radiotracers Used for Measurement of Myocardial Perfusion

Isotope	Physical Half-life (min)	Compound	Class
Cyclotron-produced			
Oxygen-15	2.1	water, butanol	diffusible
Potassium-38	7.7	chloride	extracted
Nitrogen-13	10	ammonia	extracted
Carbon-11	20.4	microspheres or macroaggregated albumin	microspheres
Generator-produced			
Rubidium-82 (parent: strontium-82)	1.3 (26 days)	chloride	extracted
Copper-62 (parent: zinc-62)	9.7 (9.3 hours)	PTSM	extracted
Gallium-68 (parent: germanium-68)	68 (288 days)	microspheres or macroaggregated albumin	microspheres

Abbreviations: PTSM = pyruvaldehyde bis N^4-methylthiosemicarbazone.

cordingly, newer approaches have incorporated corrections for partial volume and spillover effects, and the linear effects of motion with novel mathematical approaches applied to the operational flow equations themselves.[12-17]

To accurately measure the time-activity histories in blood and myocardium, tomographs that can faithfully record the high-count rates that occur after bolus intravenous administration of tracer and have high temporal-counting capabilities are required. Factors such as inaccurate random correction, the path length of positrons in tissue before annihilation, and deviation from 180° of emitted photons further complicate accurate estimation of radiotracer content.

This chapter addresses the diverse tracers available (Table 5-1) for quantification of myocardial perfusion with PET with an emphasis on quantification of perfusion in absolute terms. Clinical applications are discussed more fully in Chapter 11.

Assessment of Myocardial Blood Flow with Labeled Microspheres

Radiolabeled microspheres have long been the "gold standard" for laboratory studies of myocardial perfusion, in part because of the paucity of other quantitative approaches. Microspheres are small spheres or particles, labeled with a radioisotope, that are trapped virtually completely in the arteriolar or capillary vessels during a first pass through the vascular bed in an organ of interest.[18] To ensure adequate mixing and avoid trapping in the venous circulation, microspheres must be administered systemically (into the left atrium or left ventricle). In experimental animals, a reference flow sample is obtained by withdrawing arterial blood at a known flow rate. Blood flow is calculated by comparing radioactivity in a tissue sample (obtained postmortem) with that in the reference sample. Results with microspheres are accurate when mixing of microspheres with blood is adequate, when no aggregation or clumping occurs, when sphere size is appropriate and size and shape are uniform, when statistical considerations are fulfilled, and when corrections are applied for loss of spheres from ischemic regions.[18] Some results indicate that 15 μm microspheres (the size used predominantly in cardiovascular research) slightly overestimate the presence and extent of high-flow regions. However, smaller sized microspheres are not completely trapped by the vasculature. Microspheres may underestimate flow in absolute terms in ischemic regions.[19]

Laboratory Studies with Microspheres and Microsphere Analogs and PET

Bergmann et al. demonstrated that the distribution of gallium-68 (^{68}Ga) human albumin macroaggregates (which have an average particle size between 10 and 35 μm) estimated tomographically correlated well with flow estimated with concomitantly administered 15 μm microspheres over a wide range of flows.[20] Using correction for partial volume and spillover effects, Wisenberg and colleagues demonstrated that accurate estimates of absolute flow could be obtained with ^{68}Ga-labeled macroaggregated albumin.[21] More recently, the group at Hammersmith has labeled macroaggregated albumin with carbon-11 (^{11}C) and demonstrated that accurate estimates of flow could be obtained.[22]

Clinical Studies

Because of the need for systemic administration, the clinical applications of the microsphere approach have been limited. Selwyn et al. evaluated myocardial flow in 10 patients studied after myocardial infarction.[23] After diagnostic catheterization, 4 to 6 mCi of ^{11}C-macroaggregated human albumin (approximately 2 to 3 million particles) were injected into the apex of the left ventricle. Flow in the center of the infarct ranged from 0 to 40% of flow in remote, normal zones. Because microspheres distribute to all regions of the body and do not egress from the arterial bed and because the ^{11}C-radioisotope used has a sufficiently long half-life (20.4 minutes) to permit imaging of several regions of the body, blood flow in the brain could be estimated as well.

Because of the limitations imposed by the need for systemic administration as well as the theoretical possibility that microspheres could occlude vascular beds that may be compromised already (although no adverse effects have been reported in patients given microspheres),[3,24] use of positron-emitting radiolabeled microspheres is likely to remain limited in clinical studies. Nonetheless, the approach is straightforward and provides accurate results in patients who are undergoing invasive procedures for clinical indications.

Assessment of Perfusion with Extractable Tracers

A second approach for estimation of myocardial perfusion involves the use of tracers that are partially extracted in a single capillary transit through the vascular bed and retained by the myocardium for varying periods of time. This approach is an extension of one proposed originally by Sapirstein and is based on the assumption that an intravenously injected radiopharmaceutical, generally a cation, is taken up and released by cells throughout the organism with consistent kinetics independent of regional flow and of the metabolic status of a particular tissue.[3,24] This assumption is still made in qualitative imaging with these tracers even though none of the tracers actually fulfills the criteria. For example, all tracers in this class exhibit an inverse and nonlinear relationship between single-pass extraction and flow. Accordingly, mathematical models have been developed to account for the kinetic behavior of such tracers within myocardium. Positron-emitting tracers used with this approach include rubidium-82 (^{82}Rb) chloride, nitrogen-13 (^{13}N) ammonia, copper-62 pyruvaldehyde N^4-bis-thiosemicarbazone (^{62}Cu-PTSM), and potassium-38 (^{38}K) chloride. Each will be considered briefly.

^{82}Rb-Chloride

^{82}Rb-chloride is an attractive tracer for assessment of myocardial perfusion. It is produced from a strontium-82 generator. The half-life of the parent is 26 days; the half-life of ^{82}Rb is 76 seconds. Accordingly, sequential scans can be obtained with minimal radiation burden.

Experimental Studies

Love and Burch first suggested that the uptake of radiolabeled rubidium depended on myocardial perfusion,[25] an observation that has been corroborated extensively.[3,24] Single-pass extraction of rubidium by the heart is inversely and nonlinearly related to myocardial perfusion (Figure 5-1).[26] Selwyn et al. demonstrated that regional uptake of ^{82}Rb assessed with PET correlated only poorly with the distribution of microspheres in dogs and that extraction fraction was inversely related to flow in patients.[27] Because the absolute uptake of ^{82}Rb plateaus at flows exceeding 2 to 3 ml/min/g, net uptake at hyperemic flows is insensitive to changes in hyperemic flow. Although most metabolic and pharmacologic interventions do not significantly alter the relationships between single-pass extraction fraction of ^{82}Rb and flow,[26] ischemia and reperfusion do. Fukuyama and colleagues demonstrated that ischemia alone or ischemia followed by reperfusion reduced uptake of ^{82}Rb, not because of diminished flow per se but because of a reduction in extraction fraction, presumably

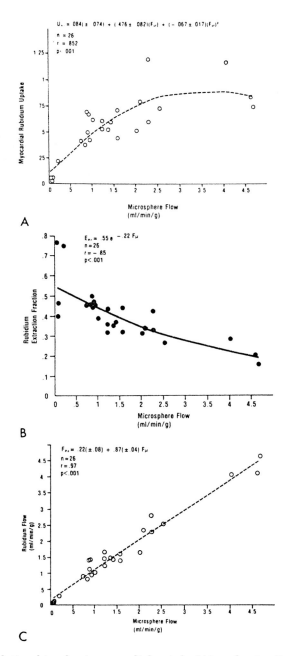

Figure 5-1. *Relationship of net myocardial uptake (A) and extraction fraction (B) of* ^{82}Rb *to flow measured with radiolabeled microspheres in dogs. Because of the inverse and nonlinear relationship between extraction fraction and flow, net myocardial uptake of tracer plateaus at flows greater than approximately 2.0 to 2.5 ml/min/g. If net uptake is corrected for this relationship, quantitative estimates of flow can be obtained (C). (Reproduced from Goldstein et al.,[26] with permission of the Society of Nuclear Medicine.)*

secondary to diminished cellular transport.[28] Wilson et al. demonstrated that net uptake and extraction are diminished even with short periods of transient occlusion.[29] Nonetheless, with the use of simple qualitative analysis, Jeremy et al. found that relative perfusion defects obtained after administration of [82]Rb correlated with those seen with microspheres.[30]

To quantify myocardial perfusion in absolute terms, the kinetics of both extraction and retention of [82]Rb must be incorporated in mathematical models.[31,32] Although some investigators have tried to apply the empirical relationship between extraction fraction and flow to quantification of myocardial perfusion in absolute terms,[26] Herrero et al. recently showed that this approach is limited.[33]

The kinetics of [82]Rb can be described accurately with a two-compartment model as shown by Mullani et al.[31] and Goldstein et al.[26] Herrero et al. recently extended this approach to tomographic estimation of perfusion in experimental animals (Figure 5-2).[32] Quantitative imaging requires dynamic scanning sequences starting at the time of onset of administration of tracer. Tissue tracer content, $C_T(t)$, can be defined by a function of arterial blood tracer concentration, $C_a(t)$, by:

$$C_T(t) = (Ae^{-\alpha t} + Be^{-\alpha t}) * C_a(t) \tag{1}$$

where the concentration of tracer in tissue ($C_T(t)$) is defined by a bi-exponential curve convolved with the arterial blood curve.

To correct PET measurements from cardiac tissue for partial volume and

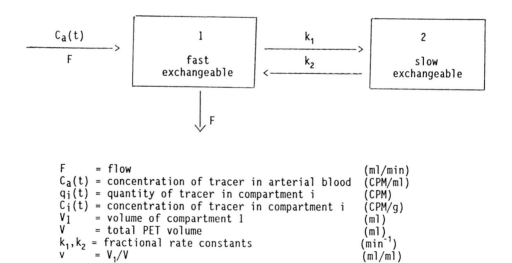

$$
\begin{array}{llll}
F & = \text{flow} & \text{(ml/min)} \\
C_a(t) & = \text{concentration of tracer in arterial blood} & \text{(CPM/ml)} \\
q_i(t) & = \text{quantity of tracer in compartment } i & \text{(CPM)} \\
C_i(t) & = \text{concentration of tracer in compartment } i & \text{(CPM/g)} \\
V_1 & = \text{volume of compartment 1} & \text{(ml)} \\
V & = \text{total PET volume} & \text{(ml)} \\
k_1, k_2 & = \text{fractional rate constants} & \text{(min}^{-1}) \\
v & = V_1/V & \text{(ml/ml)}
\end{array}
$$

Figure 5-2. *Schematic diagram of the two-compartment model used to describe the kinetic behavior [82]Rb in the myocardium. Compartment 1 represents the vascular and interstitial spaces and compartment 2 represents the intracellular space. This and similar models are used for describing the behavior of extractable tracers in the myocardium. (Reproduced from Herrero et al.,[32] with permission of the American Heart Association, Inc.)*

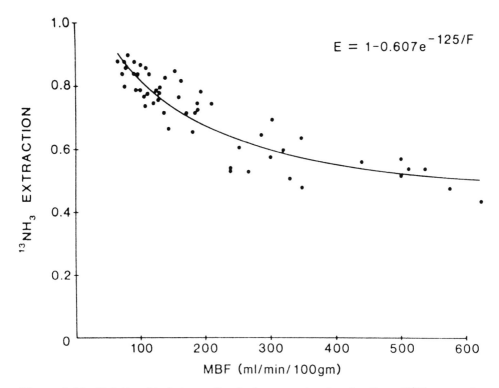

$$E = 1 - 0.607e^{-125/F}$$

Figure 5-6A. *Relationship between the single-pass extraction fraction of ^{13}N-ammonia and flow obtained after intercoronary bolus administration in dogs demonstrating the inverse, nonlinear relationship with microsphere-estimated myocardial blood flow (MBF). (Reproduced from Schelbert et al.,[43] with permission of the American Heart Association, Inc).*

in absolute terms, extraction and retention of ^{13}N-ammonia by the heart are related not only to flow but also to myocardial oxygenation and metabolism.[45-47] Because the trapping of ^{13}N-ammonia is dependent on the conversion of ammonia to glutamine by the glutamine synthetase pathway, factors that influence flux through this pathway influence tracer kinetics independent of flow. Nonetheless, some experimental approaches have demonstrated reasonably good correlations between myocardial perfusion estimated with a net uptake model and a carefully defined approach for calculating the flow-dependent extraction fraction.[43,44] For absolute quantitation, two- and three-compartment models have been used[16,17] that incorporate estimates of both the forward and backward rate constants (i.e., estimation of both extraction and retention). Use of such models requires dynamic tomographic scanning procedures to record time-activity curves in arterial blood (for the input function) and in myocardium.

More than 50% of administered ^{13}N-ammonia is degraded to metabolic intermediates (predominantly urea and the amino acid, glutamine) within 5

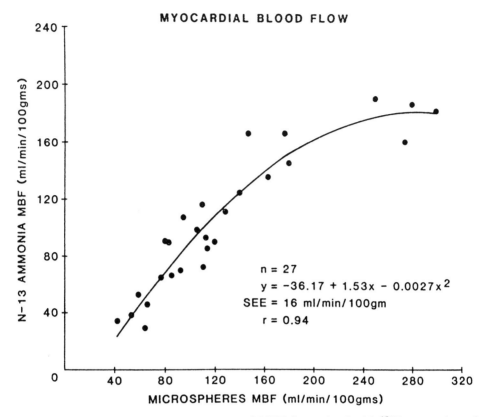

Figure 5-6B. *Relationship between regional MBF determined with ^{13}N-ammonia and PET and flow estimated with radiolabeled microspheres. When flow is greater than approximately 2 ml/min/g, net uptake plateaus and accordingly is not sensitive to flows in the hyperemic range. (Reproduced from Shah et al.,[44] with permission of The American College of Cardiology.)*

minutes after intravenous administration.[48] Although the effect of this break-down (which may vary in individual patients) as well as the magnitude of extraction of labeled metabolites by myocardium appear to be modest, both can distort quantitative estimates of perfusion.

Clinical Observations

[13]N-ammonia has been used extensively for qualitative imaging of myocardial perfusion in patients.[5-8] After administration of 10 to 15 mCi intravenously, static, 5 to 10 minute images obtained beginning 3 to 10 minutes after administration of tracer (to permit clearance of tracer from blood) clearly delineate myocardium (Figure 5-7). Although smokers or patients with lung disease have increased lung uptake of ^{13}N-ammonia, its use has permitted accurate identification of patients with coronary artery disease with a sensitivity and specificity of greater than 90% (See Chapter 11, Table 11-2). Qualitative esti-

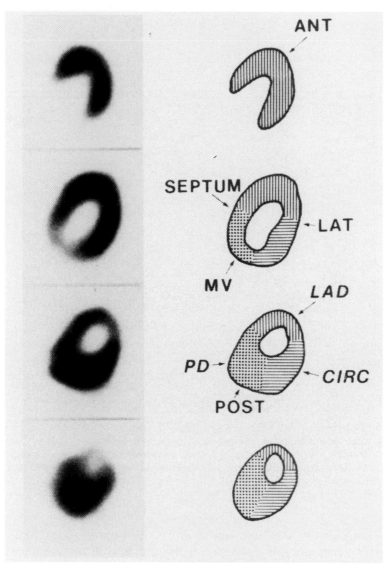

Figure 5-7. *Four contiguous transverse reconstructions of the heart obtained after the intravenous administration of* [13]*N-ammonia to a healthy human volunteer. The cross sections of the left ventricle are displayed as if viewed from below. Thus, the lateral free wall is to the right, the septum to the left, anterior is uppermost, and posterior at the bottom. The thin right ventricle is not visualized because of resolution limitations. The schematic diagram on the right delineates the anterior (ANT), lateral (LAT), and posterior (POST) myocardium and the mitral valve plane (MV). The distribution of the left anterior descending (LAD), left circumflex (CIRC), and posterior descending (PD) coronary arteries are indicated by the different cross-hatching. (Reproduced from Schelbert et al.,[6] with permission of The American Journal of Cardiology.)*

mates of myocardial perfusion at rest have been used in a number of studies of myocardial viability (See Chapter 11, Figure 11-5). For such studies, ^{13}N-ammonia is administered at rest and flow is classified simply as normal or decreased based on visual estimation of regional disparities. Obviously, this approach requires the definition of a "normal" region. Because observed counts in a region of interest can decrease simply because of wall thinning[41] (partial volume effects) (Figure 5-5), such measurements are best performed with corrections for wall thickness. Criteria for determining ischemic flows can also be based on circumferential profiles. Ischemic perfusion is classified typically as flow less than 2 standard deviations below the mean (based on percent of peak) compared with profiles obtained in healthy human volunteers.

For the diagnosis of coronary artery disease, scans are obtained at rest and again after induction of coronary hyperemia either with exercise or an intravenous vasodilator such as dipyridamole or adenosine (and a second administration of tracer). Because of the 10 minute half-life of ^{13}N, rest and hyperemia scans must be performed approximately 45 to 60 minutes apart to avoid the influence of isotope from the first administration on subsequent results.

Krivokapich et al. demonstrated that the net uptake approach was insensitive to changes in flow.[16] In 13 healthy volunteers studied at rest and during supine bicycle exercise, an average increase in flow of 1.38, as assessed by net uptake, was observed, whereas the double product increased more than 2.5-fold. Camici et al. using a modification of the net uptake approach, demonstrated that patients with hypertrophied hearts exhibit abnormal flow reserve in both the hypertrophied intraventricular septum and nonhypertrophied free wall compared with values in healthy control subjects,[49] corroborating the findings of Yoshida et al.[50] Nonetheless, judging from first principles and from laboratory and clinical data, the net uptake approach is insensitive to flow, especially at hyperemic flow rates.

Recently, Krivokapich et al.[16] and Hutchins et al.[17] have used compartmental models to assess myocardial perfusion in human subjects and to relate increased perfusion to increased myocardial work (assessed indirectly with systemic hemodynamics). For quantification of perfusion with compartmental models, dynamic scanning protocols are used. Data for model estimation is obtained in the first 1 to 4 minutes. Krivokapich et al. demonstrated a 2.2-fold increase in estimates of average perfusion (from 0.75 to 1.5 ml/min/g) in healthy subjects studied at rest and again during bicycle exercise.[16] The double product increased up to 2.8-fold but was not constant during the imaging interval. Hutchins et al. demonstrated a 4.8-fold increase in perfusion (from 0.88 to 4.17 ml/min/g) in 7 healthy subjects evaluated at rest and after intravenous infusion of dipyridamole combined with handgrip exercise.[17] In this study, flow was decreased by 5% to 10% when corrections for labeled metabolites were not applied. In both studies, corrections for partial volume and spillover effects were incorporated in the mathematical model. Should such approaches be validated in experimental animals, they would provide a promising approach for quantification of perfusion with ^{13}N-ammonia in patients.

^{62}Cu-PTSM

Copper(II)pyruvaldehyde bis (N^4-methylthiosemicarbazone) labeled with generator-produced copper-62 (^{62}Cu-PTSM) has been developed as an alternative tracer for estimates of myocardial perfusion.[51–53] This compound is lipophilic. Its single-pass uptake appears to be similar to that of ^{82}Rb and ^{13}N-ammonia (i.e., high and inversely and nonlinearly related to flow). In tumor cells, uptake of Cu-PTSM has been shown to involve diffusion of the intact complex through the cell membrane (the octanol/water partition coefficient is 100/1), with subsequent reduction of copper(II) to copper(I) by ubiquitous intracellular sulfhydryl groups. The reduced copper is believed to bind nonspecifically to intracellular macromolecules, thereby becoming trapped. In contrast to either ^{82}Rb or ^{13}N-ammonia, once extracted by the myocardium, ^{62}Cu-PTSM is essentially irreversibly bound (backdiffusion is negligible). Retention combined with the physical half-life of 9.7 minutes provide excellent counting statistics and high-quality images (Color Figure 1).

Although the 9 hour half-life of the parent, zinc-62 (t$^{1/2}$ = 9.3 hours), may be a disadvantage (because delivery would be required every 1 to 2 days), the short half-life of the parent permits acquisition of a generator only when scans are scheduled. In addition, Cu-PTSM can be labeled with a number of other single- and positron-emitting radioisotopes of copper.[51–53]

Laboratory Studies

In isolated perfused rabbit hearts, Shelton et al. demonstrated that the single-pass extraction fraction of radiolabeled Cu-PTSM was greater than 40% (in hearts perfused with crystalloid buffer at a rate of 4 to 5 ml/min/g), and that the half-life of retention was greater than 6 hours.[51] In intact dogs, these investigators demonstrated rapid arterial clearance of tracer and a high correlation between net uptake and myocardial flow estimated with radiolabeled microspheres.[52] Nonetheless, a decrease in accumulation was noted at high flows. This led Herrero et al. to develop a two-compartment model (similar to that used for ^{82}Rb or ^{13}N-ammonia) for describing the kinetics of behavior of ^{62}Cu-PTSM in myocardium. Accurate estimates of flow have been obtained with this approach.[54]

One potential problem with the use of ^{62}Cu-PTSM is that a fraction of tracer binds to erythrocytes.[52] Although binding appears to be species—dependent and is quite low in primates, a correction for tracer associated with red cells may be necessary to accurately define the arterial input function. In addition, the near 10 minute half-life would require a 45 to 60 minute delay between acquisition of scans at rest and after hyperemia (to permit sufficient decay of radioactivity from the initial administration). Since uptake of radiolabeled Cu-PTSM reflects perfusion to the brain,[55] kidneys[52] and perhaps to other organs and tumors as well, a single administration of this tracer may be used in obtaining estimates of perfusion in several organs.

Use of longer-lived copper radioisotopes may permit administration of tracer before interventions for delineation of regions of myocardium at risk.

Clinical Studies

In a preliminary report,[54] Herrero et al. show that high-quality images can be obtained with this tracer in human subjects (Color Figure 1) and that flow estimated with ^{62}Cu-PTSM and a two-compartment model correlates closely with flow estimated with ^{15}O-water. Further studies will be necessary to delineate the utility of this tracer for clinical purposes.

^{38}K

Radioisotopes of potassium have been used for assessment of myocardial perfusion in both laboratory and clinical studies predicated on avid trapping by cardiac myocytes. Potassium flux is quite sensitive to flow. The tracer clears rapidly from the blood and is extracted avidly by myocardium. In a study by Pierard et al., perfusion was evaluated with ^{38}K in patients by the comparison of decreased counts with areas with peak counts in each tomographic slice.[56] Because of the known alterations in potassium flux with ischemia followed by reperfusion,[57] validation studies will be necessary before results with this tracer can be interpreted unambiguously.

Measurement of Myocardial Perfusion with Diffusible Tracers

A third approach for estimation of myocardial perfusion entails the use of tracers that are freely diffusible within myocardium.[3,24] The advantage of this approach is that the kinetics of accumulation and clearance of tracer from myocardium are much less complex than those associated with the partially extractable tracers. It has been suggested that measurement of nutritional perfusion with diffusible tracers may permit a more valid estimation of nutritive perfusion than that obtained with inert, carbonized microspheres.[19] Positron-emitting tracers that have been used include ^{11}C-butanol and ^{15}O-water. Perfusion is quantified with a modification of equations derived by Kety for the analysis of exchange of inert gas between blood and tissue. Assessment of myocardial perfusion requires that the time-activity curves in arterial blood and in myocardium be measured (Figure 5-8).

Laboratory Results

Because of the short physical half-life of ^{15}O (2.1 minutes) and the ease of its rapid, automated production, it has been employed in most studies using the diffusible tracer approach. Bergmann et al. demonstrated that the limitations to free diffusibility of water were modest, constant, and not altered by changes in flow.[20] Thus, ^{15}O-water could be considered freely diffusible in the heart. Regional uptake of ^{15}O-water was found to correlate closely with regional uptake of microspheres.[20] The fact that ^{15}O resides in blood as well as

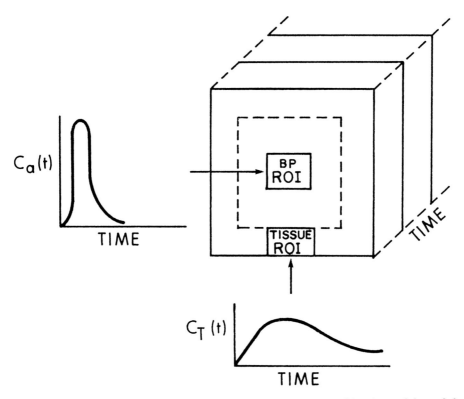

Figure 5-8. *Schematic representation of the one-compartment kinetic model used for estimation of myocardial perfusion with $H_2{}^{15}O$ and PET. For estimation of flow, the arterial input function, $C_a(t)$, and the tissue time-activity curve, $C_T(t)$, are obtained from the dynamically collected tomograms. Flow is calculated as described in detail in the text by use of partial volume and spillover corrections incorporated into the mathematical model.*

in myocardium necessitates the use of a separate scan (typically with ^{15}O-carbon monoxide) to label the blood pool to facilitate visualization of the myocardium (Figure 5-9). Care must be taken to eliminate movement or changes in physiologic status between scans. Novel approaches based on analysis of the early phase of distribution of tracer after administration of $H_2{}^{15}O$ (which reflects the first pass through the cardiac blood pool) are being developed. If successful, they would eliminate the necessity for an independent scan of vascular activity. ^{15}O-water has been used to delineate limited increases in myocardial perfusion in response to dipyridamole in animals with experimentally induced coronary stenosis[58] and demonstrated restoration of perfusion after thrombolysis.[59]

Several assumptions underlie the use of a one-compartment model for quantification of myocardial perfusion including: 1) that the uptake of tracer is flow dependent and not diffusion limited, 2) that no arteriovenous shunts or bypasses are present, 3) that the solubility of tracer is constant, and 4) that the

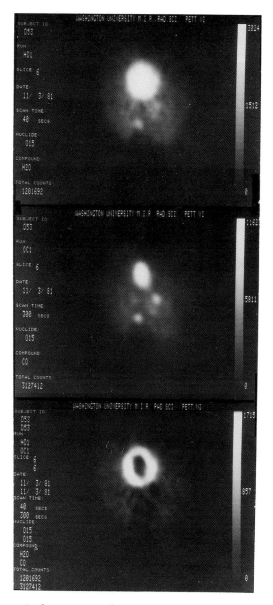

Figure 5-9. *Midventricular tomographic reconstructions obtained from a normal dog after intravenous administration of ^{15}O-water (A); after labeling the blood pool with $C^{15}O$ to define the vascular space (B); and after correcting the tomograph in A for tracer in the vascular space (C). This image represents the distribution of ^{15}O-water in the myocardium. (Reproduced from Bergmann et al.,[20] with permission of the American Heart Association, Inc.)*

flow is constant and homogeneous throughout the region interrogated during the imaging interval. It has been shown that the limitations to free diffusibility are modest, constant, and not altered by changes in flow. Exclusion of shunts or bypasses is probably valid for the heart in general. However, the distribution of a diffusible tracer such as water or butanol can differ from the distribution of microspheres. Thus, shunting cannot be excluded with certainty in all instances. Nonetheless, the single-pass diffusion of ^{15}O-water has been found to be invariant over a wide range of flows. The assumption that flow is uniform in a region is likely to be valid when small regions of interest are evaluated, but it is clearly not valid for the heart as a whole. If the assumptions are reasonably well met, regional flow can be determined by monitoring the concentration of tracer in arterial blood (the input function) and in regions of interest in tissue (Figure 5-9).

For an inert, diffusible tracer, conservation of mass exists such that the rate of change in concentration of tracer in the tissue is equal to the rate of tracer entering the tissue minus the rate of tracer leaving the tissue with respect to a given tissue volume. Therefore:

$$dC_T(t)/dt = \frac{F}{V} (C_a(t) - C_v(t)) \tag{3}$$

where:

C_T = tissue concentration of tracer (counts per gram)
F/V = flow per unit of tissue volume (milliliters per gram per minute)
C_a = arterial concentration of tracer (counts per milliliter)
C_v = venous concentration of tracer (counts per milliliter).

Kety described the relation of venous concentration of tracer to its tissue concentration assuming equilibration of tracer between blood and tissue during a single capillary passage:

$$(C_a - C_v) = m(C_a - C_T/\lambda) \tag{4}$$

where:

λ = tissue/blood partition coefficient (ml/g)
m = a diffusion constant reflecting effects of diffusion limitations and other factors tending to limit equilibration of tracer between tissue and blood:

$$m = 1 - e(-PS/F) \tag{5}$$

where PS is the product of capillary permeability and surface area (ml/min/g). For studies of $H_2^{15}O$ in myocardium, $\lambda = 0.92$ ml/g and $m = 1.0$. Substituting equation 4 into equation 3:

$$\frac{dC_T(t)}{dt} = \frac{F}{V} (C_a(t) - C_T(t)/\lambda) \tag{6}$$

Then,

$$C_T(t) = \frac{F}{V} C_a(t) * \exp\left(-\frac{Ft}{V\lambda}\right) \qquad (7)$$

where $*$ represents convolution.

Because the current generation of PET scanners cannot measure instantaneous tissue activity, scans are performed over many seconds summing the decay events occurring during the scan:

$$C_T(t_1:t_2) = \frac{F}{V} \int_{t_1}^{t_2} C_a(t) * \exp\left(-\frac{Ft}{V\lambda}\right) dt \qquad (8)$$

Averaged counts over short scan intervals are used to approximate instantaneous count rates. F/V (flow per unit volume) can be estimated by minimizing the sum of squared deviations with respect to F/V given that λ is known and $C_a(t)$ and $C_T(t)$ can be measured.

A least squares technique is used for fitting equation 8 to all data values in the interval from 0 to 90 seconds after the appearance of tracer in the left atrium. Estimates of F/V reflect both washin and washout processes. The optimal value of F/V is obtained by a direct search over the entire range of values.

The 90 second time interval has been used because the actual number of measurable counts after this interval is very small. Extending the scan time results in addition of low signal-to-noise data.[15] Simulation studies have shown that the early portion of the time-activity curve is the portion that is most sensitive to flow.

Because of the limited spatial resolution of the present generation of tomographs in relation to the thickness of myocardium and effects of cardiac motion, true tissue concentrations of radiotracer cannot be measured directly with PET. However, observed tissue and blood pool activity can be related to true tissue and blood pool tracer concentration by correcting for partial volume and spillover effects:

$$C_{T_{PET}}(t) = F_{MM} \times C_T(t) + F_{BM}C_a(t) \qquad (9)$$

where:

$$C_{a_{PET}}(t) = F_{BB} \times C_a(t) + F_{MB} \times C_T(t) \qquad (10)$$

$C_{T_{PET}}(t)$ = observed tissue activity (counts per gram)
$C_T(t)$ = true tissue activity (counts per gram)
$C_{a_{PET}}(t)$ = observed blood pool activity (counts per gram)
$C_a(t)$ = true blood pool activity (counts per gram)
F_{MM} = recovery coefficient of tissue
F_{BM} = fraction of blood activity into tissue
F_{BB} = recovery coefficient of blood pool
F_{MB} = fraction of tissue activity into blood pool.

The correction procedure requires that the true recovery coefficients and spillover factors be known. These factors can be defined analytically if the resolution of the tomograph and the blood pool and cardiac tissue dimensions are known and if no motion is present. However, when cardiac or respiratory motion is present or when inaccurate estimates of blood pool and tissue dimensions are used, or both, correction factors may be inaccurate.

To circumvent the problem of estimating correction factors with independent assessments of chamber and wall dimensions, the factors have been incorporated within the operational equations for estimating flow as follows:

$$C_{T_{PET}}(t_1 : t_2) = \int_{t_1}^{t_2} C_{t_{PET}}(t) \, dt =$$

$$F_{MM} \times \left[\frac{F}{V} \int_{t_1}^{t_2} C_a(t) * \exp\left(\frac{-Ft}{V\lambda}\right) dt \right] + F_{BM} \int_{t_1}^{t_2} C_a(t) \, dt \qquad (11)$$

where the tissue activity observed by PET can be fitted directly to the operational flow equation to estimate myocardial blood flow per unit volume (F/V) as well as F_{MM} and F_{BM} with a nonlinear least squares fitting procedure. The optimal value of F/V is obtained by a direct search over the entire range of possible flow values, with values of F_{MM} and F_{BM} estimated for each value of F/V by linear, least squares approximation. The optimal set of parameters is the set that minimizes the sum of squared deviations. By including the tissue activity correction for partial volume and spillover effects within the estimation of F/V, no a priori knowledge of F_{MM} and F_{BM} is needed, and consequently no error in calculation of these factors is introduced. Furthermore, because equation 11 characterizes the empirical relationship between true tissue activity and that measured by PET, the parameter—estimated correction fractions F_{MM} and F_{BM} include corrections for effects of linear cardiac and respiratory motion on observed positron emission tomographic counts. The approach requires the ability to obtain $C_a(t)$ directly from PET counts or that it be obtained by direct sampling of arterial blood.

To quantify myocardial perfusion, dynamic scans are obtained in 2 to 5 second frames over the 90 second interval after bolus intravenous administration of 15 to 25 mCi of ^{15}O-water. Time-activity curves of tracer are measured in arterial blood and in regions of interest. Use of the intravenous bolus approach requires a high count rate and a rapidly scanning PET instrument. Correlations between flow estimated noninvasively and that estimated with microspheres over a wide range (from 0.2 to 6.0 ml/min/g) have been close (Figure 5-10).

Recently, this approach has been modified by use of inhalation of ^{15}O-carbon dioxide (which is converted to ^{15}O-water by lung and blood carbonic anhydrase) and a more prolonged infusion protocol[60] to avoid the saturation of count capabilities of some commercial scanners. However, the inhalation approach increases radiation burden to the patient (and especially the airway) and decreases sensitivity to hyperemic flows.[61]

Labeled butanol has been used for estimation of myocardial perfusion with this approach.[61] Butanol is more lipophilic than water and theoretically more highly diffusible. A rapid synthesis scheme for ^{15}O-butanol has recently been

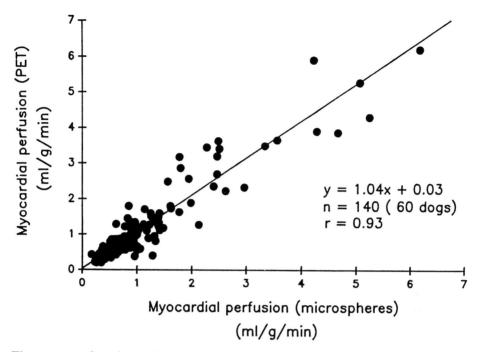

Figure 5-10. *Correlation between myocardial perfusion estimated with* ^{15}O*-water and PET and perfusion estimated with radiolabeled microspheres. The data summarize flow obtained in 60 dogs in which flow was perturbated as a result of ischemia, global low flow, reperfusion, or hyperemia after administration of dipyridamole.*

developed.[62] Future studies will be necessary to determine if the use of butanol has advantages over the use of ^{15}O-water.

Clinical Assessments of Myocardial Perfusion with ^{15}O-water

Tomographic visualization of the heart after intravenous administration of ^{15}O-water requires correction for radioactivity in the vascular compartment, accomplished in most circumstances with a separate scan after inhalation of ^{15}O-carbon monoxide (40 to 50 mCi) to label erythrocytes and delineate the vascular pool. Pixel-by-pixel correction is used to correct for labeled water residing in the blood pool and to provide images of myocardium. Our group at Washington University has developed and validated this approach and used it to characterize the efficacy of several interventions. Walsh et al. demonstrated the utility of ^{15}O-water for delineation of impaired perfusion indicative of coronary artery disease in patients[11] (See Chapter 11, Table 11-2 and Color Figure 14).

Bergmann et al. showed that myocardial perfusion could be measured in absolute terms as well.[14] The ratio of perfusion evaluated in patients at rest to that after intravenous infusion of dipyridamole averaged 1:4, comparable to the fourfold coronary flow velocity reserve reported by others using invasive

Doppler techniques. Similar results were reported by Araujo et al. who used the $C^{15}O_2$ inhalation approach.[60] Shelton et al. showed that estimates of myocardial perfusion with ^{15}O-water correlated closely with coronary flow velocity catheters.[60a] Iida et al. demonstrated decreased perfusion in patients with coronary artery disease[13] (See Chapter 11, Color Figure 15).

Walsh et al. demonstrated that, after dipyridamole, perfusion distal to a single-vessel coronary artery stenosis averaged only 64% of that in normal regions.[39] Furthermore, they demonstrated normalization of hyperemic flow after successful angioplasty. Maintenance of normal perfusion reserve was demonstrated in patients without symptoms of recurrent ischemia 7.5 months after angioplasty (Figure 5-11 and see Chapter 11, Color Figure 12). Henes et al. demonstrated normalization of myocardial perfusion in jeopardized zones

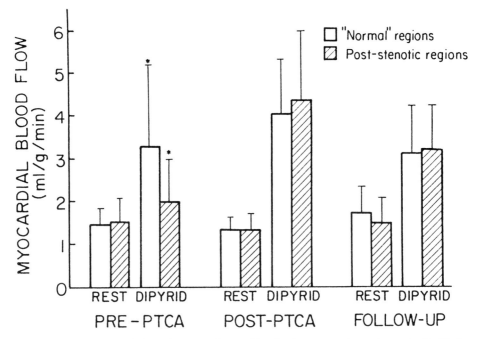

Figure 5-11. *Myocardial perfusion estimated in absolute terms in patients studied before percutaneous transluminal coronary angioplasty (PTCA), immediately after PTCA, and at long-term follow-up. Perfusion at rest and after dipyridamole (DYPYRID) are illustrated for each time point. The open bars represent flows in regions supplied by angiographically normal coronary arteries and the cross-hatched bars flows in regions subtended by the stenotic artery. Before PTCA, flow at rest is similar in the two territories. However, after pharmacologic stress, hyperemic flow in the region distal to the stenosis reaches only 64% of the flow observed in the normal region. After angioplasty, hyperemic perfusion improved in regions supplied by vessels that were dilated in the procedure. This result was unchanged in the patients without symptoms of recurrent ischemia studied an average of 7.5 months after angioplasty. This study demonstrated the power of quantitative estimates of myocardial perfusion reserve and the ability of PET to diagnose flow limitations and the efficacy of therapies designed to enhance nutritive perfusion. (Reproduced from Walsh et al.,[39] with permission of The American College of Cardiology.)*

in patients treated with thrombolytic agents within 4 hours after the onset of symptoms.[63] Sequential tomograms with ^{15}O-water proved to be helpful in characterizing changes in perfusion and its effects on myocardial metabolism (See Chapter 11, Figure 11-2).

We recently found that the hyperemic response in older adults is somewhat diminished compared with that in younger adults, perhaps because of diminished sensitivity to the vasodilator effects of dipyridamole.[64] Nevertheless, in approximately 50% of patients with chest pain but angiographically normal coronary arteries, flow at rest was higher than that in normal volunteers and perfusion reserve was markedly diminished, indicating abnormal microvascular perfusion.[65] (Color Figure 2 and Chapter 11, Figure 11-1). Impaired perfusion reserve has also been demonstrated in hearts of patients who are recipients of cardiac allografts.[66] Flow at rest is high accompanying the increased cardiac work secondary to hypertension. Patients with episodic rejection exhibit decreased maximal hyperemic flow compared with that in patients without rejection. Thus, quantification of myocardial perfusion in absolute terms has already helped to characterize the efficacy of therapeutic interventions and delineate subtle pathophysiologic mechanisms.

Unresolved Issues

Selection of Tracers

With the variety of positron-emitting tracers of perfusion available, selection may be difficult. [82]Rb is attractive because of its very short half-life and availability by generator production. Rapid scanning is feasible with this isotope minimizing clinical delays. The short half-life imposes some limitations on counting statistics and on quality of the images. Kinetics of the tracer can distort estimates of perfusion based on uptake alone—a difficulty that can be overcome by compartmental model analysis. Use of this tracer has successfully identified patients with coronary artery disease, indicating that sensitive quantitative estimates may not be necessary for clinical stratifications.

[13]N-ammonia provides images of excellent quality. If compartmental analysis does provide quantitative estimates of perfusion in absolute terms that can be validated with this tracer, it will become increasingly useful. However, breakdown of tracer in blood, extraction of labeled metabolites by the heart, and the half-life of 10 minutes are disadvantages, particularly for rapidly sequential studies.

For centers with cyclotrons, ^{15}O-water is an attractive tracer because its short physical half-life facilitates rapid sequential scanning procedures and its straightforward kinetics permit accurate quantification of myocardial perfusion in absolute terms. The necessity for a vascular pool correction for visualization of myocardium is a disadvantage.

[11]C- or ^{68}Ga-labeled microspheres require administration directly into the left heart. Nonetheless, in patients undergoing cardiac catheterization for specific indications, microspheres can yield accurate results.

^{62}Cu-PTSM and ^{38}K are presently undergoing validation studies. ^{62}Cu-PTSM is generator produced. Its prolonged retention in myocardium and its suitability for delineation of flow in multiple organs are attractive features. Disadvantages include its relatively long half-life (similar to that of ^{13}N-ammonia) and complexities attributable to binding to red cells.

Measurement of Perfusion in Regions of Low Flow

Accurate quantification of perfusion by PET in low-flow regions remains difficult. Ischemia per se limits delivery of tracer, and accordingly, the statistical accuracy of counts in low-flow regions. Parodi et al. vividly demonstrated that wall thinning, without actual changes in tracer activity, can result in an apparent perfusion defect on the tomogram when, in fact, counts per gram of tissue are unchanged[41] (Figure 5-5). Thus, partial volume corrections are essential. Qualitative images may be misleading. Tomographs with high spatial resolution may partially compensate for this effect.

Accurate quantification is necessary not only for definitive clinical diagnosis, but also for answering biologically significant questions such as whether or not a minimal level of perfusion is required to maintain myocyte viability under specific conditions and to define its magnitude.

Assessment of Perfusion Reserve

Assessment of perfusion at rest and after a hyperemic stimulus such as intravenous dipyridamole or adenosine or after a physiologic stimulus such as exercise has been used to define myocardial perfusion reserve. However, the absolute level of hyperemia that identifies patients at high risk for cardiac events is not yet clear. Lesser et al. demonstrated that patients with a coronary flow velocity reserve exceeding 3.5 to 1 (flow velocity after papaverine compared with that at rest measured with intracoronary Doppler flow probes) can be safely managed conservatively.[2] However, even with maximal exercise, myocardial perfusion rarely increases by more than two-to-threefold.[67,68] Thus, research is needed to define the level of maximal flow indicative of protection against cardiac events.

Conclusions

PET allows noninvasive quantification of regional myocardial perfusion. Perfusion imaging with PET appears to provide greater sensitivity and specificity for the diagnosis of coronary artery disease compared with conventional, single-photon scintigraphy with ^{201}Tl. However, the sensitivity achievable with scintigraphy with novel, ^{99m}Tc flow tracers and the practical utility of PET imaging for routine clinical decision making have not yet been determined.

Quantitative estimation of myocardial perfusion after maximal coronary vasodilation appears to provide the most accurate and sensitive criteria of the physiologic significance of coronary artery disease. PET is invaluable for delineation of the physiologic impact of cardiac disease on myocardial perfusion and its regulation. The availability of high-resolution, fast-scanning PET instruments has facilitated accurate measurement of tracer kinetics and the development of the physiologically based mathematical models needed for quantitative estimation of perfusion. Together, these advances are likely to improve selection of patients for invasive procedures, facilitate evaluations of the efficacy of therapeutic interventions designed to enhance nutritive perfusion, and elucidate the pathogenesis of impaired myocardial perfusion associated with diverse disorders.

Acknowledgments: The author thanks Pilar Herrero and Dr. Burton E. Sobel for review of this manuscript, Elizabeth Engeszer for editorial review, and Becky Leonard and Sue Furey for secretarial assistance. Work from the author's laboratory was supported in part by National Institutes of Health grants HL17646—Specialized Center of Research in Coronary and Vascular Disease; HL46895—Optimization of PET Estimates of Myocardial Perfusion; and by grants from the American Heart Association, Missouri Affiliate.

References

1. Marcus ML, Harrison DG, White CW, McPherson DD, Wilson RF, Kerber RE: Assessing the physiologic significance of coronary obstructions in patients: Importance of diffuse undetected atherosclerosis. Prog Cardiovasc Dis 1988; 31:39–56.
2. Lesser JR, Wilson RF, White CW: Physiologic asessment of coronary stenoses of intermediate severity can facilitate patient selection for coronary angioplasty. Coronary Artery Dis 1990; 1:697–705.
3. Bergmann SR, Fox KAA, Geltman EM, Sobel BE: Positron emission tomography of the heart. Prog Cardiovasc Dis 1985; 28:165–194.
4. Gould KL: Identifying and measuring severity of coronary artery stenosis. Quantitative coronary arteriography and positron emission tomography. Circulation 1988; 78:237–245.
5. Tamaki N, Yonekura Y, Senda M, Yamashita K, Koide H, Saji H, Hashimoto T, Fudo T, Kambara H, Kawai C, Konishi J: Value and limitation of stress thallium-201 single photon emission computed tomography: Comparison with nitrogen-13 ammonia positron tomography. J Nucl Med 1988; 29:1181–1188.
6. Schelbert HR, Wisenberg G, Phelps ME, Gould KL, Henze E, Hoffman EJ, Gomes A, Kuhl DE: Noninvasive assessment of coronary stenoses by myocardial imaging during pharmacologic coronary vasodilation. VI. Detection of coronary artery disease in human beings with intravenous N-13 ammonia and positron computed tomography. Am J Cardiol 1982; 49:1197–1206.
7. Tamaki N, Senda M, Yonekura Y, Saji H, Kodama S, Konishi Y, Ban T, Kambara H, Kawai C, Torizuka K: Dynamic positron computed tomography of the heart with a high sensitivity positron camera and nitrogen-13 ammonia. J Nucl Med 1985; 26:567–575.
8. Yonekura Y, Tamaki N, Senda M, Nohara R, Kambara H, Konishi Y, Koide H, Kureshi SA, Saji H, Ban T, Kawai C, Torizuka K: Detection of coronary artery disease with ^{13}N-ammonia and high-resolution positron-emission computed tomography. Am Heart J 1987; 113:645–654.
9. Gould KL, Goldstein RA, Mullani NA, Kirkeeide RL, Wong W-H, Tewson TJ, Berridge MS, Bolomey LA, Hartz RK, Smalling RW, Fuentes F, Nishikawa A: Noninvasive assessment of coronary stenoses by myocardial perfusion imaging during phar-

macologic coronary vasodilation. VIII. Clinical feasibility of positron cardiac imaging without a cyclotron using generator-produced rubidium-82. J Am Coll Cardiol 1986; 7:775–789.

10. Demer LL, Gould LK, Goldstein RA, Kirkeeide RL, Mullani NA, Smalling RW, Nishikawa A, Merhige ME: Assessment of coronary artery disease severity by positron emission tomography. Comparison with quantitative arteriography in 193 patients. Circulation 1989; 79:825–835.

11. Walsh MN, Bergmann SR, Steele RL, Kenzora JL, Ter-Pogossian MM, Sobel BE, Geltman EM: Delineation of impaired regional myocardial perfusion by positron emission tomography with $H_2{}^{15}O$. Circulation 1988; 78:612–620.

12. Henze E, Huang S-C, Ratib O, Hoffman E, Phelps ME, Schelbert HR: Measurements of regional tissue and blood-pool radiotracer concentrations from serial tomographic images of the heart. J Nucl Med 1983; 24:987–996.

13. Iida H, Kanno I, Takahashi A, Miura S, Murakami M, Takahashi K, Ono Y, Shishido F, Inugami A, Tomura N, Higano S, Fujita H, Sasaki H, Nakamichi H, Mizusawa S, Kondo Y, Uemura K: Measurement of absolute myocardial blood flow with $H_2{}^{15}O$ and dynamic positron-emission tomography. Circulation 1988; 78:104–115.

14. Bergmann SR, Herrero P, Markham J, Weinheimer CJ, Walsh MN: Noninvasive quantitation of myocardial blood flow in human subjects with oxygen-15-labeled water and positron emission tomography. J Am Coll Cardiol 1989; 14:639–652.

15. Herrero P, Markham J, Bergmann SR: Quantitation of myocardial blood flow with $H_2{}^{15}O$ and positron emission tomography: Assessment and error analysis of a mathematical approach. J Comp Assist Tomogr 1989; 13:862–873.

16. Krivokapich J, Smith GT, Huang S-C, Hoffman EJ, Ratib O, Phelps ME, Schelbert HR: ^{13}N ammonia myocardial imaging at rest and with exercise in normal volunteers. Circulation 1989; 80:1328–1337.

17. Hutchins GD, Schwaiger M, Rosenspire KC, Krivokapich J, Schelbert H, Kuhl DE: Noninvasive quantification of regional blood flow in the human heart using N-13 ammonia and dynamic positron emission tomographic imaging. J Am Coll Cardiol 1990; 1032–1042.

18. Heymann MA, Payne BD, Hoffman JIE, Rudolph AM: Blood flow measurements with radionuclide-labeled particles. Prog Cardiovasc Dis 1977; 20:55–78.

19. Yoshida S, Akizuki S, Gowski D, Downey JM: Discrepancy between microsphere and diffusible tracer estimates of perfusion to ischemic myocardium. Am J Physiol:Heart Circ Physiol 1985; 249:H255-H264.

20. Bergmann SR, Fox KAA, Rand AL, McElvany KD, Welch MJ, Markham J, Sobel BE: Quantification of regional myocardial blood flow in vivo with $H_2{}^{15}O$. Circulation 1984; 70:724–733.

21. Wisenberg G, Schelbert HR, Hoffman EJ, Phelps ME, Robinson GD, Selin CE, Child J, Skorton D, Kuhl DE: In vivo quantitation of regional myocardial blood flow by positron-emission computed tomography. Circulation 1981; 63:6:1248–1257.

22. Wilson RA, Shea MJ, De Landsheere CM, Turton D, Brady F, Deanfield JE, Selwyn AP: Validation of quantitation of regional myocardial blood flow in vivo with ^{11}C-labeled human albumin microspheres and positron emission tomography. Circulation 1984; 70:717–723.

23. Selwyn AP, Shea MJ, Foale R, Deanfield JE, Wilson R, De Landsheere CM, Turton DL, Brady F, Pike VW, Brookes DI: Regional myocardial and organ blood flow after myocardial infarction: Application of the microsphere principle in man. Circulation 1986; 73:433–443.

24. Bergmann SR: Positron emission tomography of the heart. In: Gerson M, Ed. *Cardiac Nuclear Medicine*. New York: McGraw-Hill, 1990; 299–335.

25. Love WD, Burch GE: Influence of the rate of coronary plasma flow on the extraction of Rb^{86} from coronary blood. Circ Res 1959; 7:24–30.

26. Goldstein RA, Mullani NA, Marani SK, Fisher DJ, Gould KL, O'Brien HA, Jr: Myocardial perfusion with rubidium-82. II. Effects of metabolic and pharmacologic interventions. J Nucl Med 1983; 24:907–915.

27. Selwyn AP, Allan RM, L'Abbate A, Horlock P, Camici P, Clark J, O'Brien HA, Grant PM: Relation between regional myocardial uptake of rubidium-82 and perfusion: Absolute reduction of cation uptake in ischemia. Am J Cardiol 1982; 50:112–121.

28. Fukuyama T, Nakamura M, Nakagaki O, Matsuguchi H, Mitsutake A, Kikuchi Y: Reduced reflow and diminished uptake of ^{86}Rb after temporary coronary occlusion. Am J Physiol:Heart Circ Physiol 1978; 234:H724-H729.

29. Wilson RA, Shea M, De Landsheere C, Deanfield J, Lammertsma AA, Jones T, Selwyn AP: Rubidium-82 myocardial uptake and extraction after transient ischemia: PET characteristics. J Comput Assist Tomogr 1987; 11:60–66.

30. Jeremy RW, Links JM, Becker LC: Progressive failure of coronary flow during reperfusion of myocardial infarction: documentation of the no reflow phenomenon with positron emission tomography. J Am Coll of Cardiol 1990; 16:695–704.

31. Mullani NA, Gould KL: First-pass measurements of regional blood flow with external detectors. J Nucl Med 1983; 24:577–581.

32. Herrero P, Markham J, Shelton ME, Bergmann SR: Implementation and evaluation of a two-compartment model for quantification of myocardial perfusion with rubidium-82 and positron emission tomography. Circ Res 1992; 70:496–507.

33. Herrero P, Markham J, Shelton ME, Weinheimer CJ, Bergmann SR: Noninvasive quantitation of regional myocardial blood flow with rubidium-82 and positron emission tomography: exploration of a mathematical model. Circulation 1990; 82:1377–1386.

34. Goldstein RA: Kinetics of rubidium-82 after coronary occlusion and reperfusion. Assessment of patency and viability in open-chested dogs. J Clin Invest 1985; 75:1131–1137.

35. Gropler RJ, Bergmann SR: Myocardial viability—what is the definition? (editorial) J Nucl Med 1991; 32:10–12.

36. Go RT, Marwick TH, MacIntyre WJ, Saha GB, Neumann DR, Underwood DA, Simpfendorfer CC: A prospective comparison of rubidium-82 PET and thallium-201 SPECT myocardial perfusion imaging utilizing a single dipyridamole stress in the diagnosis of coronary artery disease. J Nucl Med 1990; 31:1899–1905.

37. Stewart RE, Schwaiger M, Molina E, Popma J, Gacioch GM, Kalus M, Squicciarini S, al-Aouar ZR, Schork A, Kuhl DE. Comparison of rubidium-82 positron emission tomography and thallium-201 SPECT imaging for detection of coronary artery disease. Am J Cardiol 1991; 67:1303–1310.

38. Goldstein RA, Kirkeeide RL, Demer LL, Merhige M, Nishikawa A, Smalling RW, Mullani NA, Gould LK: Relation between geometric dimensions of coronary artery stenoses and myocardial perfusion reserve in man. J Clin Invest 1987; 79:1473–1478.

39. Walsh MN, Geltman EM, Steele RL, Kenzora JL, Ludbrook PA, Sobel BE, Bergmann SR: Augmented myocardial perfusion reserve after angioplasty quantified by positron emission tomography with $H_2^{15}O$. J Am Coll Cardiol 1990; 15:119–127.

40. Goldstein RA, Kirkeeide RL, Smalling RW, Nishikawa A, Merhige ME, Demer LL, Mullani NA, Gould KL: Changes in myocardial perfusion reserve after PTCA: Noninvasive assessment with positron tomography. J Nucl Med 1987; 28:1262–1267.

41. Parodi O, Schelbert HR, Schwaiger M, Hansen H, Selin C, Hoffman EJ: Cardiac emission computed tomography: Underestimation of regional tracer concentrations due to wall motion abnormalities. J Comput Assist Tomogr 1984; 8:1083–1092.

42. Gould KL, Yoshida K, Hess MJ, Haynie M, Mullani N, Smalling RW: Myocardial metabolism of fluorodeoxyglucose compared to cell membrane integrity for the potassium analogue rubidium-82 for assessing infarct size in man by PET. J Nucl Med 1991; 32:1–9.

43. Schelbert HR, Phelps ME, Huang S-C, MacDonald NS, Hansen H, Selin C, Kuhl DE: N-13 ammonia as an indicator of myocardial blood flow. Circulation 1981; 63:1259.

Chapter 6

Delineation of Myocardial Fatty Acid Metabolism with Positron Emission Tomography

René A. Lerch, M.D., Steven R. Bergmann, M.D., Ph.D., and Burton E. Sobel, M.D.

Although myocardium can utilize diverse substrates, including fatty acids, glucose, lactate, pyruvate, ketones, and amino acids, the specific pattern of substrate utilization under specific conditions depends on arterial substrate concentrations, myocardial perfusion and oxygenation, and neurohumoral stimulation, among other factors. Under normal physiologic conditions, oxidative metabolism of nonesterified (or free) fatty acids provides approximately 40% to 60% of the energy used by the heart. With the onset of ischemia, oxidation of fatty acid declines rapidly. Accordingly, characterization of the metabolism of labeled fatty acids has been a focus of cardiac positron emission tomography (PET). From a historical perspective, its characterization was of seminal importance in demonstrating: 1) that a metabolic process in myocardium could be quantified noninvasively; 2) that the extent of ischemic injury could be imaged tomographically; and 3) that cardiac PET could be implemented in critically ill patients to provide objective assessments of the efficacy of potentially therapeutic interventions.

Background

In 1965 Evans et al.[1] demonstrated that oleic acid labeled at the double bond with iodine-131 could be used to visualize the left ventricular myocardium scintigraphically. However, the tracer was extracted less extensively by myocardium than unlabeled saturated fatty acids.[2] More recently, noninvasive characterization of myocardial fatty acid metabolism by PET was accomplished with palmitate labeled with carbon-11 (^{11}C) at the carboxyl (C-1) position.[3]

From *Positron Emission Tomography of the Heart* edited by Steven R. Bergmann, MD, PhD and Burton E. Sobel, MD © 1992, Futura Publishing Inc., Mount Kisco, NY.

The single-pass extraction fraction of 1-^{11}C-palmitate is not constant. It is influenced by both residence time in the capillary bed and the rate of metabolism of fatty acid extracted into myocytes. The capillary residence time is inversely related to myocardial blood flow. Assuming a constant flux of fatty acids from the plasma into myocytes, the fraction of a bolus of tracer that crosses the capillary barrier (or single-pass extraction fraction) is inversely related to capillary flow.[10,16] The flux is dependent on the concentration gradient, which reflects plasma to intracellular fatty acid concentration differences that are, in turn, influenced by intracellular metabolism. As shown in studies in dogs, the single-pass extraction fraction decreases with inhibition of fatty acid oxidation by hypoxia.[15] Similarly, a reduction of the single-pass extraction of 1-^{11}C-palmitate occurs when mitochondrial fatty acid transfer is inhibited chemically with agents such as 2-tetradecylglycidic acid.[17] Normal values can be restored by supplementation of arterial blood with glucose, presumably because of provision of glycerol-3-phosphate for esterification of cytosolic fatty acids.[18]

In vivo, altered flow usually elicits altered metabolism. To define effects of reduced perfusion per se (with oxidative metabolism held constant) on net myocardial extraction of labeled palmitate, coronary flow was reduced stepwise in isovolumically beating isolated rabbit hearts[19] in which cardiac work was kept constant by modifying developed pressure and heart rate. Net uptake of continuously delivered ^{14}C-palmitate remained constant despite reduction of myocardial blood flow from 1.5 to 0.5 ml/min/g. Extraction fraction increased in a compensatory fashion as flow and supply decreased. With ischemia, the single-pass extraction fraction of 1-^{11}C-palmitate initially increases because of increased capillary residence time.[10,15] Because oxidative metabolism is impaired, extracted fatty acids are shunted into triglycerides or diffuse back into the coronary venous circulation. With prolonged ischemia, single-pass extraction fraction decreases, presumably because of saturation of these mechanisms.[10]

Clearance of Myocardial ^{11}C-palmitate Radioactivity

The clearance (or release) of radioactivity from myocardium after initial extraction of 1-^{11}C-palmitate in open-chest dogs has been defined.[15,20–22] In studies by our group, myocardium was perfused via an extracorporeal bypass system that permitted graded reduction of coronary flow or hypoxic perfusion with venous blood at normal flow. 1-^{11}C-palmitate was injected as a bolus directly into the cannulated coronary artery. Myocardial radioactivity was recorded with high temporal and spatial resolution with positron detectors placed on the epicardial surface.[21] The semilogarithmic plot of myocardial time-activity curves recorded under baseline conditions delineated several discrete components of clearance (Figure 6-2). The initial peak was followed by a rapid decline of the myocardial count rate representing vascular transit of nonextracted tracer. Clearance of initially extracted 1-^{11}C-palmitate exhibited 2 components consistent with incorporation of tracer into at least 2 pools with

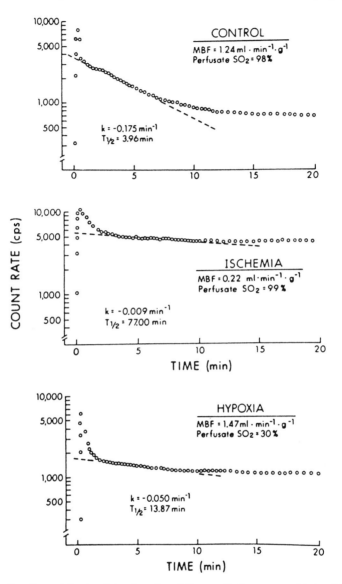

Figure 6-2. *Semilogarithmic plots of regional time-activity curves obtained in an open-chest dog with controlled perfusion of the left anterior descending coronary artery via an extracorporeal circuit. 1-^{11}C-palmitate was injected intracoronarily, and myocardial activity was monitored with a β-probe. Under control conditions (top) clearance of myocardial activity exhibits 3 components: vascular transit of nonextracted tracer, an early rapid phase evident between 3 and 7 minutes after administration of tracer (reflecting, primarily, oxidation of fatty acid to ^{11}CO$_2$), and a slower phase, evident later, (reflecting, primarily, turnover of triglyceride and phospholipid pools). With low-flow ischemia (middle panel) and with perfusion with hypoxic blood at normal flow (bottom panel), the rate of the rapid phase is markedly diminished. The dashed line represents the slope of the rapid phase. Abbreviations: MBF—myocardial blood flow; SO$_2$—hemoglobin saturation of blood entering the left anterior descending coronary artery; t$_{1/2}$—half-time of the rapid phase of ^{11}C-clearance; k—rate constant of the rapid clearance phase.(Reproduced from Lerch et al.,[20] with permission of the American Heart Association, Inc.)*

different turnover rates. A rapid clearance component (prominent between 3 and 7 minutes after injection of tracer) exhibited a rate constant (k) of 0.105 ± 0.016 (SEM) min[-1], corresponding to a biological half-time of 6.6 minutes.[20] The half-time of the slower component (most evident more than 15 minutes after injection) consistently exceeded 40 minutes.

With reduction of myocardial perfusion by 64%, the rate constant of the rapid component declined by 61%.[20] A similar reduction of clearance (by 52%) was observed when myocardium was perfused at normal flow with hypoxic blood (resulting in decreased oxygen supply comparable to that seen with ischemia). The rate constant of the slower component of clearance did not change appreciably. Thus, impairment of oxidative metabolism was reflected by slower clearance of radioactivity from myocardium during the rapid clearance phase, regardless of whether perfusion and washout of labeled metabolites were reduced concomitantly.

Definitive interpretation of residence detection clearance curves requires knowledge of the subcellular fate of the ^{11}C label. For this purpose the coronary effluent was assayed after intracoronary injection of 1-^{11}C-palmitate under control conditions and after induction of ischemia or hypoxia.[15] During the initial 10 minutes after administration of 1-^{11}C-palmitate, corresponding to the interval dominated by the rapid clearance component, 60% of initially extracted radioactivity was recovered in the coronary effluent. More than 90% of the radioactivity was in the form of [11]CO_2 (Figure 6-3). Consistent with the slower component of clearance detected externally, the overall release of radioactivity was reduced with ischemia or hypoxia. Thus, only 33% of extracted 1-^{11}C-palmitate radioactivity appeared in the coronary effluent. However, efflux of nonmetabolized 1-^{11}C-palmitate increased significantly with ischemia and hypoxia, constituting approximately 50% of label effluxing from myocardium. These results indicate that the rapid clearance under physiologic conditions reflects, primarily, release of [11]CO_2 from 1-^{11}C-palmitate that is oxidized. The slowed clearance of this rapid phase apparent with ischemia and hypoxia reflects reduced oxidative metabolism. However, the relationship between the slope of the myocardial clearance curve and the rate of oxidation of palmitate is not direct because of variable contributions of backdiffusion of nonmetabolized tracer to clearance of radioactivity.

To further elucidate the 2 components of clearance, serial myocardial biopsy samples were obtained, and the distribution of the label in subcellular lipid pools was determined[22] (see Chapter 3, Figure 3-6). Under baseline conditions, 49% of radioactivity was in the aqueous fraction within 3 minutes after injection, suggesting that rapid oxidation of a large fraction of 1-[11]C- palmitate to small, soluble products had occurred. The slower component of 1-^{11}C clearance reflected primarily 1-^{11}C-palmitate incorporated into triglycerides and phospholipids. When 1-^{11}C-palmitate was injected while myocardium was ischemic, only 13% of initially extracted activity was recovered in the aqueous phase. Thus, slower clearance of radioactivity from initially extracted 1-^{11}C-palmitate was indicative of a shift from rapid oxidation of tracer to incorporation into tissue lipids.

Despite its importance in characterization of myocardial metabolism, 1-

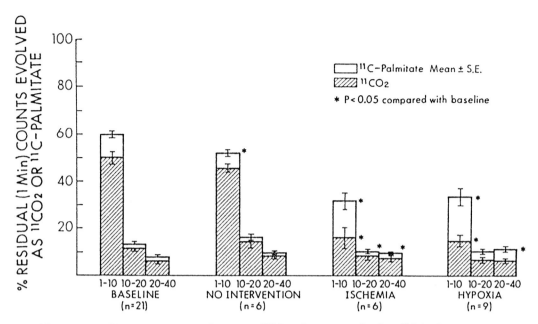

Figure 6-3. *Mean percentage of extracted ^{11}C-palmitate evolved as $^{11}CO_2$ from 1 to 40 minutes after intracoronary administration. The histogram shows that the mean percentage of extracted 1-^{11}C-palmitate evolved as $^{11}CO_2$ (cross-hatched bars) and as unaltered, backdiffusible 1-^{11}C-palmitate (open bars) in the intervals from 1–10, 10–20, and 20–40 minutes in open-chest dogs studied under baseline conditions, those with no intervention, and those subjected to low-flow ischemia or normal-flow hypoxia. The results demonstrate that under physiologic conditions, radioactivity clears the myocardium predominantly as labeled CO_2. However, under conditions of ischemia or hypoxia, a significant fraction of label leaving the myocardium egresses as backdiffused unmetabolized tracer. Accordingly, tomographic estimates of fatty acid metabolism would overestimate metabolic rate under these conditions. (Reproduced from Fox et al.,[15] with permission of the American Heart Association, Inc.)*

^{11}C-palmitate exhibits some unavoidable limitations for noninvasive characterization of metabolism. Although analysis of uptake and clearance of radioactivity after injection of 1-^{11}C-palmitate permits noninvasive recognition of altered, regional fatty acid metabolism, quantitative assessment of metabolic flux is complicated by incorporation of tracer into diverse lipid subfractions;[23] disparities between external monitoring of radioactivity and specific intracellular fluxes of metabolism of extracted 1-^{11}C-palmitate; and changes in specific lipid pool sizes.

Tomographic Assessment of Myocardial Fatty Acid Metabolism with 1-^{11}C-palmitate: Results of Studies in Experimental Animals

After intravenous injection of 1-^{11}C-palmitate in anesthetized, closed-chest dogs, uptake and clearance of myocardial radioactivity quantified by PET was found to be homogenous throughout the left ventricular myocardium.[9] Sequential PET scans delineated a characteristic biexponential pattern of clearance.[9] The clearance rate constant for the rapid component (most evident between 5 and 15 minutes after administration of tracer) averaged 0.060 ± 0.005 (SEM) min,[-1] corresponding to a half-time of 11.6 minutes. In normal myocardium of fasted dogs, $46 \pm 18\%$ of extracted 1-^{11}C-palmitate was incorporated into the fast turnover pool. The magnitude of the early clearance component and the overall clearance rate increased with pacing-induced tachycardia, consistent with augmented fatty acid oxidation.[14] Conversely, they decreased after intravenous infusion of glucose because a larger fraction of extracted 1-^{11}C-palmitate was being initially incorporated into lipid pools turning over slowly[12] (Figure 6-4).

Effects of Coronary Stenosis

To determine whether the metabolic consequences of coronary stenosis are reflected by altered myocardial kinetics of 1-^{11}C-palmitate, coronary stenoses of specific extent were induced in dogs 24 to 48 hours before tomography.[9] The initial distribution of 1-^{11}C-palmitate radioactivity was not significantly altered by coronary stenosis. When the reduction of coronary diameter was $< 70\%$, the early, rapid component of 1-^{11}C clearance remained homogenous throughout the left ventricular myocardium. However, when stenosis exceeded 70%, clearance in the myocardium distal to the stenosis was reduced markedly. In other studies,[14] 1-^{11}C-palmitate was injected in dogs subjected to atrial pacing and coronary stenosis severe enough to abolish the hyperemic response. Clearance and initial accumulation of 1-^{11}C-palmitate were reduced in the compromised myocardium. Thus, regions distal to critical coronary stenosis can be localized tomographically with 1-^{11}C-palmitate.

Myocardial Infarction

With complete coronary occlusion, regional uptake of 1-^{11}C-palmitate is reduced. To determine whether PET permits determination of infarct size, we injected 1-^{11}C-palmitate intravenously in dogs 48 hours after coronary occlusion,[11] an interval selected to ensure completion of infarction in the jeopardized zones.[24] Infarct size was estimated tomographically by summation of the number of volume elements (voxels) that contained less than 50% of maximal myocardial radioactivity. A close correlation was found between infarct size estimated tomographically and histochemically ($r = 0.97$) and between tomographic estimates and those based on direct measurement of creatine kinase depletion ($r = 0.93$) (Figure 6-5). Furthermore, in transmural biopsy samples from regions of infarction, depression of accumulation of concomitantly administered ^{14}C-palmitate correlated closely with the extent of depletion of myocardial creatine kinase ($r = 0.92$). Unfortunately, however, when myocardial infarction is *evolving*, tomographic static imaging with 1-^{11}C-palmitate cannot differentiate reversibly from irreversibly injured tissue.[25]

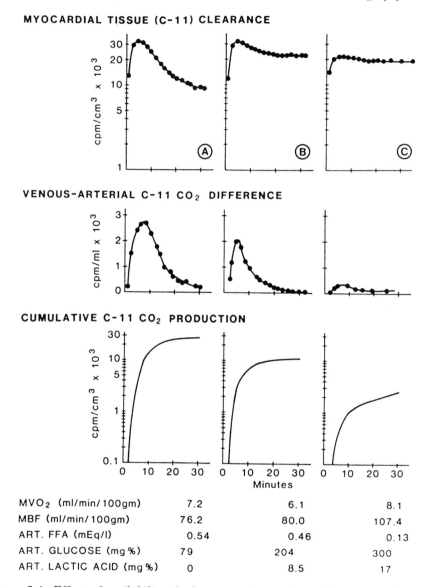

Figure 6-4. *Effects of availability of substrate on the uptake and clearance of ^{11}C-radioactivity by myocardium. Studies A and B were obtained in the same dog under control conditions and after administration of glucose and insulin. Study C was performed in another dog given glucose and insulin. The corresponding myocardial blood flow, oxygen consumption, and arterial substrate concentrations in plasma are shown at the bottom. Myocardial oxygen consumption was comparable in all 3 studies even though arterial free fatty acid concentrations were progressively lower from A to C. Conversely, glucose and lactate increased. The magnitude and slope of the rapid phase were associated with a decreased [11]CO$_2$ efflux as well as lower amounts of total [11]CO$_2$ produced (as shown by the cumulative [11]CO$_2$ production curves in the lower panel). Thus, the kinetics of ^{11}C-palmitate in the heart are markedly influenced by the pattern of substrate use. (Reproduced with permission from Schelbert et al.[12])*

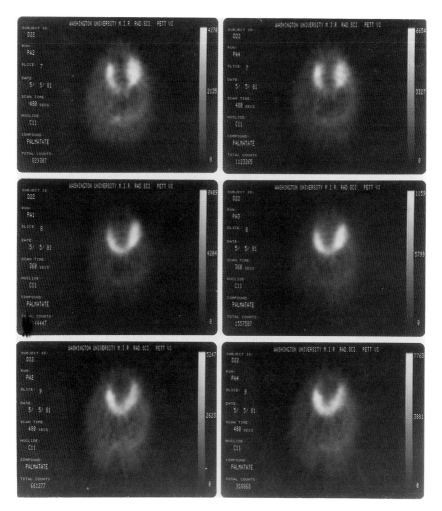

Figure 6-6B. *Three contiguous midventricular transverse tomograms obtained before (left) and after (right) thrombolysis. In the dog studied, the initial tomogram was obtained 6 hours after occlusion. Thrombolysis was then induced with intracoronary streptokinase. The second scan was obtained 1½ hours after the initial tomogram. In contrast to the case in dogs with reperfusion early after occlusion, in dogs with reperfusion later, no significant alteration in either the distribution or concentration of 1-^{11}C-palmitate in the jeopardized regions was evident, indicating lack of salvage when thrombolysis was delayed. (Reproduced with permission from Bergmann et al.[26].)*

hearts subjected to 60 minutes of no-flow ischemia leading to irreversible injury, extraction and oxidation of ^{14}C-palmitate recovers initially to nearly normal values early after reperfusion.[29] Furthermore, in irreversibly injured myocardium of canine hearts, accumulation of labeled heptadecanoic acid 1 hour after reperfusion is substantial.[30] Thus, the amount of viable myocardium may be overestimated by PET with 1-^{11}C-palmitate early after reperfusion.[25] This

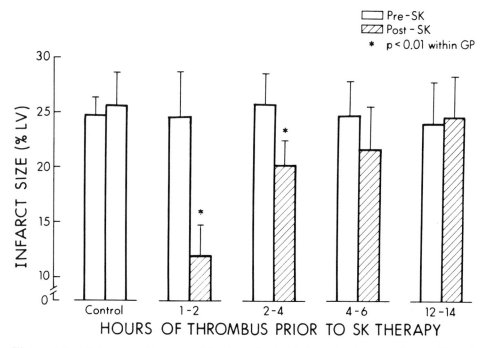

Figure 6-7. *Histogram of tomographically estimated infarct size in intact dogs subjected to persistent occlusion (control) or to ischemia of selected duration before intracoronary streptokinase. Infarct size refers to the extent of compromised zones based on the number of pixels containing less than 50% of peak left ventricular myocardial activity divided by the total number of pixels in the left ventricular wall. Values indicate the mean ± standard error. Abbreviations: SK–streptokinase. The results are consistent with strikingly beneficial effects of early reperfusion on metabolic salvage. (Reproduced with permission from Bergmann et al.[26])*

may explain the greater amount of 1-^{11}C-palmitate uptake in canine myocardium after 1 hour as compared with 4 weeks after reperfusion.

The second consideration concerns myocardial release of labeled CO_2. When a bolus of [14]C- or ^{11}C-labeled palmitate is administered via the coronary arteries during the first 30 minutes after reperfusion in isolated hearts[31] or in vivo,[32] release of labeled CO_2 is diminished. However, under steady-state conditions with continuous infusion of ^{14}C-palmitate and sequential determinations of release of [14]CO_2 from perfused hearts,[31,33] oxidation of exogenous palmitate is seen to be reduced only briefly, with complete recovery within 15 to 30 minutes. A possible explanation for these apparently discordant observations is that after reperfusion, a larger fraction of extracted fatty acids is initially incorporated into triglycerides before oxidation.

Despite these limitations, PET with 1-^{11}C-palmitate has been extremely helpful for evaluation of interventions designed to limit infarct size. It helped to demonstrate the recovery of nutritive blood flow and myocardial metabolism after thrombolysis with tissue-type plasminogen activator,[34] and to document enhancement of myocardial salvage with calcium-channel blockers after reperfusion.[35]

Metabolic Imaging with ^{11}C-palmitate in Patients

For applications in clinical research, usually 10 to 20 mCi of 1-^{11}C-palmitate bound to albumin is injected intravenously. Within 4 to 8 minutes, the left ventricular myocardium can be delineated.[36] Regional time-activity curves demonstrate biexponential clearance, with the rapid component prominent during the first 10 to 20 minutes.[37,38]

Analogous to observations in experimental animals, the rate of rapid clearance of 1-^{11}C-palmitate from normal myocardium in human subjects is dependent on concentrations of substrates in plasma and on cardiac work. The average clearance half-time in normal human hearts is prolonged from 19.1 ± 7.2 (SD) to 27.8 ± 5.7 minutes ($p < 0.01$) after ingestion of 50 g of glucose,[39] which results in decreased concentrations of fatty acids in plasma secondary to diminished lipolysis. It increases significantly ($t_{1/2}$ declining from 22.2 ± 5.2 [SD] to 13.4 ± 2.5 minutes [$p < 0.01$]) with pacing.[38] Conversely, it is prolonged ($t_{1/2}$ increasing from 22.5 ± 2.6 [SEM] to 75.6 ± 31.1 minutes) by dynamic bicycle exercise, probably reflecting the marked increases in concentrations of lactate in arterial blood seen with dynamic exercise and the consequent reduction of fatty acid oxidation.[37]

Coronary Artery Disease

Myocardial Infarction

PET with 1-^{11}C-palmitate has been used to detect abnormal myocardial metabolism in patients with myocardial infarction (Figure 6-8). Tomographic examinations performed between 2 and 10 days after the onset of symptoms in 21 patients with electrocardiographically and enzymatically documented transmural myocardial infarction[36] delineated a defect in uptake of tracer corresponding to the electrocardiographic locus of infarction in each case. Among 24 other patients with electrocardiographically identified nontransmural infarction, a defect was noted in 23 (96%).[40] Among 13 patients with documented acute, initial transmural myocardial infarctions, the extent of necrosis estimated tomographically correlated closely with infarct size estimated from serial changes in plasma MB-creatine kinase activity[36] (Figure 6-5). Repeat tomographic estimates of infarct size 1 month later correlated with initial estimates.

Sequential tomography with 1-^{11}C-palmitate has been used for clinical assessment of the efficacy of therapeutic interventions designed to reduce infarct size.[41,42] Thus, among 21 patients with acute myocardial infarction studied immediately after admission and again after 1 week, apparent infarct size was reduced by an average of 16% after treatment with oral nifedipine but did not change in controls.[41] In another example, 19 patients with acute myocardial infarction were studied immediately before and 48 to 78 hours after throm-

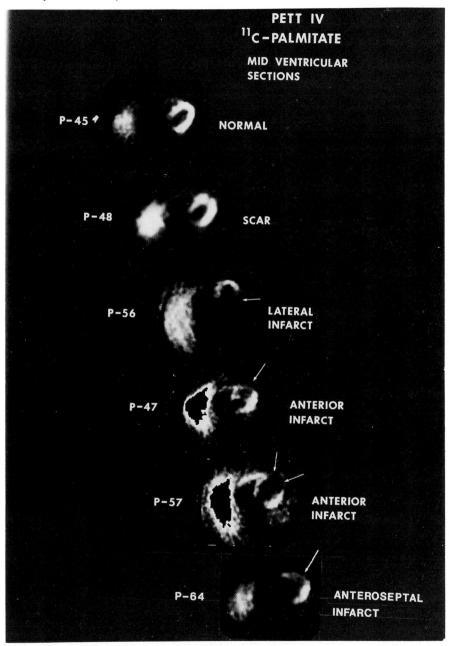

Figure 6-8. *PET reconstructions obtained at the midventricular level after administration of 1-^{11}C-palmitate in a normal subject and in patients with myocardial infarctions at specific loci (determined by analysis of the images and of the electrocardiograms in each case). The left ventricular free wall is to the right, anterior is to the top, and the septum is to the left. The liver, which accumulates fatty acids, is seen to the extreme left. The mitral valve plane is to the bottom. (Reproduced from Ter-Pogossian et al.,[36] with permission of the American Heart Association, Inc.)*

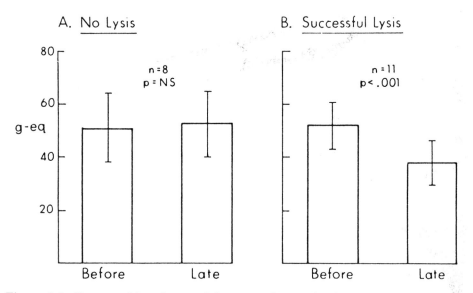

Figure 6-9. *Tomographic estimates of the extent of jeopardized myocardium before and after infusion of streptokinase or tissue-type plasminogen activator (t-PA) in 19 patients with evolving myocardial infarction. (A) represents results from 8 patients in whom thrombolysis was not successful, and (B) represents data from 11 patients with reperfusion. With successful thrombolysis, significant improvement was evident for the group as a whole (see Color Figure 17). (Reproduced from Sobel et al.,* [42] *with permission of the American Heart Association, Inc.)*

bolysis with either intracoronary streptokinase or intravenous tissue-type plasminogen activator.[42] (see Color Figure 17). Recanalization was documented angiographically in 11 patients in whom the extent of the 1-^{11}C-palmitate uptake defect decreased by 29%; no change occurred in 8 patients with persistent occlusion (Figure 6-9).

Ischemia without infarction

To determine whether alterations of fatty acid metabolism induced by reversible ischemia could be detected, 10 patients with angiographically documented coronary stenosis of greater than 70% were studied.[38] Both uptake and clearance of ^{11}C-radioactivity were homogenous at rest in 8 subjects without a history of myocardial infarction. After acceleration of heart rate by pacing from 65 ± 12 (SD) to 102 ± 15 beats/min, ischemia was evident in 70%, as judged from wall motion abnormalities detected echocardiographically. The rapidity of initial ^{11}C-clearance increased in both normal and ischemic zones. However, the increase was less pronounced in regions supplied by the stenotic vessel[38] (Figure 6-10). Conversely, the clearance half-time was prolonged in patients and controls subjected to dynamic bicycle exercise,[37] consistent with inhibition of fatty acid oxidation as a result of the increased arterial plasma concentration of lactate.

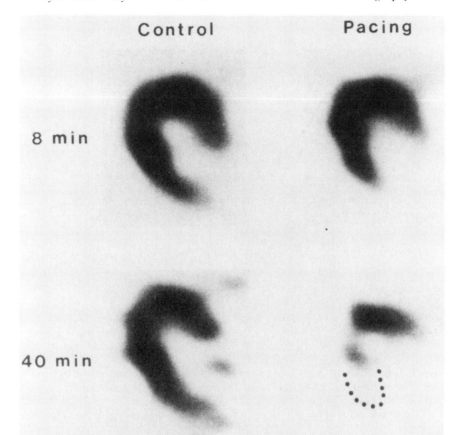

Figure 6-10A. *Midventricular reconstructions after administration of 1-^{11}C-palmitate under control conditions (left) and with atrial pacing (right) in a patient with a 90% stenosis of the left anterior descending coronary artery. Images are oriented with the anterior wall at the upper left, the septum at the upper right, and the lateral wall at the lower left. The 8-minute images (top) reflect initial uptake of tracer, and the 40-minute images (bottom) reflect clearance of radioactivity from the myocardium. Uptake is homogenous both at rest and with pacing. Although clearance of radioactivity was homogeneous at rest, it became heterogeneous with pacing. The delayed clearance (greater myocardial retention) in the anteroseptal myocardium reflected impairment of beta-oxidation with pacing in myocardium supplied by the stenotic coronary artery.*

Cardiomyopathy

Dilated Cardiomyopathy

Fatty acid oxidation is reduced in isolated hearts and homogenates from hearts of cardiomyopathic hamsters.[43,44] Impaired oxidation may contribute to the physiologic dysfunction.[45,46]

When PET with 1-^{11}C-palmitate was performed in 17 patients with dilated cardiomyopathy,[47] marked spatial heterogeneity of initial myocardial 1-^{11}C-palmitate uptake was evident. Multiple small regions with reduced radioactivity were seen, in contrast to extensive, homogeneous defects in patients with

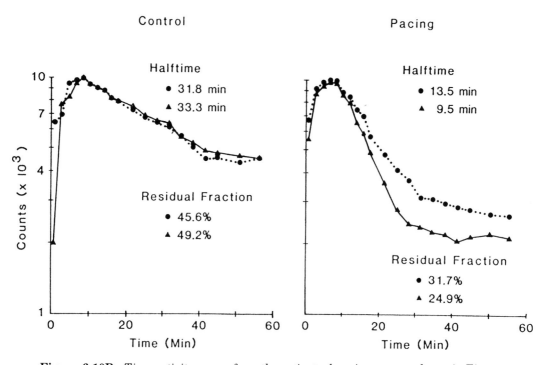

Figure 6-10B. *Time-activity curves from the patient whose images are shown in Figure 6-10A. Normal myocardium is represented by triangles and the anteroseptal myocardium (myocardium at risk) by the closed circles. Under control circumstances, the clearance half-times and residual fractions were similar. In contrast, with pacing, the clearance half-time was protracted in the jeopardized region compared with normal myocardium. Note, however, that during pacing overall clearance, reflective of myocardial metabolism of fatty acids, was increased in both regions. (Reproduced from Grover-McKay et al.,[38] with permission of the American Heart Association, Inc.)*

ischemic cardiomyopathy and comparable depression of ejection fraction[48] (Figure 6-11).

With fasting, clearance of myocardial 1-^{11}C-palmitate radioactivity is similar in control subjects and patients with dilated cardiomyopathy. However, the response of myocardial clearance of 1-^{11}C-palmitate to oral administration of glucose differs in the 2 groups. The rate of the rapid clearance component decreases in controls. However, it remains the same or increases in patients.[39] Presently, the factors responsible for the differences and pathophysiologic significance of altered kinetics of 1-^{11}C-palmitate clearance from myocardium in patients with dilated cardiomyopathy are not clear. Apparent variations in regional count density could be related to heterogeneity of wall motion and wall thickness rather than actual variation in uptake. However, the abnormal response of 1-^{11}C-clearance to glucose points toward a metabolic explanation:[39] the variations may reflect effects on regional tracer kinetics attributable to either patchy fibrosis or altered fatty acid metabolism in still viable but metabolically compromised myocytes.

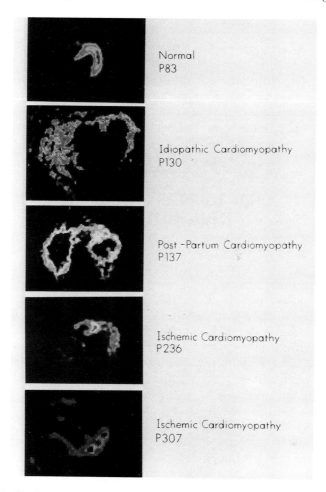

Figure 6-11. *Midventricular tomograms obtained from patients with cardiomyopathy of diverse causes after administration of 1-*[11]*C-palmitate. Patients with nonischemic cardiomyopathy exhibit spatial heterogeneity of accumulation of this tracer. Image orientation is similar to Figure 6-8. (Reproduced with permission from Bergmann et al.)*[55]

Cardiomyopathy Secondary to Inherited Metabolic Disease

Recently, hearts of patients with long-chain acyl-CoA dehydrogenase deficiency have been characterized by PET. Long-chain acyl-CoA dehydrogenase catalyzes the initial step in myocardial fatty acid oxidation. Genetic deficiency of the enzyme is associated with cardiomyopathy with varying manifestations. The ratio of myocardial clearance of ^{11}C-palmitate to that of ^{11}C-acetate (reflecting the relative oxidation rates of long- compared with short-chain fatty acids) is markedly decreased in patients with this genetic abnormality and the extent of depression of the ratio correlates with the clinical severity of the cardiomyopathy.[49]

Hypertrophic Cardiomyopathy

Alterations of fatty acid metabolism, including a reduction of myocardial carnitine content,[43] have been observed in hearts of animals with hereditary cardiac hypertrophy. In patients with echocardiographic criteria of hypertrophic cardiomyopathy, uptake of 1-^{11}C-palmitate (but not its clearance) is reduced by an average of 29% in the septum relative to uptake in the lateral wall.[50] Because the reduction corresponds spatially and quantitatively to the reduction of accumulation of [13]NH$_3$ and ^{18}F-glucose delineated tomographically, fibrosis may be responsible.

Other Fatty Acids Labeled with Positron-emitting Radionuclides

Fatty acid tracers have been modified to facilitate trapping in the tissue (for use in defining parameters needed in mathematical modeling) and by labeling with radionuclides other than [11]C. Livini et al.[51] synthetized 1- ^{11}C-beta-methyl-heptadecanoic acid (1-^{11}C-BMHA) by introducing a methyl group at the 3 position to truncate β-oxidation. Its single-pass extraction fraction in canine hearts averaged 19.8 ± 9.8% (SD) after intracoronary injection. Egress from myocardium was slower than that of 1-^{11}C-palmitate, but trapping was not complete. Within 20 minutes, 17% of the label egressed as [11]CO$_2$, and 25% backdiffused.[52] Dimethylation in the beta position was not helpful, as evidenced by the low uptake of 1-^{11}C-3,3-dimethyl-heptadecanoic acid.[53]

To avoid the need for an on-site cyclotron, fatty acids have been labeled with fluorine-18 (^{18}F). Metabolism of such compounds varies as a function of the length of the carbon chain.[54] When (^{18}F)-17-fluoro-heptadecanoic acid is used, free fluoride ([18]F-) is the predominant metabolite in myocardium. (^{18}F)-16-fluoro-hexadecanoic acid gives rise to a different water-soluble labeled metabolite, presumably (^{18}F)-fluorocitric acid.

Conclusions

PET with 1-^{11}C-palmitate has permitted identification, localization, and assessment of the extent of regional abnormalities of fatty acid metabolism indicative of ischemia, infarction, and myopathic disease. Delayed clearance in a region supplied by a stenotic vessel is indicative of reduced fatty acid oxidation. However, interpretation may be clouded by multiple potential metabolic fates of the ^{11}C label.

Under standardized conditions in hearts of experimental animals, the rate of clearance of 1-^{11}C-palmitate activity correlates with myocardial oxygen consumption. However, measurement of total oxidative metabolic flux in hearts of patients is not possible with the use of 1-^{11}C-palmitate alone because of contributions to overall oxidative metabolism from other substrates. Nevertheless, PET with 1-^{11}C-palmitate does permit noninvasive characterization of the influence on myocardial metabolism of work load, nutritional state, and age.

PET with ^{11}C-labeled fatty acids has made a substantial contribution in clinical research. It provided a foundation for the use of diverse tracers of metabolism and demonstrated the feasibility of quantitative assessment of cardiac metabolism noninvasively. Future applications in clinical decision making may be facilitated by use of tracers of fatty acid metabolism with a relatively long physical half-life and the use of agents that can be trapped in myocardium, thereby permitting tomographic delineation of regions initially at risk despite pharmacologic or mechanical coronary revascularization soon after administration of the tracer.

References

1. Evans JR, Gunton RW, Baker RG, Beanlands DS, Spears JC. Use of radioiodinated fatty acid for photoscans of the heart. Circ Res 1965; 16:1–10.
2. Poe ND, Robinson GD, MacDonald NS. Myocardial extraction of labeled long-chain fatty acid analogs. Proc Soc Exp Biol Med 1975; 148:215–218.
3. Welch MJ, Dence CS, Marshall DR, Kilbourn MR. Remote system for production of carbon-11 labeled palmitic acid. J Labelled Comp Radiopharm 1983; 20:1087–1095.
4. Carlsten A, Hallgren B, Jagenburg R, Svanborg A, Werko L. Myocardial arteriovenous differences of individual free fatty acids in healthy human individuals. Metabolism 1963; 12:1063–1071.
5. Vasdev SC, Kako KJ. Incorporation of fatty acids into rat heart lipids. In vivo and in vitro study. J Mol Cell Cardiol 1977; 9:617–631.
6. Oram JF, Bennetch SL, Neely JR. Regulation of fatty acid utilization in isolated perfused rat hearts. J Biol Chem 1973; 248:5299–5309.
7. Evans JR, Opie LH, Shipp JC. Metabolism of palmitic acid in perfused rat heart. Am J Physiol 1963; 205:766–770.
8. Veerkamp JH, Moerkerk HTB. Peroxisomal fatty acid oxidation in rat and human tissues. Effect of nutritional state, clofibrate treatment and postnatal development in the rat. Biochim Biophys Acta 1986; 875:301–310.
9. Lerch RA, Ambos HD, Bergmann SR, Welch MJ, Ter-Pogossian MM, Sobel BE. Localization of viable, ischemic myocardium by positron-emission tomography with ^{11}C-palmitate. Circulation 1981; 64:689–699.
10. Weiss ES, Hoffman EJ, Phelps ME, Welch MJ, Henry PD, Ter-Pogossian MM, Sobel BE. External detection and visualization of myocardial ischemia with ^{11}C-substrates in vivo and in vitro. Circ Res 1976; 39:24–32.
11. Weiss ES, Ahmed SA, Welch MJ, Williamson JR, Ter-Pogossian MM, Sobel BE. Quantification of infarction in cross sections of canine myocardium in vivo with positron emission transaxial tomography and ^{11}C-palmitate. Circulation 1977; 55:66–73.
12. Schelbert HR, Henze E, Schön HR, Keen R, Hansen H, Selin C, Huang SC, Barrio JR, Phelps ME. C-11 palmitate for the noninvasive evaluation of regional myocardial fatty acid metabolism with positron computed tomography. III. In vivo demonstration of the effects of substrate availability on myocardial metabolism. Am Heart J 1983; 105:492–504.
13. Schwaiger M, Fishbein MC, Block M, Wijns W, Selin C, Phelps ME, Schelbert HR. Metabolic and ultrastructural abnormalities during ischemia in canine myocardium: Noninvasive assessment by positron emission tomography. J Mol Cell Cardiol 1987; 19:259–269.
14. Schelbert HR, Henze E, Keen R, Schön HR, Hansen H, Selin C, Huang SC, Barrio JR, Phelps ME. C-11 palmitate for the noninvasive evaluation of regional myocardial fatty acid metabolism with positron-computed tomography. IV. In vivo evaluation of acute demand-induced ischemia in dogs. Am Heart J 1983; 106:736–750.

15. Fox KAA, Abendschein DR, Ambos HD, Sobel BE, Bergmann SR. Efflux of metabolized and nonmetabolized fatty acid from canine myocardium. Implications for quantifying myocardial metabolism tomographically. Circ Res 1985; 57:232–243.

16. Schön HR, Schelbert HR, Robinson G, Najafi A, Huang SC, Hansen H, Barrio J, Kuhl DE, Phelps ME. C-11 labeled palmitic acid for the noninvasive evaluation of regional myocardial fatty acid metabolism with positron-computed tomography. I. Kinetics of C-11 palmitic acid in normal myocardium. Am Heart J 1981; 103:532-547.

17. Wyns W, Schwaiger M, Huang S-C, Buxton DB, Hansen H, Selin C, Keen R, Phelps ME, Schelbert HR. Effects of inhibition of fatty acid oxidation on myocardial kinetics of ^{11}C-labeled palmitate. Circ Res 1989; 65:1787–1797.

18. Denton RM, Randle PJ. Measurement of flow of carbon atoms from glucose and glycogen glucose to glyceride glycerol and glycerol in rat heart and epididymal adipose tissue. Biochem J 1967; 104:423–434.

19. Fox KAA, Nomura H, Sobel BE, Bergmann SR. Consistent substrate utilization despite reduced flow in hearts with maintained work. Am J Physiol 1983; 244:H799-H806.

20. Lerch RA, Bergmann SR, Ambos HD, Welch MJ, Ter-Pogossian MM, Sobel BE. Effect of flow-independent reduction of metabolism on regional myocardial clearance of ^{11}C-palmitate. Circulation 1982; 65:731–738.

21. Lerch RA, Ambos HD, Bergmann SR, Sobel BE, Ter-Pogossian MM. Kinetics of positron emitters in vivo characterized with a beta probe. Am J Physiol 1982; 242:H62-H67.

22. Rosamond TL, Abendschein DR, Sobel BE, Bergmann SR, Fox KAA. The metabolic fate of radiolabeled palmitate in ischemic canine myocardium: Implications for positron emission tomography. J Nucl Med 1987; 28:1322–1329.

23. Schelbert HR, Phelps ME. Positron computed tomography for the in vivo assessment of regional myocardial function. J Mol Cell Cardiol 1984; 16:683–693.

24. Jennings RB, Reimer KA. Factors involved in salvaging ischemic myocardium: Effect of reperfusion of arterial blood. Circulation 1983; 68:(Suppl I):I-25-I-36.

25. Knabb RM, Bergmann SR, Fox KAA, Sobel BE. The temporal pattern of recovery of myocardial perfusion and metabolism delineated by positron emission tomography after coronary thrombolysis. J Nucl Med 1987; 28:1563–1570.

26. Bergmann SR, Lerch RA, Fox KAA, Ludbrook PA, Welch MJ, Ter-Pogossian MM, Sobel BE. Temporal dependence of beneficial effects of coronary thrombolysis characterized by positron tomography. Am J Med 1982; 73:573–581.

27. Schwaiger M, Schelbert HR, Ellison D, Hansen H, Yeatman L, Vinten-Johansen J, Selin C, Barrio J, Phelps ME. Sustained regional abnormalities in cardiac metabolism after transient ischemia in the chronic dog model. J Am Coll Cardiol 1985; 6:336–347.

28. Schwaiger M, Schelbert HR, Keen R, Vinten-Johansen J, Hansen H, Selin C, Barrio J, Huang SC, Phelps ME. Retention and clearance of ^{11}C-palmitic acid in ischemic and reperfused canine myocardium. J Am Coll Cardiol 1985; 6:311–320.

29. Görge G, Chatelain P, Schaper J, Lerch R. Effect of increasing degrees of ischemic injury on myocardial oxidative metabolism early after reperfusion in isolated rat hearts. Circ Res 1991; 68:1681–1692.

30. Chappuis F, Meier B, Belenger J, Bläuenstein P, Lerch R. Early assessment of tissue viability with radioiodinated heptadecanoic acid in reperfused canine myocardium. Comparison with thallium-201. Am Heart J 1990; 119:833–841.

31. Chatelain P, Lüthy P, Papageorgiou I, Lerch R. Free fatty acid metabolism in "stunned" myocardium. Circulation 1986; 74(Suppl. II):II-67 (abstract).

32. Fox KAA, Abendschein DR, Sobel BE. Persistent impairment of myocardial metabolism and clearance rate of labeled fatty acid after brief ischemia: Implications for positron emission tomography (PET). J Am Coll Cardiol 1985; 5:451 (abstract).

33. Liedtke AJ, Demaison L, Eggleston AM, Cohen LM, Nellis SH. Changes in substrate metabolism and effects of excess fatty acids in reperfused myocardium. Circ Res 1988; 62:535–542.

34. Bergmann SR, Fox KAA, Ter-Pogossian MM, Sobel BE, Collen D. Clot-selective coronary thrombolysis with tissue-type plasminogen activator. Science 1983; 220:1181–1183.
35. Knabb RM, Rosamond TL, Fox KAA, Sobel BE, Bergmann SR. Enhancement of salvage of reperfused ischemic myocardium by diltiazem. J Am Coll Cardiol 1986; 8:861–871.
36. Ter-Pogossian MM, Klein MS, Markham J, Roberts R, Sobel BE. Regional assessment of myocardial metabolic integrity in vivo by positron-emission tomography with ^{11}C-labeled palmitate. Circulation 1980; 61:242–255.
37. Geltman EM, Kaiserauer S, Walsh MN, Ehsani AA. Effect of maximal and submaximal exercise on myocardial ^{11}C-palmitate clearance assessed with positron emission tomography. J Am Coll Cardiol 1988; 11:12A (abstract).
38. Grover-McKay M, Schelbert HR, Schwaiger M, Sochor H, Guzy PM, Krivokapich J, Child JS, Phelps ME. Identification of impaired metabolic reserve by atrial pacing in patients with significant coronary artery stenosis. Circulation 1986; 74:281–292.
39. Schelbert HR, Henze E, Sochor H, Grossman RG, Huang S-C, Barrio JR, Schwaiger M, Phelps ME. Effects of substrate availability on myocardial C-11 palmitate kinetics by positron emission tomography in normal subjects and patients with ventricular dysfunction. Am Heart J 1986; 111:1055–1064.
40. Geltman EM, Biello D, Welch MJ, Ter-Pogossian MM, Roberts R, Sobel BE. Characterization of nontransmural myocardial infarction by positron-emission tomography. Circulation 1982; 65:747–755.
41. Jaffe AS, Biello DR, Sobel BE, Geltman EM. Enhancement of metabolism of jeopardized myocardium by nifedipine. Int J Cardiol 1987; 15:77–89.
42. Sobel BE, Geltman EM, Tiefenbrunn AJ, Jaffe AS, Spadaro JJ, Ter-Pogossian MM, Collen D, Ludbrook PA. Improvement of regional myocardial metabolism after coronary thrombolysis induced with tissue-type plasminogen activator or streptokinase. Circulation 1984; 69:983–990.
43. Whitmer JT. Energy metabolism and mechanical function in perfused hearts of syrian hamsters with dilated or hypertrophic cardiomyopathy. J Mol Cell Cardiol 1986; 18:307–317.
44. Kako, Thornton MJ, Heggveit HA. Depressed fatty acid and acetate oxidation and other metabolic defects in homogenates from hearts of hamsters with hereditary cardiomyopathy. Circ Res 1974; 34:570–580.
45. Wittels B, Spann JF. Defective lipid metabolism in the failing heart. J Clin Invest 1968; 47:1787–1794.
46. Chapoy PR, Angelini C, Brown WJ, Stiff JE, Shug AL, Cederbaum SD. Systemic carnitine deficiency—A treatable inherited lipid storage disease presenting as Reye's syndrome. New Engl J Med 1980; 303:1389–1394.
47. Geltman EM, Smith JL, Beecher D, Ludbrook PA, Ter-Pogossian MM, Sobel BE. Altered regional myocardial metabolism in congestive cardiomyopathy detected by positron tomography. Am J Med 1983; 74:773–785.
48. Eisenberg JD, Sobel BE, Geltman EM. Differentiation of ischemic from nonischemic cardiomyopathy with positron emission tomography. Am J Cardiol 1987; 59:1410–1414.
49. Kelly DP, Hartman JJ, Herrero P, Sobel BE, Bergmann SR: Detection of the specific impairment of cardiac fatty acid oxidation in patients with long chain acyl-CoA dehydrogenase deficiency by positron emission tomography (PET). Circulation 1991; 84:Supp.II:630 (abstract).
50. Grover-McKay M, Schwaiger M, Krivokapich J, Perloff JK, Phelps ME, Schelbert HR. Regional myocardial blood flow and metabolism at rest in mildly symptomatic patients with hypertrophic cardiomyopathy. J Am Coll Cardiol 1989; 13:317–324 1989.
51. Livini E, Elmaleh DR, Levy S, Brownell GL, Strauss WH. Beta-methyl(1-^{11}C)heptadecanoic acid: A new myocardial metabolic tracer for positron emission tomography. J Nucl Med 1982; 23:169–175.

52. Abendschein DR, Fox KAA, Ambos HD, Sobel BE, Bergmann SR. Metabolism of beta-methyl[1-^{11}C]heptadecanoic acid in canine myocardium. Intl J Radiat Appl Instrum, Nucl Med Biol 1987; 14:579–585.
53. Jones GS, Livini E, Strauss W, Hanson RN, Elmaleh DR. Synthesis and biological evaluation of 1-(^{11}C)-3,3–dimethylheptadecanoic acid. 1988; J Nucl Med 29:68–72.
54. Knust EJ, Kupfernagel C, Stöcklin G. Long-chain F-18 fatty acids for the study of regional metabolism in heart and liver; odd-even effects of metabolism in mice. J Nucl Med 1979; 20:1170–1175.
55. Bergmann SR, Fox KAA, Geltman EM, Sobel BE. Positron emission tomography of the heart. Prog Cardiovasc Dis 1985; 28:165–194.

Chapter 7

Assessment of Myocardial Viability with Tracers of Blood Flow and Metabolism of Glucose

Gerold Porenta, M.D., Ph.D., Johannes Czernin, M.D., and Heinrich R. Schelbert, M.D., Ph.D.

Modern therapy of coronary artery disease increasingly uses interventional strategies aimed at restoring adequate blood flow to ischemic myocardial segments. Thrombolytic agents, percutaneous transluminal coronary angioplasty (PTCA), and coronary artery bypass surgery have significantly reduced the mortality of patients in the settings of acute myocardial infarction[1,2] and chronic coronary artery disease.[3] However, the selection of individual patients for such interventional revascularization and the delineation of the risk/benefit ratio requires a careful assessment of coronary anatomy, cardiac function and myocardial perfusion, and the presence of ischemically compromised but viable myocardium.

Revascularization procedures attempt to salvage ischemically injured dysfunctional myocardium that is still metabolically active. Frequently, these myocardial regions regain contractile function after restoration of adequate perfusion. In contrast, dysfunctional myocardial regions consisting mostly of scar tissue without signs of metabolic activity are usually found to have suffered irreversible damage so that contractile function in these regions will not improve despite revascularization. Thus, definition of metabolic activity in dysfunctional myocardium identifies tissue as potentially salvageable, thereby providing information pertinent to the risk/benefit ratio of revascularization procedures.

Coronary angiography, radionuclide perfusion imaging, radionuclide ven-

This work was supported in part by the Director of the Office of Energy Research, Office of Health and Environmental Research, Washington, D.C., by Grants HL 29845 and HL 33177, from the National Institutes of Health, Bethesda, Maryland, and by an Investigative Group Award by the Greater Los Angeles Affiliate of the American Heart Association, Los Angeles, California.

From *Positron Emission Tomography of the Heart* edited by Steven R. Bergmann, MD, PhD and Burton E. Sobel, MD © 1992, Futura Publishing Inc., Mount Kisco, NY.

Topol et al. may be attributable to a transient unspecific adrenergic response of myocardium during the perioperative period.

Thus, hibernating myocardium is characterized by hypoperfusion with impairment of contractile function that is potentially reversible. However, the actual time course of events leading to development of hibernating myocardium and to functional recovery after reperfusion has not been systemically investigated and may not be uniform. Furthermore, cellular and molecular mechanisms responsible for this phenomenon remain to be elucidated.

Stunned Myocardium

In contrast to hibernating myocardium, the concept of stunned myocardium is supported primarily by laboratory observations in experiments focusing on the sequence of myocardial reactions after complete occlusion and reperfusion of a coronary vessel. It has been well documented in these experiments that the recovery of contractile function in postischemic myocardial segments can lag behind the restoration of blood flow.[11-13]

In a study by Heyndrickx et al.,[11] myocardium that had been subjected to a 15 minute period of total ischemia showed postischemic ventricular dysfunction for at least 6 hours. Ellis et al.[12] occluded the left anterior descending arteries of dogs for 2 hours and observed prolonged functional impairment for at least 2 weeks after reperfusion. Bush et al.[13] compared the recovery of left ventricular segmental function after 2 and 4 hour periods of occlusion of the left anterior descending artery. They reported that reperfusion, when instituted 2 hours after occlusion, resulted in improvement in wall motion after 1 month, whereas no improvement in contractile function could be demonstrated after a 4 hour occlusion. These findings demonstrate that the time to recovery of function correlates with the severity of ischemic injury, as defined in these studies by the duration of sustained total ischemia. Moreover, myocardial tissue that has been subjected to total ischemia for at least 4 hours seems to be destined for necrotic damage.

In dogs, Murry et al.[14] demonstrated that preconditioning of the myocardium with multiple brief ischemic periods slows the rate of utilization of adenosine triphosphate (ATP) and delays ultrastructural damage during a subsequent sustained ischemic period. In agreement with these results in canine experiments, Geft et al.[15] reported a beneficial effect of intermittent episodes of reperfusion during coronary occlusion. However, they also noted that multiple brief periods of ischemia had a cumulative effect and caused necrosis even though one single ischemic episode by itself did not. Therefore, in addition to severity, time course and type of ischemic insult also determine the fate of ischemically injured myocardium.

In patients, myocardial stunning probably occurs during variant angina, unstable angina, acute myocardial infarction with early reperfusion, and open heart surgery. It has been shown in patients with acute myocardial infarction and successful thrombolysis that ischemic wall motion abnormalities do not revert immediately after restoration of normal myocardial perfusion, but gradually improve over time.[16,17]

Table 7-1
Myocardial Tissue States as Classified by Perfusion,
Metabolism, and Reversible Dysfunction

Tissue State	Perfusion	Metabolism	Reversible Dysfunction
Normal	normal	maintained	N.A.
Viable			
Stunned	normal	maintained	+
Hibernating	reduced	maintained	+
Necrotic	reduced	impaired	−

Although the cellular mechanisms responsible for myocardial stunning have not been elucidated completely, metabolic changes involving calcium transport in sarcoplasmatic reticulum,[18] nucleotide metabolism,[19] and the generation of free radicals[20] have been implicated.

Table 7-1 summarizes the patterns of perfusion, metabolism, and contractile function differentiating normal and viable (hibernating or stunned) myocardium from necrotic tissue.

Advantages of Metabolic Imaging

Measures of myocardial function and perfusion do not accurately delineate viable from nonviable myocardial tissue since contractile dysfunction and hypoperfusion are common in both necrotic and in hibernating myocardium. In contrast, presence or absence of metabolic activity in ischemically injured myocardium indicates the reversibility, or lack thereof, of impairment of myocardial contractile function. However, attempts have been made to determine tissue viability indirectly from more detailed investigations of contractile function or myocardial perfusion.

Viable myocardium has been reported to respond with an improvement in wall motion to different interventions such as exercise, postextrasystolic potentiation, or drugs with positive inotropic effects.[21–23] Consequently, its detection in a clinical setting has been attempted with established diagnostic techniques that permit the monitoring of wall motion at rest and during different interventions designed to improve regional wall motion.

Myocardial perfusion has been considered to be an indirect indicator of tissue viability. Ischemically injured hypoperfused myocardium can only maintain metabolic activity if myocardial perfusion, even though decreased, is sufficient to deliver a minimal amount of basic nutrients and remove toxic metabolic products such as lactate and hydrogen ions. Accordingly, it has been suggested that the degree of myocardial hypoperfusion is indirect evidence of myocardial viability.[24,25]

Although imaging techniques assessing myocardial contractile function or myocardial perfusion may hold promise in the assessment of viable myocardium, their clinical value in groups of patients in which adequate therapy critically depends on an accurate assessment of viability still remains undetermined.

In contrast, PET imaging of myocardial metabolism has been established as a valuable and important clinical tool that has also been validated in prospective clinical trials.

PET imaging can be used to detect and quantify changes in myocardial oxidative metabolism with tracers of glucose metabolism, β-oxidation, and citric acid cycle activity, although clinical experience in the assessment of myocardial viability has primarily been established with PET imaging of glucose metabolism.

A short summary of glucose metabolism provides the rationale for the use of metabolic imaging of glycolytic activity as an indicator of viable myocardium. The initial sequence of glycolysis occurs in the cytoplasm and leads to the formation of pyruvate. During these enzymatic steps, 2 moles of ATP are generated anaerobically for every mole of glucose metabolized. Pyruvate can then enter the citric acid cycle in the mitochondria where aerobic oxidative phosphorylation is used to produce 36 moles of ATP for every mole of glucose. Compared with fatty acid utilization, glycolysis can generate 17% more ATP for an equal amount of oxygen used.[26] Thus in ischemic tissue with a limited supply of oxygen, glycolysis becomes an especially attractive pathway for the generation of high-energy phosphates.

Compatible with these metabolic findings, ischemic tissue has been shown to exhibit increased glucose utilization compared with normal tissue.[27] Thus, imaging methods capable of measuring myocardial glucose utilization are helpful in delineating ischemically compromised tissue.

Imaging of Glucose Metabolism by PET

18-Fluorodeoxyglucose (FDG), a glucose analog marked with the positron-emitting isotope fluorine-18 (^{18}F), has been used to image myocardial glucose metabolism by PET.[28,29] After intravenous injection, FDG traces myocardial uptake and intracellular phosphorylation of glucose by hexokinase. Phosphorylated FDG is a poor substrate for further steps in the glycolytic pathway and is dephosphorylated only at a very slow rate. Since the cell membrane is impermeable to FDG-phosphate, it is effectively trapped within the myocardium. Therefore, the ^{18}F concentration measured noninvasively as count density directly represents myocardial glucose utilization without the need for adjustments for tracer metabolism or myocardial washout.

Although static imaging of FDG yields a qualitative assessment of glucose utilization, it does not fully exploit the quantitative capability of PET. To obtain quantitative estimates of regional metabolic rates of glucose metabolism, dynamic image acquisition and principles of tracer kinetic modeling have to be used. Figure 7-1 illustrates a compartment model of FDG kinetics that has been used successfully for quantitative analysis. Model fitting by nonlinear regression analysis or parametric imaging based on a modified Patlak analysis

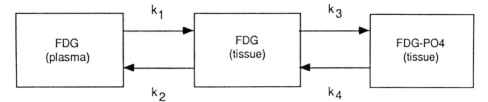

Figure 7-1. *Compartmental model of myocardial FDG kinetics. After intravenous injection, FDG distributes in the plasma compartment and is taken up by myocardial tissue (k_1). Subsequently, FDG can either diffuse back into the extracellular space (k_2) or be phosphorylated by hexokinase (k_3) to FDG-phosphate, which is a poor substrate for further steps in the glycolytic pathway. Because dephosphorylation (k_4) is very slow, FDG-phosphate becomes effectively trapped within the myocardial cell. Principles of tracer kinetic modeling applied to noninvasive PET measurements of time-activity curves of ^{18}F activity in the plasma and tissue compartments allow estimation of regional exogenous myocardial glucose utilization rates in units of micromoles of glucose/gram tissue/minute.*

can be used to compute estimates of regional exogenous glucose utilization in units of micromoles of glucose/gram of tissue/minute.[30,31]

Dynamic PET imaging and tracer kinetic modeling can be used to quantitate myocardial glucose utilization, but image analysis typically involves several hours of computer processing time and operator interaction. Therefore, quantitative image analysis usually is restricted to research studies, while clinical investigations with an emphasis on patient throughput employ either visual analysis or a semiquantitative circumferential profile analysis of static FDG images. However, the distribution of relative ^{18}F activity depicted on static FDG images contains insufficient information to allow accurate assessment of myocardial viability because it cannot be determined whether areas with a high relative ^{18}F concentration reflect increased glucose metabolism attributable to ischemically injured tissue, with areas of less activity reflecting the normal state, or whether these areas reflect normal metabolic activity, with decreased activity corresponding to scar tissue. Thus in patients, PET images of resting myocardial perfusion are obtained in addition to static FDG images.

Patterns of Myocardial Perfusion and Glucose Utilization

A comparison of myocardial perfusion and glucose metabolism in corresponding myocardial segments of PET images can identify three different patterns of clinical significance: areas with both normal perfusion and normal glucose metabolism (normal pattern, Figure 7-2), areas with normal or augmented glucose metabolism but reduced perfusion (flow/metabolism mismatch pattern, Figure 7-3), and areas with a concomitant decrease in both perfusion and glucose metabolism (flow/metabolism match pattern, Figure 7-4).

Presence or absence of these patterns has been correlated with signs of myocardial ischemia and infarction and, clinically more relevant, with reversi-

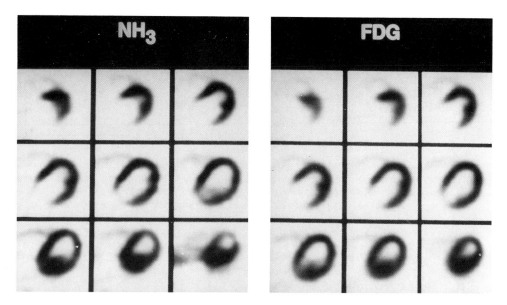

Figure 7-2. *Transaxial PET images obtained with* ^{13}N*-ammonia and* ^{18}F*-deoxyglucose as tracers of myocardial perfusion and glucose metabolism in a normal volunteer. Image planes continue from the base (top left) to the apex (bottom right) of the heart. Image orientation: left—septal (patient right); top—anterior; right—lateral (patient left); bottom—inferior.*

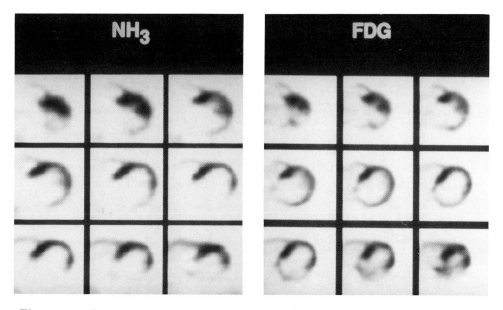

Figure 7-3. *Transaxial PET images obtained with* ^{13}N*-ammonia and* ^{18}F*-deoxyglucose in a patient with coronary artery disease (image orientation as in Figure 2). Note the blood flow/glucose metabolism mismatch pattern (relatively maintained* ^{18}F *activity in areas of reduced* ^{13}N *activity) in the lateral posterolateral, inferior, and posteroseptal segments indicating the presence of hypoperfused myocardium with maintained metabolic activity. The images were obtained 1 month after thrombolysis for acute inferoposterior myocardial infarction. Coronary angiography revealed two-vessel disease with significant 90% stenoses in both the right dominant coronary artery (the infarct related vessel) and the circumflex artery. Global ejection fraction was 40%.*

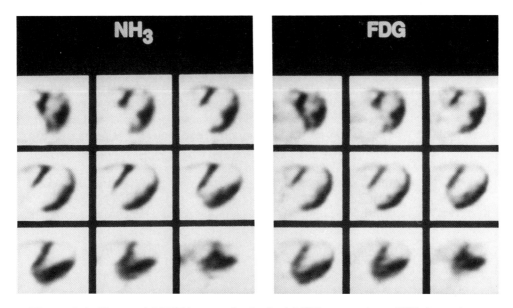

Figure 7-4. *Transaxial PET images obtained with* ¹³*N-ammonia and* ¹⁸*F-deoxyglucose in a patient with ischemic cardiomyopathy (image orientation as in Figure 2). Note the matched decrease of myocardial perfusion and glucose metabolism in the anterior wall and apex. Coronary angiography revealed two-vessel disease with complete occlusion of the left anterior descending artery and a high-grade (80%) stenosis of the circumflex artery. Global ejection fraction was 20%.*

ble and irreversible dysfunction. The flow/metabolism mismatch and flow/metabolism match patterns have been referred to as "PET ischemia" and "PET infarct," respectively, since the former has been observed in ischemic tissue and the latter in infarcted tissue. Reversible dysfunction has been observed in normal areas and in areas of flow/metabolism mismatch on PET images, but irreversible dysfunction is invariably associated with a pattern of PET infarction. Since reversible dysfunction is the hallmark of myocardial viability, myocardial segments appearing normal or ischemic on PET images correspond to viable segments, whereas segments with PET infarction reflect nonviable scar tissue. It is tempting to speculate that dysfunctional myocardial segments with normal perfusion and metabolism correspond to "stunned" tissue and that PET ischemia reflects myocardial hibernation; however, currently there is not sufficient evidence to prove this hypothesis.

Patterns of PET-normal, PET-ischemic, and PET-infarcted tissue have been demonstrated in patients with chronic coronary artery disease,[25,32] in patients after acute myocardial infarctions with or without thrombolytic therapy,[33,34] and in patients with exercise-induced ischemia.[35]

Marshall et al.[32] examined 15 patients with a history of myocardial infarction a mean of 3 weeks after the acute event. Fourteen regions were associated with a flow/metabolism match, but an additional 11 showed a flow/metabolism mismatch associated with postinfarction angina, transient ischemic electrocardiographic (ECG) changes during angina, and wall motion abnormalities. Moreover, the myocardial tissue exhibiting a flow/metabolism mismatch pattern on PET imaging was supplied by coronary arteries with arteriographically evident severe, flow-limiting stenoses.

Tamaki et al.[25] studied 28 patients with chronic coronary artery disease at least 2 months after an acute infarction. In 13 of 22 patients with a flow/metabolism mismatch on PET imaging, a corresponding exercise-induced perfusion defect was detected on thallium imaging, corroborating the correlation between the presence of ischemically compromised myocardium and the flow/metabolism mismatch pattern.

Schwaiger et al.[33] examined 13 patients with acute myocardial infarction within 72 hours of the onset of symptoms. Among 32 myocardial segments with decreased myocardial perfusion, 16 (50%) demonstrated a concordant decrease in glucose utilization (PET infarct), while 16 (50%) exhibited a flow/metabolism mismatch (PET ischemia). All 5 patients with postinfarction angina had evidence of PET ischemia, while none of the patients without signs of PET ischemia experienced postinfarction chest pain. Patent infarct-related vessels supplied 8 of 10 PET-ischemic segments, while 10 of 13 segments with PET infarction were located in the territory of an occluded infarct-related vessel. These findings are consistent with the presence of ischemically injured yet viable myocardial tissue in areas of flow/metabolism mismatch after acute myocardial infarction.

Pierard et al.[34] correlated findings from PET imaging and echocardiography in 17 patients early (1 week) and late (9 months) after an acute anterior myocardial infarction. These patients had received thrombolytic therapy within 3 hours after the onset of chest pain. While an improvement in wall motion was observed in 5 of 11 patients in whom viable myocardium was demonstrated by PET in the area of infarction at 1 week, wall motion abnormalities persisted to the time of the late study in all 6 patients in whom PET infarction was evident. These results indicate that myocardial tissue exhibiting PET infarction has suffered irreversible ischemic injury.

Twelve patients with chronic coronary artery disease and stable angina were examined at rest and approximately 1 hour after exercise testing by Camici et al.[35] using rubidium-82 (^{82}Rb) and FDG as tracers of myocardial perfusion and glucose utilization. Exercise-induced ischemia as demonstrated by serial flow measurements before, during, and after bicycle stress testing was associated with increased myocardial glucose utilization (flow/metabolism mismatch) in postischemic myocardial segments. In the nonischemic areas, FDG uptake in patients was comparable to that in normal volunteers. Thus, enhanced glucose utilization reflecting prolonged metabolic changes in myocardial metabolism can occur in response to transient ischemia.

Focusing on chronic coronary artery disease, other investigations tested the prognostic significance of PET imaging in predicting functional improvements after elective reperfusion therapy.[36,37]

Tillisch et al.[36] studied myocardial viability with PET in 17 patients before bypass surgery and compared the findings to improvements in regional wall motion evaluated before and 12 to 18 weeks after surgery. Sixty-seven segments that showed contractile dysfunction before surgery were successfully revascularized. Eighty-five percent of 41 segments that were PET-normal or PET-ischemic before surgery did exhibit significant improvement in wall motion after surgery. However, only 8% of the remaining 26 segments that were PET infarcted before surgery exhibited improved contractile function after surgery. Moreover, while the global ejection fractions of patients with less than two segments with mismatch or PET did not improve after surgery, ejection fraction did improve significantly in patients with at least two such segments. Thus, the amount of tissue characterized as ischemic on PET imaging seems to reflect the capacity of functional improvement that can be expected after revascularization.

Tamaki et al.[37] performed PET imaging in 22 patients before attempted revascularization and related the observed PET patterns to the functional outcome assessed 6 weeks after the intervention. Of forty-six dysfunctional segments, 23 were PET-normal or PET-ischemic before revascularization; the other 23 showed PET infarction. Eighteen of 23 (78%) of the segments determined to be viable by PET exhibited improved contractile function; 18 of 23 (78%) PET-infarcted segments remained dysfunctional.

The moderate differences in positive (85% and 78%) and negative predictive accuracy (92% and 78%) observed in these two studies can be explained to some extent by differences in glucose loading. Tamaki et al. studied their patients in the fasted state; Tillisch et al. used oral glucose loading. As outlined below, the former approach tends to be more sensitive yet less specific for the detection of viable myocardium.

In summary, PET imaging by use of tracers of blood flow and glucose utilization is able (1) to differentiate ischemically injured but viable myocardium from necrotic nonviable scar tissue, and (2) to predict the reversibility of contractile dysfunction that can be expected subsequent to successful revascularization procedures.

Methods for Imaging Myocardial Viability by PET

Image Acquisition

Images of relative myocardial perfusion and glucose metabolism needed for the assessment of viability by PET should preferably be obtained during a single imaging session. In this manner, differences in patient positioning between scans are minimized, so that corresponding myocardial areas can easily be identified on both image sets. After proper patient positioning, a transmission scan with a positron-emitting isotope of external source is obtained to allow for accurate attenuation correction of subsequently acquired emission images. If appropriate, glucose loading can be undertaken before or during the transmission scan.

The half-lives of tracers of flow and glucose metabolism determine the imaging sequence. Positron emitters generate pairs of photons with an energy of 511 keV. Thus, if two studies with positron-emitting substances are scheduled to be performed in temporal sequence, a time period sufficiently long (four to five half-lives) for the decay of the first tracer has to be allowed before the acquisition of the second image can commence. Since the half-lives of positron-emitting flow tracers range from 1 to 10 minutes, compared with the 109 minute half-life of FDG, flow images should be obtained before FDG images.

Myocardial perfusion can be assessed by use of various tracer substances, including nitrogen-13 (^{13}N)-ammonia, ^{82}Rb, and oxygen-15 (^{15}O)-water. At present, an ideal flow tracer satisfying all theoretical and practical constraints associated with PET imaging is not yet available, so that experience of the imaging center and isotope delivery methods (cyclotron versus generator) frequently determine the selection of the flow tracer. For the PET assessment of myocardial viability, the most experience has been accumulated with static images of myocardial ^{13}N activity acquired for 20 minutes after the intravenous injection of ^{13}N-ammonia.

After the activity of the flow tracer has decayed to background level, FDG can be injected intravenously. For quantitation of metabolic rates, dynamic image acquisition has to be initiated concurrent with the FDG injection. If only qualitative images are desired, the injection of FDG can actually immediately follow the acquisition of flow images, with FDG imaging performed 1 hour later when the activity of the flow tracer has decayed away. This shorter acquisition protocol can help to decrease the examination time.

Under special circumstances, the comparably long half-life of FDG obviates the need for an on-site cyclotron. The imaging center can be located at some distance from the cyclotron and FDG can be supplied once or twice daily. Using generator-produced flow tracers such as ^{82}Rb and FDG delivered from a regional cyclotron, mobile PET imaging centers serving regional hospitals at regularly scheduled intervals have already been successfully launched. Alternatively, combining single-photon emission computed tomographic (SPECT) imaging of myocardial perfusion with PET imaging of glucose metabolism might also allow for tomographic visualization of flow/metabolism patterns. Thus, it is conceivable that the assessment of myocardial viability will be possible at regional hospitals without the need to install a complete PET center including a cyclotron and a radiochemistry division.

Efforts have been made to adjust standard gamma camera equipment to image 511 keV photons that are generated by positron annihilation. Höflin et al.[38] reported preliminary findings of thallium/FDG imaging for the detection of flow/metabolism mismatches by use of a seven-pinhole collimator tomographic gamma camera with adjustments in collimation and shielding. Williams et al.[39] demonstrated the feasibility of use of a mobile gamma camera with a parallel-hole rotating tungsten collimator to image cardiac FDG activity in three standard planar views. However, the diagnostic performance and clinical utility of these approaches remain to be determined.

Patient-related Issues

To obtain FDG images of good diagnostic quality the dietary state of the patient and a possible diabetic condition have to be considered.

Dietary State

The dietary state has a profound influence on myocardial glucose utilization. Unlike the brain, which relies on a constant and adequate glucose supply to fulfill its metabolic demand, the heart can switch between different substrates to satisfy its energy requirements. After an overnight fast, normal myocardium preferentially consumes lipids, so that carbohydrates account for only 40% of the energy generated by oxidative metabolism. After a meal rich in carbohydrates, with the associated increase in plasma glucose and insulin levels, glucose becomes the preferred energy substrate.[26]

Whereas dietary conditions significantly affect glucose metabolism and thus signal intensity of FDG activity in normal myocardium, ischemic myocardium preferentially uses glucose as its fuel substrate independent of substrate availability. Thus, dietary conditions influence substrate selection in ischemic myocardium less than they do in normal myocardium.

FDG imaging can be performed in patients in the fasting state or after oral administration of a glucose load. If imaging is conducted in the fasting patient, normal myocardium will appear very faint, whereas ischemic myocardium with an increased contribution of glycolysis will appear as increased activity. Thus, fasting potentially increases the contrast between normal and ischemic myocardium, enhancing diagnostic sensitivity. However, in our experience, FDG images obtained in fasting patients are frequently associated with insufficient count statistics, precluding a diagnostic reading. Moreover, increased sensitivity of testing in the fasting patient can lead to overestimation of the amount of viable myocardium because small islands of viable tissue with a high count rate may mimic a more extensive flow/metabolism mismatch.

Alternatively, FDG imaging can be conducted after a standardized oral glucose load. Although glucose loading tends to equalize the differences in glucose metabolism in normal and ischemic segments and consequently lowers diagnostic sensitivity, it improves image quality significantly and increases diagnostic specificity. Berry et al.[40] used visual image interpretation to assess the effects of glucose loading on image quality in one group of 26 patients given an oral glucose load of 50 g and one group of 27 patients who had fasted. They reported that 88% and 14% of images from the respective groups had minimal or no blood pool activity, 77% and 11% were of excellent quality, and 85% and 56% were clinically interpretable. Another advantage of FDG imaging after glucose loading arises from the homogeneous tracer uptake in normal myocardium, while an increased FDG uptake has been shown in the lateral and posterolateral wall in the fasted state.[41]

In our laboratory we have found improved image quality and higher specificity to be of considerable importance for accurate diagnostic readings, so that we currently recommend that glucose loading be used when conducting FDG imaging with the objective of assessment of myocardial viability. However, a controlled study of the effects of glucose loading in one patient group has not yet been accomplished.

diagnostic readout and the comparison of patient data with normal data base values is achieved with more consistency. Moreover, vascular territories can be outlined on the polar maps, facilitating comparisons between multiple studies for the same patient and between studies for different patients (Color Figure 3).

In the future, quantitative polar maps of cardiac perfusion and glucose utilization will facilitate the accurate assessment of extent and severity of reductions in myocardial blood flow and improve the capability to delineate hypoperfused myocardial tissue with maintained or relatively enhanced glucose metabolism.

PET Imaging in Comparison with Alternate Methods of Assessment of Myocardial Viability

In addition to PET, other diagnostic modalities and clinical indicators have been used to assess myocardial viability, with varying degrees of success.

Angina

Typical angina, a clearly defined clinical symptom, is commonly considered an indication of myocardial ischemia. However, presence or absence of angina does not consistently correlate with presence or absence of viable tissue as assessed by PET. While a correlation between angina and PET viability has been demonstrated in patients after an acute infarction,[32,33] these findings could not be corroborated in other studies focusing on patients with depressed left ventricular function.

Brunken et al.[42] studied 20 patients with chronic coronary artery disease and depressed left ventricular function (ejection fraction 35 ± 12%). Six of 11 patients with documented PET ischemia experienced angina, as did 5 of 9 patients without signs of PET ischemia. Similarly, in a subsequent study by the same group,[43] the incidence of angina was not different in the patients with PET ischemia (8/16, 50%) than in those without signs of PET ischemia (5/11, 45%). Again, in both patient groups left ventricular ejection fraction was poor (30% versus 34%). Thus, presence or absence of angina is inadequate to discern the subgroup of patients with coronary artery disease and severely depressed ventricular function that would benefit from reperfusion therapy.

Electrocardiography

The electrocardiogram, a virtually universally available diagnostic tool, continues to be used extensively for the assessment of myocardial viability. The presence of Q waves has traditionally been taken as reliable evidence that the corresponding myocardial tissue is in fact necrotic. However, studies investigating the relationship between ECG findings and myocardial viability do not support this hypothesis and argue against the clinical strategy of correlating the presence of Q waves with irreversible myocardial dysfunction.

Using ventricular unloading with nitroglycerin, Banka et al.[44] demonstrated reversible asynergy in 44% of myocardial segments showing Q waves on the electrocardiogram. Comparing PET imaging with ECG findings, Brunken et al.[42] found that 54% of segments with Q waves were classified as viable by PET. Hashimoto et al.[45] compared patients with Q wave and non-Q wave infarcts by use of PET with ammonia and FDG. Ninety-one percent of 11 patients after non-Q wave infarctions had viable tissue in the area of the infarct by PET, whereas in 11 patients with Q wave infarcts viable myocardium was visualized in 36%, indicating that Q waves are not reliable indicators of transmural infarction.

Thus, when ECG findings indicative of scar tissue are the sole evidence of irreversible tissue injury, attempts to reperfuse akinetic myocardial segments should not be abandoned.

Responses of Wall Motion to Inotropic Stimulation or Changes in Ventricular Loading Conditions

In studies in dogs, dysfunctional but viable myocardium after acute ischemic injury has been shown to respond to inotropic stimulation with functional improvement.[21–23] Therefore, diagnostic techniques that allow monitoring of cardiac wall motion or wall thickening have been combined with interventions such as exercise,[46] inotropic drugs,[34] nitroglycerin,[47] or postextrasystolic potentiation[48,22] in an attempt to differentiate viable from necrotic tissue in patients as well. If reversible asynergy is elicited by an intervention, viable myocardium is assumed to be present.

Rozanski et al.[46] performed exercise and postexercise radionuclide ventriculography in 53 patients before bypass surgery and follow-up radionuclide ventriculography at rest postoperatively. Preoperative ejection fraction was 52 $\pm$ 10%. Fifty-seven of 124 segments with resting myocardial asynergy showed reversible asynergy after exercise; 52 of these segments also exhibited improved resting wall motion after surgery (91% positive predictive accuracy). Conversely, no improvement in function after surgery was observed in 56 of 67 segments with irreversible preoperative asynergy (negative predictive accuracy of 84%).

Thus, in patients with normal or slightly reduced global ventricular function, postexercise radionuclide ventriculography can be used to predict reversible myocardial asynergy. However, in patients with severe depression of left ventricular function or immediately after thrombolysis, the applicability of this method is probably limited because exercise will generally not be tolerated well enough to achieve an adequate stimulus. In a routine clinical setting, this approach has not been widely used.

Hamby et al.[48] compared the response of hypokinetic myocardial areas to postextrasystolic potentiation in 24 patients with normal or slightly decreased ejection fractions undergoing bypass surgery. In 14 of 15 patients an improve-on a second day are further disadvantages of the routine use of 24 hour delay imaging.

These last two shortcomings do not apply to another modified thallium protocol aimed at enhancing thallium redistribution: the reinjection of a second thallium dose preceding the acquisition of the delayed images. Dilsizian et al.[24] studied 100 patients with angiographically proven coronary artery disease by use of a SPECT thallium protocol with three acquisition periods: poststress, 3 to 4 hours later, and after the reinjection of a second thallium dose. They reported that 49% of the defects appearing fixed on the 4 hour redistribution images improved on the reinjection images, and average relative thallium uptake significantly increased from 56 ± 12% to 64 ± 10% between the 4 hour and reinjection images.

In a subgroup of 20 patients who underwent revascularization by angioplasty, a fixed defect on the reinjection images obtained before the intervention was invariably associated with abnormal thallium uptake and abnormal regional wall motion after angioplasty.

The average ejection fraction for all patients in this study was 44 ± 12% (range 16% to 69%), with only 50% of all patients falling below the normal range. A separate analysis for patients with severely reduced ventricular function was not presented. Thus, the value of a reinjection protocol for the detection of viable myocardium in patients with poor left ventricular function remains undetermined. Moreover, while radionuclide ventriculography was performed in all patients, the incidence of thallium redistribution after reinjection in dysfunctional myocardial segments was not included in the results presented. Since myocardial areas that maintain contractile function are clearly viable, the predictive value of a thallium reinjection protocol with respect to dysfunctional segments is of greater clinical interest than an average value for all segments. Thus, while thallium reinjection enhances the overall detection of thallium redistribution, its diagnostic utility with respect to dysfunctional myocardial segments remains unclear.

Ohtani et al.[56] also investigated the value of thallium reinjection for prediction of improvement in perfusion and wall motion in 24 patients undergoing bypass surgery. Exercise thallium imaging and radionuclide angiography were performed before and 4 to 8 weeks after surgery. Reinjection images that had been obtained after the 3 hour delayed images during the preoperative thallium study had positive and negative predictive accuracies of 79% and 82% for postoperative improvement in perfusion and of 73% and 75% for improvement in wall motion. However, because data about global ventricular function were omitted in this report, it remains unknown whether these predictive values apply to patients with preserved and/or those with depressed left ventricular function. Furthermore, the negative predictive accuracy reported in this study was considerably lower than the value reported by Dilsizian et al.[24] Thus, further studies are needed to characterize in more detail the prognostic value of the thallium reinjection protocol.

To facilitate a comparison of the results discussed above, Tables 7-2 through 7-4 list values for positive and negative predictive accuracies of thallium imaging for the assessment of myocardial viability.

Table 7-2
Accuracy of PET Imaging for Prediction of
Functional Improvement after Revascularization

Study	Type	Predictive Accuracy (%)	
		+	−
Tillisch (1986)	PET	85	92
Tamaki (1989)	PET	78	78

In a recent article, Moore et al.[57] provided experimental evidence that thallium kinetics in stunned and normal dog myocardium are not significantly different. Accordingly, these authors argue that thallium kinetics remain unchanged until irreversible tissue damage occurs. Thus, thallium imaging should be able to accurately delineate normal and stunned myocardium. However, stunned myocardium as investigated in their study is only a subgroup of dysfunctional but viable myocardium, and it is conceivable that hibernating myocardium or other still-unrecognized states from which it is possible to regain contractile function after reperfusion result in disturbances in energy-dependent thallium uptake with maintenance of glucose utilization. Presumably these regions would be undetectable by thallium imaging and may account for the observed differences between PET and thallium assessments of viability and predictions of postinterventional improvement.

Table 7-3
Accuracy of Completely or Partially Reversible Defects on Exercise
Thallium Imaging for Prediction of Improvement or Normalization of
Myocardial Perfusion after Revascularization

Study	Procedure	Type	Delayed Image	Predictive Accuracy (%)	
				+	−
Gibson (1983)	CABG	Planar	4 hr	88	55
Liu (1985)	PTCA	Planar	4 hr	86	19
Kiat (1988)	CABG + PTCA	SPECT	4 hr	85	28
			24 hr	90	63
Dilsizian (1990)	PTCA	SPECT	RI, 4 hr		100
Ohtani (1990)	CABG	SPECT	RI, 3 hr	79	82

RI = thallium reinjection before delayed imaging;

CABG = coronary artery bypass grafting.

Table 7-4
Accuracy of Completely or Partially Reversible Defects on Exercise
Thallium Imaging for Assessment of Myocardial Viability as Evaluated by
PET FDG Imaging

Study	Type	Delayed Image	Predictive Accuracy (%) +	Predictive Accuracy (%) −
Brunken (1987)	Planar	4 hr	73	42
Tamaki (1988)	SPECT	3 hr	95	62
Brunken (1988)	SPECT	24 hr	66	47
Brunken (1989)	SPECT	4 hr	73	53

Isonitrile Imaging

Recently, technetium-99m (^{99m}Tc)-labeled compounds have been introduced as a new class of perfusion tracers with improved dosimetry, energy spectrum, and tissue kinetics compared with thallium. The use of Tc-MIBI (2-methoxy isobutyl isonitrile), an isonitrile compound, as a flow tracer has been validated in studies with thallium and it has been approved by the Food and Drug Administration. MIBI imaging also allows the assessment of regional wall motion,[58] so that myocardial perfusion and contractile function can be evaluated simultaneously in identical anatomic segments. Expectations have also been raised that isonitriles may be useful for the assessment of myocardial viability: a mild reduction in blood flow may be indicative of tissue viability while severely reduced myocardial uptake of MIBI should indicate scar tissue.

Sinusas et al.[59] examined myocardial uptake of thallium and MIBI under conditions of low flow and postischemic dysfunction in a canine model. They found that MIBI and thallium uptake were similar under the conditions studied and that both closely paralleled flow alterations. These data suggest that the assessment of viability by MIBI is subject to the same limitations as that by thallium. Rocco et al.[60] confirmed that MIBI is probably not an ideal tracer of myocardial viability. Using planar imaging, they compared perfusion scores in 8 patients undergoing coronary artery bypass surgery and found that 12 of 13 segments with a reduced MIBI score exhibited improved perfusion after surgery. However, 5 of 5 segments that had been assigned a score of 0, indicating markedly reduced MIBI uptake and therefore nonviable myocardium, also demonstrated improvement after surgery.

Thus, MIBI, to date the most important isonitrile compound, has been established as a valuable flow tracer but does not seem to qualify as an adequate marker of viability.

Magnetic Resonance Spectroscopy

Magnetic resonance spectroscopy is a noninvasive imaging technique capable of measuring the time course of magnetic spins in certain atoms after an external magnetic excitation. Several atomic nuclei abundant in human tissues are particularly appropriate for clinical investigations. In a recent review article,[61] Higgins pointed out that magnetic resonance spectroscopy potentially can provide a noninvasive evaluation of metabolic aspects of myocardial physiology and myocardial disease. In particular, phosphorus-31(^{31}P) spectroscopy, capable of interrogating high-energy phosphate metabolism, shows promise for the differentiation of reversibly and irreversibly injured myocardium.[62]

Schaefer et al.[63] demonstrated the feasibility of ^{31}P spectroscopic imaging in patients with congestive cardiomyopathy and left ventricular hypertrophy. However, the clinical significance of spectroscopic results remains to be determined before the diagnostic modality can be adopted for routine use.

In summary, diagnostic modalities other than PET often underestimate the amount of viable myocardium actually present. The absence of angina or the presence of Q waves on the electrocardiogram have an established poor negative predictive accuracy of viability, and the predictive value of reversible asynergy elicited by different interventions has so far been established only for patients with preserved global ventricular function.

Thallium studies with various delayed imaging and/or reinjection protocols continue to be used in the assessment of viability. Although the presence of early or late redistribution has a high positive predictive accuracy for postinterventional functional improvement, the negative predictive accuracy has consistently been shown to be significantly less than that of PET. At present, thallium reinjection appears to improve negative predictive accuracy, but additional studies are needed to firmly establish its clinical value, especially in patients with depressed left ventricular function.

Isonitrile imaging has only recently been introduced for clinical use. Research data obtained so far indicate that uptake of isonitriles parallels blood flow and seems to be inadequate for the assessment of viability.

Magnetic resonance spectroscopy, while offering considerable promise for a noninvasive determination of viability, has not yet fully evolved technologically and consequently has not yet been used extensively for clinical, cardiac diagnostic imaging of perfusion or metabolism.

Indications for Clinical PET Imaging for Assessment of Myocardial Viability

Patient Selection

Limited availability and considerations of cost effectiveness prohibit the indiscriminate use of PET imaging and necessitate the careful selection of patients (Table 7-5). Accordingly, patients with normal or only slightly reduced global ventricular function are not considered candidates for PET imaging of myocardial viability; the absence of myocardial dysfunction obviously indicates that myocardial viability is maintained and that surgical risk is not increased.

In contrast, clinical management of patients with more extensive myocardial dysfunction can critically depend on the differentiation between reversible

Table 7-5
Clinical Indications for PET Imaging with Use of Tracers of Myocardial
Perfusion and Glucose Metabolism

Assessment of potentially reversible contractile dysfunction in patients with
depressed left ventricular function
Differential diagnosis between idiopathic and ischemic cardiomyopathy
Assignment of patients to the most appropriate treatment early after acute
myocardial infarction
Assessment of reperfusion interventions in patients with chronic coronary
artery disease

and irreversible dysfunction because both the surgical risk during revascularization procedures and associated potential benefits increase with decreasing left ventricular function. The contribution of metabolic imaging is therefore essential, particularly in patients with severely depressed ventricular function in whom it is the only available method for accurate assessment of the amount of viable and salvageable myocardium.

Assessment of Potentially Reversible Contractile Dysfunction in Patients with Depressed Ventricular Function

Patients with severe left ventricular dysfunction resulting from coronary artery disease are frequently not considered candidates for bypass surgery. Indeed, multiple infarctions can irreversibly damage the left ventricle to such an extent that medical therapy or cardiac transplantation are the only therapeutic options. However, Akins et al.[64] have reported on 2 patients in whom surgery was initially not advised on the basis of poor ventricular function and absence of angina but in whom ejection fraction (from 15% to 30%) and New York Heart Association (NYHA) classification (NYHA IV to NYHA II) significantly improved after surgery. In these patients, partial reversibility of defects on radionuclide thallium perfusion scans had been interpreted as evidence of viability and had contributed to a reversal of the initial decision against surgery. Subsequent studies have corroborated these observations and emphasized the benefit of coronary artery bypass surgery in patients with severely depressed left ventricular function.[65–67]

Tillisch et al.[36] demonstrated that left ventricular ejection fraction improved from 30 ± 11% to 45 ± 14% in 11 patients in whom PET had revealed a significant fraction of dysfunctional myocardium to be viable. These data suggest that PET imaging can provide an estimate of the functional improvement to be expected after bypass surgery and can thus be used advantageously for risk stratification and clinical decision making. However, while the clinical significance of large flow/metabolism mismatches has been established, the prognostic value of small areas of mismatch such as those frequently visualized in the peri-infarct zone remains to be determined.

In patients with severely depressed contractile function of unclear cause, PET imaging has been shown to correctly differentiate between idiopathic and ischemic cardiomyopathy,[68] indicating that it can be used in the evaluation of patients for cardiac transplantation and to select patients that may profit from revascularization instead of cardiac replacement therapy.

Selection of the Most Appropriate Treatment Early After Acute Myocardial Infarction

PET ischemia appears early after myocardial infarction in patients undergoing conservative treatment.[33] Seventy-two hours after the acute event, 16 of 32 (50%) hypoperfused and dysfunctional myocardial segments did show maintained glucose utilization. When studied with echocardiography 6 weeks later without interceding reperfusion therapy, 8 of these viable segments exhibited improved function, in 2 segments function had deteriorated, and in 6 segments there was no change. In contrast, no functional improvement was seen in the segments exhibiting PET infarction.

These data illustrate that the fate of ischemically injured yet viable myocardial tissue as visualized by PET early after acute infarction varies. In terms of myocardial states, recovery of contractile function is consistent with the presence of stunned myocardium, prolonged wall motion abnormality could reflect hibernating myocardium, and deterioration of wall motion presumably indicates development of scar tissue. Characterization of ischemically injured myocardium by PET can therefore be used in the assignment of patients to conservative treatment or to proper revascularization procedures aimed at altering the natural course of ischemic injury.

It should be noted, however, that the absence of a flow/metabolism mismatch in dysfunctional segments very early after myocardial infarction does not necessarily negate the possibility of reversible dysfunction. Animal experiments have shown that a mismatch that may not be seen within 3 hours of reperfusion, may be detected 24 hours after the acute event.[69] Thus, it appears that the diagnostic value of PET may be suboptimal when images are acquired within 1 day of the acute ischemic event.

As conservative treatment of myocardial infarction is increasingly abandoned in favor of more aggressive interventional strategies, assessing the success of reperfusion therapy and decisions regarding further therapy gain more importance. While the benefit of early thrombolytic therapy or PTCA has been clearly established in several multicenter trials including a large cohort of patients, the clinical assessment of success early after the institution of reperfusion therapy has remained difficult in individual patients. Pierard et al.[34] reported that after intravenous thrombolysis in 17 patients with anterior myocardial infarction early PET imaging identified five patients with a normal flow/metabolism pattern, six patients with a flow/metabolism mismatch, and six patients with a concordant decrease in flow and glucose utilization.

Thus, detection of viability in asynergic myocardial segments by PET can expedite treatment and guide decisions regarding therapy in postreperfusion patients. If limited success of an initial attempt at reperfusion can be verified by PET, additional therapeutic strategies to relieve the remaining ischemic burden can be scheduled without further delay.

Assessment of Interventions Designed to Restore Perfusion in Patients with Chronic Coronary Artery Disease

The success of revascularization after PTCA or bypass surgery can be assessed by PET imaging. Tamaki et al.[37] concluded in their study of 22 patients that the new FDG uptake after bypass surgery observed in 5 asynergic segments may be a specific marker of bypass graft occlusion. Nienaber et al.[70] showed that the recovery of myocardial metabolism as assessed by PET precedes improvements in wall motion abnormalities. Thus, initial evidence suggests that PET imaging can be used early after interventional therapy to establish its success and predict functional recovery of revascularized myocardium. However, more detailed studies are needed to establish the precise role PET imaging can play in clinical risk stratification after revascularization procedures.

In summary, clinical PET imaging is currently used primarily for the assessment of severity of disease to enable and facilitate the most appropriate treatment choices. In addition, PET imaging can be used in the noninvasive diagnostic workup of patients with coronary artery disease when other noninvasive techniques have yielded inconclusive data.

Future Outlook

PET imaging of myocardial viability by use of tracers of perfusion and glucose metabolism has been adopted for routine clinical use in several medical centers. The currently somewhat higher costs of PET imaging compared with other diagnostic techniques are offset by the additional and often critically important information it provides about myocardial viability, information that cannot be obtained with other diagnostic modalities.

While the presence of PET ischemia has been proven to be a highly reliable predictor of postintervention contractile improvement, insufficient data about the natural time course of appearance and disappearance of this pattern are currently available. Larger clinical trials are needed to explore PET patterns of myocardial hibernation and stunning and to develop clinical decision aids to determine the nature and timing of the most appropriate therapeutic strategy.

State-of-the-art PET scanners allow the simultaneous acquisition of 15 to 31 transaxial image planes spaced densely enough so that image processing algorithms can conduct image reorientation yielding standardized views of the heart. Polar map displays already widely used in cardiac SPECT imaging will thus also improve the quality of PET images. True three-dimensional image acquisition yielding homogeneous spatial resolution in all three directions is currently already possible in research laboratories and the clinical implementation of adequate algorithms will allow generation of a high-resolution, truly three-dimensional representation of cardiac perfusion and metabolism.

Moreover, gated PET imaging in which images of the heart are captured in different phases of the cardiac cycle will help in the precise correlation of cardiac wall motion with perfusion and metabolism. This will provide a very detailed view of the sequence of events leading from nutritional perfusion to substrate metabolism and cardiac contraction.

PET imaging is likely to make a significant contribution to clinical noninvasive cardiac imaging. It offers exciting possibilities for the in-depth exploration of cardiac pathophysiology.

Acknowledgments: We thank Ron Sumida and his staff for their technical assistance in image acquisition and Wendy Wilson for the preparation of the illustrations.

References

1. GISSI. Long-term effects of intravenous thrombolysis in acute myocardial infarction: final report of the GISSI study. Lancet 1987; 2:871–874.
2. Bates ER, Califf RM, Stack RS, Aronson L, George BS, Candela RJ, Kereiakes DJ, Abbottsmith CW, Anderson L, Pitt B, O'Neill WW, Topol EJ. Thrombolysis and angioplasty in myocardial infarction (TAMI-1) trial: influence of infarct location on arterial patency, left ventricular function and mortality. J Am Coll Cardiol 1989; 13:8–12.
3. Rahimtoola S. A perspective on the three large multicenter randomized clinical trials of coronary bypass surgery for chronic stable angina. Circulation 1985; 72(suppl V):V-123-V-135.
4. Braunwald E, Kloner R. The stunned myocardium: prolonged, postischemic ventricular dysfunction. Circulation 1982; 66:1146–1149.
5. Kloner RA, Przyklenk K, Patel B. Altered myocardial states: the stunned and hibernating myocardium. Am J Med 1989; 68(suppl 1A):14–22.
6. Braunwald E, Rutherford JD. Reversible ischemic left ventricular dysfunction: evidence for the "hibernating myocardium." J Am Coll Cardiol 1986; 6:1467–1470.
7. Rahimtoola SH. The hibernating myocardium. Am Heart J 1989; 117:211–219.
8. Matsuzaki M, Gallagher KP, Kemper WS, White F, Ross J. Sustained regional dysfunction produced by prolonged coronary stenosis: gradual recovery after reperfusion. Circulation 1983; 68:170–182.
9. Topol E, Weiss JL, Guzman P, et al. Immediate improvement of dysfunctional myocardial segments after coronary revascularization: detection by intraoperative transesophageal echocardiography. J Am Coll Cardiol 1984; 6:1123–1134.
10. Johnson AD, O'Rourke RA, Karliner JS, Burian C. Effect of myocardial revascularization on systolic time intervals in patients with left ventricular dysfunction. Circulation 1972; 45(suppl I):I-91.
11. Heyndrickx GR, Millard RW, McRitchie RJ, Maroko PR, Vatner SF. Regional myocardial functional and electrophysiological alterations after brief coronary artery occlusion in conscious dogs. J Clin Invest 1975; 56:978–985.
12. Ellis SG, Henschke CI, Sandor T, Wynne J, Braunwald E, Kloner RA. Time course of functional and biochemical recovery of myocardium salvaged by reperfusion. J Am Coll Cardiol 1983; 1:1047–1055.
13. Bush LR, Buja ML, Samowitz W, Rude RE, Wathen M, Tilton GD, Willerson JT. Recovery of left ventricular segmental function after long-term reperfusion following temporary coronary occlusion in conscious dogs. Circ Res 1983; 53:248–263.
14. Murry CE, Richard VJ, Reimer KA, Jennings RB. Ischemic preconditioning slows

energy metabolism and delays ultrastructural damage during a sustained ischemic episode. Circ Res 1990; 66:913–931.

15. Geft IL, Fishbein MC, Ninomiya K, Hashida J, Chaux E, Yano J, Y-Rit J, Genov T, Shell W, Ganz W. Intermittent brief periods of ischemia have a cumulative effect and may cause myocardial necrosis. Circulation 1982; 66:1150–1153.

16. Anderson J, Marshall H, Bray BE, Lutz JR, Frederick PR, Yanowitz FG, Datz FL, Klausner SC, Hagan AD. A randomized trial of intracoronary streptokinase in the treatment of acute myocardial infarction. N Engl J Med 1983; 308:1312–318.

17. Stack RS, Phillips HR, Grierson DS, Behar VS, Kong Y, Peter Rh, Swain JL, Greenfield JC Jr. Functional improvement of jeopardized myocardium following intracoronary streptokinase infusion in acute myocardial infarction. J Clin Invest 1983; 72:84–95.

18. Krause SM, Jacobus WE, Becker LC. Alterations in cardiac sarcoplasmic reticulum calcium transport in the postischemic "stunned" myocardium. Circ Res 1989; 65:526–530.

19. Jennings RB, Steenbergen C. Nucleotide metabolism and cellular damage in myocardial ischemia. Annu Rev Physiol 1985; 47:727–749.

20. Bolli R. Oxygen-derived free radicals and postischemic myocardial dysfunction ("stunned myocardium"). J Am Coll Cardiol 1988; 12:239–249.

21. Ellis SG, Wynne J, Braunwald E, Henschke CI, Sandor T, Kloner RA. Response of reperfusion-salvaged, stunned myocardium to inotropic stimulation. Am Heart J 1984; 107:13–19.

22. Becker LC, Levine JH, DiPaula AF, Guarnieri T, Aversano T. Reversal of dysfunction in postischemic stunned myocardium by epinephrine and postextrasystolic potentiation. J Am Coll Cardiol 1986; 7:580–589.

23. Buda A, Zotz R, Gallagher KP. The effect of inotropic stimulation on normal and ischemic myocardium after coronary occlusion. Circulation 1987; 76:163–172.

24. Dilsizian V, Rocco TP, Freedman NMT, Leon MB, Bonow RO. Enhanced detection of ischemic but viable myocardium by the reinjection of thallium after stress-redistribution imaging. N Engl J Med 1990; 323:141–146.

25. Tamaki N, Yonekura Y, Yamashita K, Senda M, Saji H, Hashimoto T, Kambara FTH, Kawai C, Ban T, Konishi J. Relation of left ventricular perfusion and wall motion with metabolic activity in persistent defects on Thallium-201 tomography in healed myocardial infarction. Am J Cardiol 1988; 62:202–208.

26. Opie LH. *The Heart: Physiology, Metabolism, Pharmacology, and Therapy*. London: Grune and Stratton, 1984.

27. Jennings RB, Reimer KA, Mayer S. Total ischemia in dog hearts, in vitro: 1. Comparison of high energy phosphate production, utilization, and depletion, and of adenine nucleotide catabolism in total ischemia in vitro vs. severe ischemia in vivo. Circ Res 1981; 49:892–900.

28. Phelps ME, Hoffman EJ, Selin CE, Huang SC, Robinson G, MacDonald N, Schelbert H, Kuhl DE. Investigation of [18-F]2–fluoro 2-deoxyglucose for the measure of myocardial glucose metabolism. J Nucl Med 1978; 19:1311–1319.

29. Ratib O, Phelps ME, Huang SC, Henze E, Selin CE, Schelbert H. Positron tomography with deoxyglucose for estimating local myocardial glucose metabolism. J Nucl Med 1982; 23:577–586.

30. Gambhir SS, Schwaiger M, Huang SC, Krivokapich J, Schelbert HR, Nienaber CA, Phelps ME. Simple noninvasive quantification method for measuring myocardial glucose utilization in humans employing positron emission tomography and fluorine-18 deoxyglucose. J Nucl Med 1989; 30:359–366.

31. Choi Y, Hawkins RA, Huang SC, Gambhir SS, Phelps ME, Schelbert HR. Parametric images of myocardial glucose utilization generated from dynamic cardiac FDG-PET studies (abstract). J Nucl Med 1989; 30:735.

32. Marshall RC, Tillisch JH, Phelps ME, Huang SC, Carson R, Henze E, Schelbert HR. Identification and differentiation of resting myocardial ischemia and infarction in man with positron computed tomography F-18 labeled fluorodeoxyglucose and N-13 ammonia. Circulation 1983; 67:766–778.

33. Schwaiger M, Brunken R, Grover-McKay M, Krivokapich J, Child J, Tillisch JH, Phelps ME, Schelbert HR. Regional myocardial metabolism in patients with acute myocardial infarction assessed by positron emission tomography. J Am Coll Cardiol 1986; 8:800–808.

34. Pierard LA, DeLandsheere CM, Berthe C, Rigo P, Kulbertus HE. Identification of viable myocardium by echocardiography during dobutamine infusion in patients with myocardial infarction after thrombolytic therapy: comparison with positron emission tomography. J Am Coll Cardiol 1990; 15:1021–1031.

35. Camici P, Araujo LI, Spinks T, Lammertsma AA, Kaski JC, Shea MJ, Selwyn AP, Jones T, Maseri A. Increased uptake of F-18 fluorodeoxyglucose in postischemic myocardium of patients with exercise-induced angina. Circulation 1986; 74:81–88.

36. Tillisch J, Brunken R, Marshall R, Schwaiger M, Mandelkern M, Phelps M, Schelbert H. Reversibility of cardiac wall motion abnormalities predicted by positron tomography. N Engl J Med 1986; 314:884–888.

37. Tamaki N, Yonekura Y, Yamashita K, Saji H, Magata Y, Senda M, Konishi Y, Hirata K, Ban T, Konishi J. Positron emission tomography using fluorine-18 deoxyglucose in the evaluation of coronary artery bypass grafting. Am J Cardiol 1989; 64:860–865.

38. Höflin F, Lederman H, Noelpp U, Weinreich R, Rösler H. Routine 18-F-2-deoxy-fluoro-D-Glucose (18-F-FDG) myocardial tomography using a normal large field of view gamma-camera. Angiology 1989; 49:1058–1064.

39. Williams KA, Garvin AA, Stark VL, Holohan KM. Planar imaging of myocardial glucose metabolism and perfusion imaging for detection of residual viability after acute myocardial infarction: correlation with angiographic presence of arterial flow and wall motion (abstract). J Nucl Med 1990; 31(suppl):842.

40. Berry JJ, Hanson MW, Coates D, Hamblen S, Hoffman JM, Coleman RE. FDG cardiac PET image quality is critically affected by glucose loading (abstract). J Nucl Med 1990; 31:840.

41. Gropler RJ, Siegel BA, Lee KJ, Moerlein SM, Perry DJ, Bergmann SR, Gletman EM. Nonuniformity in myocardial accumulation of fluorine-18-fluorodeoxyglucose in normal fasted humans. J Nucl Med 1990; 31:1749–1756.

42. Brunken R, Tillisch J, Schwaiger M, Child JS, Marshall R, Mandelkern M, Phelps ME, Schelbert HR. Regional perfusion, glucose metabolism and wall motion in chronic electrocardiographic Q-wave infarctions. Evidence for persistence of viable tissue in some infarct regions by positron emission tomography. Circulation 1986; 73:951–963.

43. Brunken R, Kottou S, Nienaber C, Schwaiger M, Ratib OM, Phelps ME, Schelbert HR. PET detection of viable tissue in myocardial segments with persistent defects at Tl-201 SPECT. Radiology 1989; 172:65–73.

44. Banka VS, Bodenheimer MM, Helfant RH. Determinants of reversible asynergy: effect of pathological Q waves, coronary collaterals, and anatomic location. Circulation 1974; 50:714–719.

45. Hashimoto T, Kambara H, Fudo T, Hayashi M, Tamaki S, Tokunaga S, Tamaki N, Yonekura Y, Konishi J, Kawai C. Non-Q wave versus Q wave myocardial infarction: regional myocardial metabolism and blood flow assessed by positron emission tomography. J Am Coll Cardiol 1988; 12:88–93.

46. Rozanski A, Berman D, Gray R, Diamond G, Raymond M, Prause J, Maddahi J, Swan HJ, Matloff J. Preoperative prediction of reversible myocardial asynergy by postexercise radionuclide ventriculography. N Eng J Med 1982; 307:212–216.

47. Helfant RH, Pine R, Meister SG, Feldman MS, Trout RG, Banka VS. Nitroglycerin to unmask reversible asynergy: correlation with postcoronary bypass ventriculography. Circulation 1974; 50:108–113.

48. Hamby RI, Aintablian A, Wisoff G, Hartstein ML. Response of the left ventricle in coronary artery disease to postextrasystolic potentiation. Circulation 1975; 51:428–435.

49. Gibson RS, Watson DD, Taylor GJ, Crosby IK, Wellons HL, Holt ND, Beller GA.

Prospective assessment of regional myocardial perfusion before and after coronary revascularization surgery by quantitative thallium-201 scintigraphy. J Am Coll Cardiol 1983; 1:804–815.

50. Liu P, Kiess MC, Okada RD, Block PC, Strauss HW, Pohost GM, Boucher CA. The persistent defect on exercise thallium imaging and its fate after myocardial revascularization: does it represent scar or ischemia? Am Heart J 1985; 110:996–1001.

51. Kiat H, Berman DS, Maddahi J, Yang LD, Van Train K, Rozanski A, Friedman J. Late reversibility of tomographic myocardial thallium-201 defects: an accurate marker of myocardial viability. J Am Coll Cardiol 1988; 12:1456–1463.

52. Brunken R, Schwaiger M, Grover-McKay M, Phelps ME, Tillisch J, Schelbert HR. Positron emission tomography detects tissue metabolic activity in myocardial segments with persistent thallium perfusion defects. J Am Coll Cardiol 1987; 10:557–567.

53. Brunken RB, Mody FV, Hawkins RA, Phelps ME, Schelbert HR. Positron tomography detects glucose metabolism in segments with 24 hour tomographic thallium defects. Circulation 1988; 78(suppl):II-91.

54. Dilsizian V, Rocco TP, Freedman NM, Lean MB, Bonow RO. Enhanced detection of ischemic but viable myocardium by the reinjection of thallium after stress-redistribution imaging. N Engl J Med 1990; 323:141–146.

55. Watson DD, Smith WH, Lillywhite RC, Beller GA. Quantitative analysis of Tl-201 redistribution at 24 hours compared to 2 and 4 hours post injection (abstract). J Nucl Med 1990; 31:763.

56. Ohtani H, Tamaki N, Yonekura Y, Mohiuddin IH, Hirata K, Ban T, Konishi J. Value of thallium-201 reinjection after delayed SPECT imaging for predicting reversible ischemia after coronary artery bypass grafting. Am J Cardiol 1990; 66:394–399.

57. Moore CA, Cannon J, Watson DD, Kaul S, Beller GA. Thallium-201 kinetics in stunned myocardium characterized by severe postischemic systolic dysfunction. Circulation 1990; 81:1622–1632.

58. Villanueva-Meyer J, Mena I, Narahara KA. Simultaneous assessment of left ventricular wall motion and myocardial reperfusion with technetium-99m-methoxy isobutyl isonitrile at stress and rest in patients with angina: comparison with thallium-201 SPECT. J Nucl Med 1990; 31:457–463.

59. Sinusas AJ, Watson DD, Cannon JM, Beller GA. Effect of ischemia and postischemic dysfunction on myocardial uptake of technetium-99m-labelled methoxyisobutyl isonitrile and thallium-201. J Am Coll Cardiol 1989; 14:1785–1793.

60. Rocco TP, Dilsizian V, Strauss HW, Boucher CA. Technetium-99m isonitrile myocardial uptake at rest. II. relation to clinical markers of potential viability. J Am Coll Cardiol 1989; 14:1678–1684.

61. Higgins CB, Saeed M, Wendland M, Chew WM. Magnetic resonance spectroscopy of the heart: overview of studies in animals and man. Invest Radiol 1989; 24:962–968.

62. Wolfe CL, Moseley ME, Wikstrom MG, Sievers RE, Wendland MF, Dupon JW, Finkbeiner WE, Lipton MJ, Parmley WW, Brasch RC. Assessment of myocardial salvage after ischemia and reperfusion using magnetic resonance imaging and spectroscopy. Circulation 1989; 80:969–982.

63. Schaefer S, Gober J, Schwartz GG, Twieg DB, Weiner MW, Massie B. In vivo phosphorus-31 spectroscopic imaging in patients with global myocardial disease. Am J Cardiol 1990; 65:1154–1161.

64. Akins CW, Pohost GM, Desanctis RW, Block PC. Selection of angina-free patients with severe left ventricular dysfunction for myocardial revascularization. Am J Cardiol 1980; 46:695–700.

65. Alderman EL, Fisher LD, Litwin P, Kaiser GC, Myers WO, Maynard C, Levine F, Schloss M. Results of coronary artery surgery in patients with poor left ventricular function (CASS). Circulation 1983; 68:785–795.

66. Passamani E, Davis KB, Gillespie MJ, Killip T. A randomized trial of coronary

artery bypass surgery: survival of patients with a low ejection fraction. N Engl J Med 1985; 312:1665–1671.

67. Bounous EP, Mark DB, Pollock BG, Hlatky MA, Harrell Jr. HE, Lee KL, Rankin S, Wechsler AS, Pryor DB, Califf RM. Surgical survival benefits for coronary disease patients with left ventricular dysfunction. Circulation 1988; 73(suppl I):I-151-I-157.

68. Mody VF, Brunken RC, Stevenson WL, Nienaber CA, Phelps ME, Schelbert HR. Can positron emission tomography distinguish dilated from ischemic cardiomyopathy? (abstract). Circulation 1988; 78(suppl II):II-92.

69. Buxton DB, Vaghaiwalla Mody F, Krivokapich J, Phelps ME, Schelbert HR. Quantitative measurement of sustained metabolic abnormalities in reperfused canine myocardium (abstract). J Nucl Med 1990; 31:795.

70. Nienaber C, Brunken R, Sherman T, et al. Recovery of myocardial metabolism by PET precedes improvement of ischemic wall motion after PTCA (abstract). J Am Coll Cardiol 1988; 13:28A.

Chapter 8

Assessment of Myocardial Amino Acid and Protein Metabolism with the Use of Amino Acids Labeled with Positron-Emitting Radionuclides

Janine Krivokapich, M.D.

Amino acids play pivotal roles in the detoxification of ammonia and in the transfer of reducing equivalents from the cytosol into mitochondria. In addition, amino acids are a source of energy because the oxidative degradation of amino acids can eventually lead to pyruvate, acetyl-CoA, or directly to the tricarboxylic acid (TCA) cycle, as outlined in Figure 8-1. However, not all amino acids are oxidized in the myocardium.

The various roles of amino acids in cardiac metabolism will be reviewed in this chapter with emphasis on their use in conjunction with positron emission tomography (PET). In addition, selected aspects of protein metabolism will be reviewed as they pertain to the heart and the use of positron emission isotopes for the characterization of myocardial protein synthesis.

Myocardial Amino Acid Metabolism

Ammonia

Ammonia is produced from the catabolism of amino acids and nucleic acids. Three reactions result in the removal of free ammonia: the first uses the enzyme glutamate dehydrogenase and results in the formation of the amino acid gluta-

Part of the work reviewed in this chapter was supported by the National Institutes of Health Grant HL 36232 and the U.S. Department of Energy Contract DE-AC03-76-SF00012.

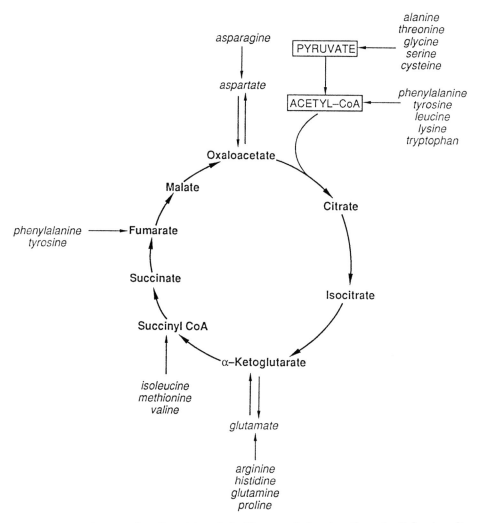

Figure 8-1. *The tricarboxylic acid cycle is illustrated showing the potential entry sites of the amino acids into this cycle. Not all tissues can metabolize every amino acid. Phenylalanine and tyrosine, for example, are essentially not metabolized by myocardium.*

mate, the second is catalyzed by glutamine synthetase and combines ammonia with glutamate to yield glutamine, and the third is the first step in the synthesis of urea, which permits the excretion of ammonia into urine. The relative contributions of these three reactions, diagrammed below, to the trapping of ammonia in myocardial cells have not been defined:

1. NH_3 + α-ketoglutarate $\longleftrightarrow$ glutamate.
2. NH_3 + glutamate + ATP $\rightarrow$ glutamine + ADP + P_1
3. NH_3 + CO_2 + 2 ATP + H_2O $\rightarrow$ carbamyl phosphate

Nitrogen-13 (^{13}N)-labeled ammonia was first introduced as a myocardial imaging agent almost two decades ago[1,2] and has been used extensively as a tracer of myocardial perfusion.[3–5] Bergmann et al.[6] used the isolated perfused rabbit heart and Schelbert et al.[7,8] used a canine model to demonstrate the dependence of myocardial uptake of ^{13}N-ammonia on flow and metabolism.

To delineate the fate of exogenously delivered ^{13}N-ammonia in myocardium, ^{13}N-ammonia was delivered via artery to isolated perfused rabbit interventricular septa.[9,10] Chemical analysis of myocardium 6 minutes after an injection of the tracer revealed that approximately two-thirds of the radioactivity was present in ^{13}N-labeled glutamine and that one-fourth was present as free ^{13}N-ammonia (Table 8-1). The small amount of remaining ^{13}N-radioactivity was detected predominantly in the precipitated protein pellet or in ^{13}N-glutamate and ^{13}N-aspartate. Most of the radioactivity in the effluent was in the chemical form of ^{13}N-ammonia, with less than 15% detected as ^{13}N-glutamine. These results indicated that the predominant mechanism by which ^{13}N radioactivity is retained in myocardial tissue, permitting myocardial imaging after the administration of ^{13}N-ammonia, is the formation of ^{13}N-glutamine from endogenous glutamate via the glutamine synthetase reaction. These findings were consistent with those of Bergmann[6] and Schelbert[7] and their colleagues, who found that perfusion with the glutamine synthetase inhibitor, methionine sulfoximine, resulted in a decrease in the retention of radioactivity in the myocardium after injection of ^{13}N-ammonia. These results were important because glutamine synthetase had been reported to be absent from myocardium.[11]

To determine directly whether the trapping of ^{13}N-ammonia in myocardium results, for the most part, from the action of glutamine synthetase via reaction 2 above, interventricular septa were perfused with methionine sulfoximine before injection of ^{13}N-ammonia.[10] The resulting marked reduction in ^{13}N retention was due to a significant reduction in the formation of ^{13}N-glutamine in tissue. Inhibition of the glutamine synthetase reaction did not divert ^{13}N-ammonia to one of the alternate pathways for its retention, however.

It must be emphasized that these studies explored only the fate of exogenously delivered ^{13}N-ammonia. It is possible that the formation of glutamate via reaction 1 or the formation of urea, which begins with reaction 3, may play an important role in the detoxification of endogenously produced ammonia.

Table 8-1
The Percentage Distribution in Tissue and
in Effluent of ^{13}N 6 Minutes after Injection
of ^{13}N-ammonia

Amino Acid	Tissue %	Effluent %
^{13}N-glutamine	67 ± 19	11 ± 4
^{13}N-ammonia	27 ± 19	88 ± 4
Protein pellet	6 ± 1	9 ± 3

Smirnov et al.[12] have observed urea synthesis in isolated rat hearts. Definitive studies to explore these possibilities have not yet been completed.

Glutamine

Glutamine plays an important role in the myocardium as a reservoir for potentially toxic ammonia, as delineated above. Its concentration is significantly higher than that of any other amino acid, except the amino acid analog taurine. The majority of ^{13}N-labeled glutamine delivered arterially to interventricular rabbit septa is retained in myocardium as ^{13}N-glutamine.[10] Myocardial tissue also has been shown to contain a small quantity of free ^{13}N-ammonia, which indicates the presence of glutaminase or an equivalent enzyme in myocardium because the glutamine synthetase reaction is not reversible. The retention fraction of ^{13}N derived from ^{13}N-labeled glutamine is approximately 20%, which is significantly lower than that of ^{13}N-ammonia (~32%), suggesting that ^{13}N-glutamine is much less permeable than ^{13}N-ammonia. In addition, the clearance of ^{13}N-glutamine delivered exogenously is significantly faster than that of ^{13}N-glutamine endogenously produced from exogenous ^{13}N-ammonia. These data are consistent with compartmentation of myocardial glutamine.

Henze et al.[13] measured the retention fraction of ^{13}N-glutamine delivered into the left anterior descending artery of dogs under control conditions and after induction of ischemia. They found that, in contrast to the high retention fraction (80%) of ^{13}N-ammonia in dogs, the retention fraction for ^{13}N-glutamine was only 10% to 12% under control conditions. With low-flow ischemia, however, this value increased significantly to 20% to 22%. Retention of ^{13}N-glutamine was not affected by addition of the transaminase inhibitor aminooxyacetic acid. These results suggest that a combination of a flow tracer and ^{13}N-glutamine might be useful for the metabolic definition of ischemia with PET.

Glutamate, Aspartate, and Alanine

Glutamate is the second most abundant amino acid in myocardium. It plays an important role in maintaining myocardial nitrogen balance and linking nitrogen metabolism with the TCA cycle because it participates in most of the transamination reactions in myocardial tissue. Alanine and aspartate, the third and fourth most abundant amino acids in myocardium, also participate in transamination reactions. Aspartate and alanine aminotransferase are the 2 most important aminotransferases in myocardium and catalyze the following freely reversible reactions, respectively:

    4. α-ketoglutarate + aspartate ⟷ glutamate + oxaloacetate
    5. α-ketoglutarate + alanine ⟷ glutamate + pyruvate

Glutamate and aspartate, via reaction 4, play important roles in the malate-aspartate shuttle, necessary for the critically important function of transfer of

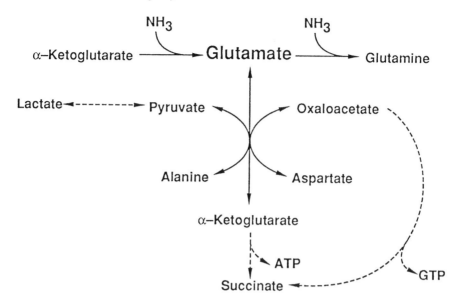

Figure 8-2. *The central role of glutamate in nitrogen metabolism as well as in substrate level phosphorylation is illustrated. Specific reactions are detailed in the text.*

reducing equivalents from the cytosol to mitochondria in the heart.[14,15] Glutamate combines with ammonia to yield glutamine via the glutamine synthetase reaction and is important in the detoxification of ammonia (reaction 2). This reaction may be particularly important in maintaining homeostasis with ischemia or anoxia, when production of ammonia is increased. The central role of glutamate in myocardial metabolism and the interrelationships between the reactions described above are illustrated in Figure 8-2.

Initial analysis of the myocardial exchange of amino acids in human subjects indicated that glutamate was the only naturally occurring amino acid that was extracted by the myocardium.[16,17] Moreover, glutamate was found to be extracted at a higher rate in patients with coronary artery disease.[16,17] Alanine was observed to be the only measured amino acid (glutamine levels were not measured) released by myocardium, and its release was found to be more extensive in patients with coronary artery disease. A more recent study showed that, in patients with coronary artery disease, increased myocardial extraction of glutamate and increased release of both glutamine and alanine occurred at rest compared with values in patients without coronary artery disease.[18] Furthermore, extraction of glutamate was correlated closely with extraction of glucose and lactate, as well as with the detoxification of ammonia through production of glutamine. The increase in glutamate extraction was thought to be related to increased activity of the malate-aspartate cycle resulting from increased myocardial uptake and oxidation of lactate and glucose in hearts of patients with chronic ischemic coronary artery disease.[18] Thus, ischemia may result in specific adaptations in myocardial metabolism of amino acids.

synthetase. This is despite the fact that injection of ^{13}N-ammonia results in the rapid incorporation of ^{13}N into ^{13}N-glutamine, using glutamate as a substrate, with little or none of the ^{13}N label detected in glutamate, aspartate, or alanine. The available data emphasize the complexities of compartmentalization of amino acids in the cell.

Amino acid concentrations in tissue and effluent from rabbit interventricular septa injected with ^{13}N-glutamate indicate that the efflux of alanine is more than 3 times greater than that of glutamate, glutamine, and aspartate.[30] This finding is consistent with the hypothesis that alanine efflux is the major mechanism for removal of amino groups from myocardium.

In studies in rabbit septa it has been observed that anoxia does not affect the retention fraction of ^{13}N-glutamate but does significantly change the distribution of the ^{13}N label.[30] The ^{13}N-alanine distribution increases dramatically from 12% to 39% and ^{13}N-glutamine distribution increases modestly from 4.6% to 6.3% (Table 8-2), whereas ^{13}N-glutamate distribution decreases from 70% to 40% and ^{13}N-aspartate distribution falls from 11% to 5%. Tissue levels of glutamate and aspartate decrease, and those of alanine increase. These results indicate increased production of glycolytically derived pyruvate that combines with ^{13}N-glutamate via reaction 5 to produce ^{13}N-alanine and α-ketoglutarate. As noted previously, α-ketoglutarate and aspartate can enter the TCA cycle at two separate sites and participate in substrate level phosphorylation producing high-energy phosphate compounds and succinate. In addition, ^{13}N-glutamine synthesis may be stimulated modestly, presumably because of excess production of ammonia with anoxia.

In contrast to the results with ^{13}N-glutamate in rabbit septa, anoxia significantly reduces the retention fraction of the ^{13}N label from ^{13}N-ammonia, but does not change the distribution of ^{13}N in tissue, which is found predominantly in the form of ^{13}N-glutamine.[30] Thus, the ^{13}N from labeled glutamate and ammonia is retained by different mechanisms that are differentially affected by anoxia. The demonstration that during oxygen deprivation myocardial ^{13}N-ammonia uptake is decreased without a similar decrease in the uptake of ^{13}N-glutamate is in accord with results obtained with myocardial ischemia in dogs.[13] The results support the notion that a combination of a flow tracer, such as ^{13}N-ammonia, and a putative metabolic marker, ^{13}N-glutamate, might be useful for identification of myocardial ischemia in human subjects with the use of PET.

Knapp[31] and Zimmerman[32] and their colleagues pursued this line of investigation in patients with coronary artery disease. They imaged patients with a planar gamma camera after injection of the flow tracer thallium-201 (^{201}Tl) at peak exercise and after injection of ^{13}N-glutamate at the same exercise level. In 35% to 40% of the patients studied, a mismatch pattern consisting of a relative increase in ^{13}N uptake in an area of decreased ^{201}Tl uptake was observed. These results suggested that ^{13}N-glutamate had potential as a metabolic tracer of use in the detection of ischemia.

PET imaging of ^{13}N-glutamate uptake with exercise has been directly compared with ^{13}N-ammonia imaging under the same conditions in patients

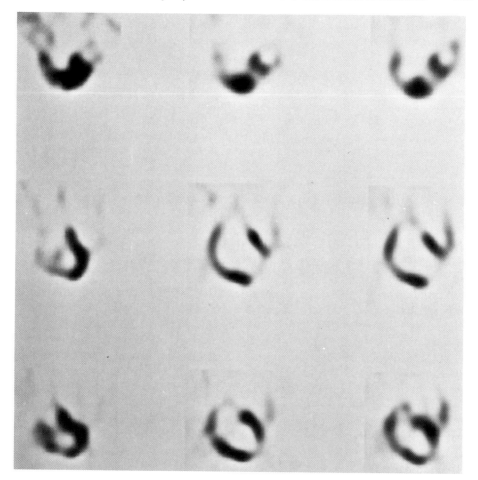

Figure 8-3. *Tomographic images from three planes from a patient with a 100% left anterior descending artery occlusion. The right ventricle appears at the upper left of the image, the interventricular septum is in the middle, the anterior wall is superior, and the lateral wall is on the right side of each image. ^{13}N-glutamate (^{13}N-Glu, top) and ^{13}N-ammonia (^{13}NH$_3$, middle) images were obtained under conditions of similar exercise stress. ^{18}F-fluorodeoxyglucose (FDG, bottom) was injected after the second exercise period. Similar anterior defects are observed on both the ^{13}N-glutamate and ^{13}N-ammonia images, with a marked increase in accumulation of ^{18}F-fluorodeoxyglucose in the anterior wall extending into the anterior interventricular septum. The mismatched ^{13}N-ammonia and ^{18}F-fluorodeoxyglucose defects are consistent with ischemia. There is no evidence of increased uptake of ^{13}N-glutamate in the ischemic region. Instead, ^{13}N-glutamate uptake parallels the uptake of the flow tracer.*

with suspected coronary artery disease (Figure 8-3).[33] In 12 of 17 patients studied, reductions in ^{13}N-ammonia uptake occurred in the distribution of a stenosed coronary artery. In each patient, ^{13}N-glutamate uptake with exercise paralleled ^{13}N-ammonia uptake with exercise. Eleven of these patients underwent imaging with fluorine-18 (^{18}F)-fluorodeoxyglucose after exercise. In 7, a ^{18}F-fluorodeoxyglucose/^{13}N-ammonia mismatch consistent with myocardial ischemia was observed. Thus, despite the presence of myocardial ischemia demonstrated with ^{18}F-fluorodeoxyglucose, there was no evidence that ^{13}N-glutamate uptake was enhanced in the same distribution. This study therefore failed to document the usefulness of ^{13}N-glutamate as a metabolic marker of ischemia. Instead, in this study, ^{13}N-glutamate appeared to behave as a flow marker similar to ^{13}N-ammonia.[33] This result can be explained, in part, by the very high uptake of ^{13}N-glutamate by human myocardium, which is even higher than that of ^{13}N-ammonia, in contrast to the much lower uptake of ^{13}N-glutamate in hearts of rabbits and dogs. It is not possible to directly compare these results[33] with those of others[31,32] to resolve the discrepancies because of differences in imaging modalities (PET vs planar gamma camera imaging) and in flow tracers used (^{13}N-ammonia vs ^{201}Tl).

^{13}N-labeled alanine, aspartate, glutamine, and leucine, as well as ^{13}N-glutamate, exhibit increased retention fractions of the ^{13}N label with ischemia in dogs.[13,34] However, only ^{13}N-glutamate imaging of human myocardium has been explored with PET to date.

In addition to labeling amino acids with ^{13}N, it is possible to label one of the carbons with the positron emitter carbon-11 (^{11}C). This has been accomplished with aspartic acid, which was labeled at the first carbon.[35] The retention fraction of ^{11}C-aspartate after intracoronary injection in dogs was only 13%. ^{11}C radioactivity cleared the myocardium rapidly and measurements of ^{11}C-carbon dioxide in the blood indicated that ^{11}C-aspartate was assimilated rapidly in the TCA cycle. These data suggest that ^{11}C-aspartate may be a useful tracer for assessment of TCA cycle activity. In pilot experiments with PET imaging with ^{11}C-aspartate, the retention fraction was much higher in rhesus monkeys than in dogs. Thus, as is the case for ^{13}N-glutamate, the retention fraction of ^{11}C-aspartate may be relatively high in humans. The utility of ^{11}C-aspartate for imaging myocardial metabolism with PET in human subjects has not yet been investigated.

Branched-Chain Amino Acids

In addition to being protein building blocks, the branched-chain amino acids, leucine, isoleucine, and valine, enter the TCA cycle after first being transaminated with α-ketoglutarate to yield glutamic acid and the respective α-ketoacid. All 3 α-ketoacids are then oxidized with the release of carbon dioxide and NADH. Valine and isoleucine enter the TCA cycle at the succinyl-CoA step and leucine enters at the acetyl-CoA step. Leucine, but not valine or isoleucine, has been shown to stimulate protein synthesis and inhibit protein degradation in modified Langendorff rat heart preparations.[36] No other amino acid studied has this same effect in this preparation. The effect of leucine on protein synthesis and degradation is similar to that of insulin but of less magnitude. Mechanisms responsible have not yet been elucidated.

Leucine and valine have been labeled with ^{13}N and leucine has been labeled with ^{11}C at the first (carboxyl) carbon.[37] The retention fractions of ^{13}N-leucine and ^{13}N-valine in canine myocardium are 25% and 17%, respectively, under control conditions. The retention fractions of both ^{13}N amino acids are significantly reduced in the presence of the nonspecific transaminase inhibitor aminooxyacetate, and the clearance half-times of the retained fraction are markedly shortened. These data emphasize the importance of transaminase reactions in the retention of these amino acids. Low-flow ischemia, on the other hand, results in significantly increased retention fractions for both ^{13}N-leucine and ^{13}N-valine, without a change in the clearance half-times.[37] Further investigation is required to explain this phenomenon, but it is possible that the increased retention is related to the influence of leucine and valine on increasing the levels of TCA cycle intermediates at a time when they have become depleted. As with ^{13}N-glutamate, properly labeled branch chain amino acids could be used as metabolic markers of ischemia. However, given the marked variation in the uptake of amino acids in different species, studies with these amino acids in human subjects are necessary to address this possibility.

The retention fraction of ^{11}C-leucine in canine myocardium is only 15%, compared with the 25% retention fraction observed for ^{13}N-leucine.[37] The time-activity curves for ^{11}C-leucine are similar to those for ^{11}C-aspartate.[35] The more rapid clearance of ^{11}C compared with ^{13}N from leucine is secondary to the decarboxylation of ^{11}C-leucine, which yields ^{11}C-carbon dioxide that, as with ^{11}C-aspartate, freely diffuses from the myocardium. The rapid removal of the radioactive label from ^{11}C-leucine that has been metabolized is an advantage when incorporation of ^{11}C-leucine into protein is being measured because the ^{11}C label that remains in tissue is largely trapped in proteins.

Myocardial Protein Metabolism

Myocardial proteins are in a dynamic state of continuous synthesis and continuous degradation. Both are energy-requiring processes, although they account for only a small portion of the total oxygen requirement expenditure of myocardial cells. Myocardial viability is intimately linked to protein metabolism. Approximately one-sixth of the wet weight of the heart is accounted for by protein,[38] and 50% of the total myocardial protein complement is in myofibrils, predominantly in actin and myosin.[38] Mitochondrial proteins comprise approximately 25% of myocytic protein. Proteins play a critical role in maintaining the structural integrity of myocardium and in enzymatic reactions. A complex and intricate system has evolved that controls the concentrations of specific proteins in the cellular and extracellular spaces of the heart. Ultimately, concentrations at any time are a result of the two competing processes, synthesis and degradation. Under steady-state conditions, a balance between the two must exist. The rate of turnover is protein specific. On average, the myocardial protein pool turns over every 1 to 2 weeks.

Protein Synthesis

Amino acids, the building blocks of proteins, are present both cellularly and extracellularly. Some intracellular amino acids are synthesized. Some arise only from breakdown of protein. Many are imported from the extracellular space by various transport mechanisms, most notably the alanine-(A-system) and the leucine-preferred systems (L-system). Several transport systems are energy dependent. However, physiologic intracellular concentrations of amino acids do not appear to be a rate-limiting step in protein synthesis.

Amino acids destined for incorporation into protein are acylated and coupled to specific transfer RNAs (tRNAs) by the enzymatic action of aminoacyl-tRNA synthetases, the immediate precursors of protein metabolism. Several labeled amino acids, including phenylalanine, tyrosine, valine, lysine, and leucine, have been used as tracers of myocardial protein metabolism. An ideal amino acid for this purpose would not be synthesized or degraded by myocardium.

Protein synthesis begins with transcription of DNA to form messenger RNA (mRNA) specific for a given protein. The mRNA is transported into the cytoplasm, where it attaches itself to ribosomes in preparation for assembly of polypeptide chains. An initiation factor begins translation of the mRNA codons into amino acid sequences. An elongation factor facilitates the formation of peptide bonds between successive amino acids. When protein synthesis is completed, a termination factor facilitates release of newly synthesized peptide chains from the RNA complex.

Protein Degradation

The breakdown of proteins is largely an all or none process and occurs primarily by hydrolysis of peptide bonds via proteolytic enzymes present within the cell. There are two major pathways for protein degradation.[38,39] The first is basal or microautophagy and entails the continual, random removal of proteins from their individual cellular pools into microvesicles with degradation by lysosomal particle enzymes. Larger proteins exhibit more rapid turnover by this mechanism than do smaller proteins. A second mechanism, accelerated proteolysis or macroautophagy, involves sequestration of a region of cytoplasm into membrane-limited vacuoles that fuse with lysosomes, inducing complete protein degradation through the action of lysosomal proteases. A third mechanism of protein degradation, which does not involve lysosomes, has been noted with myofibrillar proteins and involves a calcium-dependent proteinase present at the Z lines of myofibrils.[38,39] All three processes result in the release of free amino acids into the cytoplasm where they can be reutilized in protein synthesis or in other chemical reactions.

Quantification of Protein Metabolism

Traditionally, myocardial protein synthesis and degradation have been quantified in vitro and in vivo after administration of amino acids labeled with carbon-14 (^{14}C) or hydrogen-3 (^{3}H). However, the specific activity of the labeled amino acid in the specific protein synthesis precursor pool is difficult to measure. Approximations are usually made from measurements of specific activity in the extracellular or intracellular space.[40] On occasion, the relative rates of synthesis of two different cardiac proteins are compared, obviating the need for determination of the specific activity of the precursor pool.

When specifically measuring protein degradation, a problem encountered is that it is difficult to correct for reutilization of labeled amino acids into new proteins. The degree of reutilization of an amino acid depends both on the specific amino acid and its concentration in the intracellular space.[40]Protein degradation is often estimated as the difference between cardiac growth and protein synthesis. Turnover rates of protein can also be measured, particularly under steady-state conditions when the rates of synthesis and degradation are equal. Under these conditions, turnover can be equated with the fractional rate of degradation.[41]

Most studies assess synthesis and degradation of the total protein pool in the heart, rather than that of an individual protein. Results reflect contributions from the whole myocardial tissue, which includes a mixture of myocytes, fibroblasts, and endothelial cells, as well as the interstitial space. Despite these confounding difficulties, much has been learned regarding myocardial protein metabolism under basal conditions, stress, and in response to hormonal stimulation.

Protein Metabolism in Cardiac Hypertrophy

Effects of Increased Afterload

Long-term increases in afterload result in an increase in myocardial protein content and ventricular hypertrophy. With hypertrophy, the number of contractile units is increased and wall stress is thereby normalized.[42] Myocardial protein metabolism has been assessed with the use of [14]C- or ^{3}H-labeled amino acids such as phenylalanine, tyrosine, lysine, or leucine to delineate mechanisms underlying development of hypertrophy.

Results in vitro show that increased afterload leads to a rapid increase in protein synthesis[40,43] and that the acceleration of synthesis is not attributable directly to increased coronary flow, intraventricular pressure development, or oxygen consumption. Apparently, it is related to stretching of the ventricular wall as a result of elevated aortic pressure (the "garden hose effect").[44] The positive effect of stretch on protein synthesis was first described in quiescent papillary muscles.[45]

A biochemical signal linking stretch of the myocardium to increased protein synthesis has been sought. Sodium influx has been shown to be important in the stimulation of growth in many cell types.[46] Studies by Kent et al. with ferret papillary muscles have explored the possibility that increased afterload stimulated sodium influx via stretch-activated sodium channels, and that increased sodium influx is a signal to increase protein synthesis.[47] Measurement of protein synthesis at varying degrees of passive and/or active tension in quiescent and contracting muscles revealed that rates of protein synthesis increased in proportion to total tension, regardless of whether the muscle contracted. The rate of sodium-24 ([24]Na) uptake correlated directly with the total tension development. Pharmacologic interventions with inotropic agents, all of which increase tension development but have diverse effects on sodium influx, demonstrated that those agents that increased ^{24}Na influx also increased protein synthesis. Inotropic interventions that decreased ^{24}Na influx, despite increasing tension development, decreased protein synthesis. Thus, myocardial protein synthesis was consistently correlated with sodium influx, but not with tension development.[47] Accordingly, stretch-dependent sodium influx may be an important signal in processes leading to cell growth.[47]

Investigation of the direct effect of an increased afterload on protein degradation has been particularly difficult and has produced differing results. It is complicated by the presence of the focal myocardial necrosis that results from acute introduction of stress of this kind. Presently, the consensus is that the rate of degradation is not consistently or significantly changed early after the induction of physiologic stress. However, once a new steady-state is reached, degradation increases to parallel the increased synthesis.[40,43]

Effects of Increased Preload or Volume Loading

Although hypertrophy is a frequent accompaniment of chronic volume loading of the ventricle, it has not been possible to detect increased protein synthesis in its initial phases.[40] Thus, there is a distinct temporal difference in the development of hypertrophy in the presence of the two different loading conditions most often studied (increased afterload and increased preload).

Protein Metabolism with Physiologic, Rapid Growth

The study of protein metabolism under conditions in which pathologically induced hypertrophy develops secondary to increased afterload is hampered because focal necrosis may develop, mechanical performance may be impaired, and/or high-energy phosphate content may be reduced.[48] The newborn pig heart has been used for study of development of cardiac hypertrophy[48] because the left ventricle grows much more rapidly than the right in the neonates, presumably in response to the higher physiologic afterload imposed on the left ventricle after parturition. During the first 10 days, the rate of accumulation of protein (not synthesis) is 3 times greater in the left compared with the right ventricular free wall.[48] Measurement of the rate of protein synthesis with ^{14}C-labeled phenylalanine after 5 days of life demonstrates a twofold difference between the left and right ventricular walls. The increase reflects both greater efficiency of protein synthesis (nmol phenylalanine incorporated/mg RNA/hr) and greater capacity in terms of the amount of RNA to be translated.[48]

Manifestations of Thyroxine-Induced Hypertrophy

Administration of thyroid hormone has been used to induce cardiac hypertrophy. In rabbits studied with ^{3}H-leucine, high doses of thyroxine were shown to markedly accelerate both protein synthesis and degradation, with acceleration of synthesis predominating.[49] Cardiac growth and increased protein synthesis have been induced with physiologic doses of thyroxine given to hypothyroid rats.[50] In both models, mechanical function and high-energy phosphate levels were preserved and focal necrosis was absent.[43,48] In rats, the hypertrophic effect of thyroxine can be blocked by propranolol.[51] Thyroxine does not elicit hypertrophy in orthotopically transplanted, nonworking hearts even though the native heart in situ responds with significant hypertrophy.[51] Thus, it seems likely that the effects of thyroid hormone on protein metabolism are secondary to the increased cardiac work induced by peripheral responses to the hormone.

Protein Synthetic Capacity

Rapid cardiac growth with increased protein synthesis induced by thyroid hormone and other interventions has been associated with increases in total RNA and accelerated synthesis of ribosomes.[43] Thus, the increased protein synthesis appears to be supported by or dependent on an increased capacity for protein synthesis.

Hormonal Effects on Myocardial Protein Metabolism

Compared with perfusion without insulin, addition of insulin to the perfusate of Langendorff rat heart preparations results in a marked increase in the rate of protein synthesis, as determined with ^{14}C-phenylalanine. Insulin stimulates peptide chain initiation and inhibits protein degradation.[52,53] Catecholamines such as isoproterenol and phenylephrine, along with glucagon, also inhibit protein degradation.[54]

Glucocorticoids exhibit catabolic effects on skeletal muscle. Studies on the effects of glucocorticoids on cardiac protein synthesis have not yielded consistent results. Clark et al.[55] treated rats with dexamethasone and reported an early increase in protein synthesis that was greater than an accompanying increase in protein degradation. However, Czerwinski et al.[56] found that rats treated with hydrocortisone for 15 days initially exhibited cardiac enlargement, but the cardiac enlargement was not maintained at 15 days. During the anabolic phase of the glucocorticoid effect, no evidence of stimulation of total protein or of myosin heavy-chain synthesis was obtained.[56] Moreover, after approximately 1 week, the total protein and myosin heavy-chain synthesis rates were markedly reduced. This change preceded the cardiac muscle loss by ≥ 1 week.[56] More work is required to clarify the direct effects of glucocorticoids on ventricular muscle.

Effects of Fasting on Myocardial Protein Metabolism

Results of studies with ^{3}H-leucine in rabbits demonstrate that prolonged fasting profoundly inhibits protein synthesis in vivo, including the synthesis of actin and myosin.[57] In addition, the fractional rate of degradation is increased.[57] Fasting of rats decreases protein synthesis, particularly in the myofibrillar fraction.[58] Studies in vitro demonstrate that the rate of actin synthesis in vitro is more reduced than that of myosin in the heart, but not in skeletal muscle.[59]

Effects of Ischemia, Hypoxia, Anoxia, and Cardiac Arrest on Myocardial Protein Metabolism

Protein synthesis is inhibited in vitro by anoxia in isolated rat hearts. Incorporation of intracellular amino acids into proteins is prevented.[60] Inhibition of protein synthesis occurs also in isolated anoxic rabbit right ventricular papillary muscle preparations.[61] Perfusion of anoxic muscle with 15 mM glucose does not attenuate the inhibition, despite the fact that tissue levels of high-energy phosphates are similar to those in control muscles.[61] In contrast, in preparations without increased glucose in the perfusate, in which mild hypoxia results in a reduction of high-energy phosphate levels, protein synthesis is normal.[61] These results concur with those of studies of protein synthesis in rat hearts in vivo in which mild hypoxia (10% ambient oxygen for 24 hours) did not inhibit protein synthesis, but severe hypoxia (5% ambient oxygen for 1 to 2 hours) did.[58] Furthermore, decreased synthesis has been observed in all three subcellular protein fractions studied: soluble, myofibrillar, and stromal. Thus, the effect of oxygen deprivation on cardiac protein synthesis did not correlate directly with overall high-energy phosphate stores.

Chua et al. studied the effects of anoxia (0% oxygen), hypoxia (30% oxygen), and low-flow ischemia on protein degradation (with ^{14}C-phenylalanine in rat hearts).[62] Protein degradation was inhibited in each case. In contrast to the case in controls, insulin had no additional inhibitory effect on protein degradation. Although high-energy phosphate levels were decreased by anoxia and ischemia, they did not decrease with hypoxia. Again, a dissociation between high-energy phosphate stores and protein degradation rates was evident.[62]

The effects of metabolites that accumulate with hypoxia, such as lactate and hydrogen ion, have been examined.[62] Both lowering of pH to 7.0 and the addition of 50 mM lactate to aerobic or anoxic hearts resulted in inhibition of protein degradation.[62] Thus, inhibition of protein degradation by hypoxia is likely to be multifactorial.

Effects of cardiac arrest on protein synthesis have been studied in guinea pig hearts in vitro that were arrested with 16 mEq/liter K+ but perfused aerobically.[63] No decrease in protein synthesis occurred. In contrast, when hearts were arrested by hypocalcemia, marked inhibition of protein synthesis and degradation ensued.[40] Cardiac arrest induced by the introduction of anoxia, in the presence of 4 mEq/liter K+ in the perfusate, occurred in 30 to 40 minutes and was associated with a reduction in both high-energy phosphate stores and protein synthetic rates. However, when anoxia was accompanied by perfusion with 16 mEq/liter K+, cardiac arrest was immediate and neither high-energy phosphates nor protein synthesis declined.[63] Thus, integrity of protein synthesis during anoxia is maintained by the presence of high concentrations of potassium. This is one reason why cardioplegic solutions used in cardiac surgery contain high concentrations of potassium.

Effects of Heart Muscle Contraction on Myocardial Protein Metabolism

Increases in afterload often result in increased contractile performance. Acetaldehyde, a metabolite of ethanol that transiently increases contractile performance and heart rate inhibits, rather than stimulates, myocardial protein synthesis.[64] Perfusion with calcium in concentrations that increase contractility does not increase myocardial protein synthesis.[64]

To determine whether decreased contractile activity contributes to the inhibition of protein degradation observed under conditions of reduced oxygen supply in the rat heart, tetrodotoxin, which stops contractile activity, has been added to perfusates. Protein degradation was not affected.[62] Furthermore, in guinea pig hearts perfused with an aerobic perfusate to which high K^+ was added to induce arrest, protein synthesis did not decrease,[63] indicating that protein synthesis in normal myocardium is not dependent on contraction of the heart—at least in the short term.

Effects of Ethanol on Myocardial Protein Metabolism

Pathophysiologic mechanisms responsible for development of conditions such as alcohol-induced cardiomyopathy have not yet been defined. In vitro, ethanol in concentrations that inhibit hepatic protein synthesis do not inhibit cardiac protein synthesis.[40] However, the primary metabolite of ethanol, acetaldehyde, despite its positive inotropic and chronotropic effects on the heart, does inhibit protein synthesis.[40] The concentrations of acetaldehyde that inhibit protein synthesis occur in vivo with only moderate intoxication. Interestingly, effects of this metabolite on protein synthesis persist even when chronotropic and inotropic effects are blocked by a β-adrenergic blocker.[40] Thus, the effect of acetaldehyde on protein synthesis may contribute to the development of alcohol-induced heart disease.

Regulation of Cardiac Protein Metabolism

Much investigation now focuses on the regulation of protein synthesis and degradation. How is gene expression modulated? What are the specific biochemical triggers and inhibitors of altered synthesis and degradation?

Stimulation of gene expression in the heart is extremely rapid. It can occur within 30 minutes.[42] In guinea pig hearts subjected to increased left ventricular afterload, protein synthesis increased by 80% within 3 hours after the induction of physiologic stress.[64] Most of the increase occurs in soluble and myofibrillar fractions. Myosin synthesis increases in this interval, but the rate of synthesis of collagen and of myoglobin does not change.[64]

Muscles of diverse types contain similar proteins (but in different proportions). In dogs, the average half-time of ventricular protein synthesis is 8.4 ± 0.3 days compared with 12.2 ± 1.1 days for synthesis in diaphragm (a predominantly red tonic fiber-type muscle) and 18.1 ± 0.8 days for vastus

use in studies of brain protein metabolism because a substantial amount of the compound is hydroxylated to tyrosine.[71]

If it can be established that positron-labeled amino acids can be used with PET, and an appropriate tracer kinetic model for estimation of protein synthesis in the heart validated, the applications will be broad. Viability of myocardial cells is obviously dependent on protein synthesis. Altered protein synthesis may well underlie conditions such as cardiac failure. Elucidation of protein synthesis in human studies in vivo offers promise for clarification of pathophysiology and development of improved therapeutic approaches based on their impact on objective end points that are presently elusive.

References

1. Hunter WW, Monahan WG. ^{13}N-ammonia: a new physiologic radiotracer for molecular medicine. J Nucl Med 1971; 12:368 (abstract).
2. Harper PV, Lathrop KA, Krizek H, Lembares N, Stark V, Hoffer PB. Clinical feasibility of myocardial imaging with ^{13}NH$_3$. J Nucl Med 1972; 13:278–280.
3. Gould KL, Schelbert HR, Phelps ME, Hoffman EJ. Noninvasive assessment of coronary stenoses with myocardial perfusion imaging during pharmacologic coronary vasodilation. V. Detection of 47 percent diameter coronary stenosis with intravenous nitrogen-13 ammonia and emission-computed tomography in intact dogs. Am J Cardiol 1979; 43:200–208.
4. Phelps ME, Hoffman EJ, Coleman RE, et al. Tomographic images of blood pool and perfusion in brain and heart. J Nucl Med 1976; 17:603–612.
5. Walsh WF, Harper PV, Resnekov L, Fill H. Noninvasive evaluations of regional myocardial perfusion in 112 patients using mobile scintillation camera and intravenous nitrogen-13 labeled ammonia. Circulation 1976; 54:1811–1814.
6. Bergmann SR, Hack S, Tewson T, Welch MJ, Sobel BE. The dependence of accumulation of ^{13}NH$_3$ by myocardium on metabolic factors and its implication of quantitative assessment of perfusion. Circulation 1980; 61:34–43.
7. Schelbert HR, Phelps ME, Hoffman EJ, Huang SC, Selin CE, Kuhl DE. Regional myocardial perfusion assessed with N-13 labeled ammonia and positron emission computerized axial tomography. Am J Cardiol 1979; 43:209–218.
8. Schelbert HR, Phelps ME, Huang SC, et al. N-13 ammonia as an indicator of myocardial blood flow. Factors influencing its uptake and retention in myocardium. Circulation 1981; 63:1259–1272.
9. Krivokapich J, Huang SC, Phelps ME, MacDonald NS, Shine KI. Dependence of ^{13}NH$_3$ myocardial extraction and clearance on flow and metabolism. Am J Physiol 1982; 242:H536–542.
10. Krivokapich J, Barrio JR, Phelps ME, et al. Kinetic characterization of ^{13}NH$_3$ and [^{13}N]glutamine metabolism in rabbit heart. Am J Physiol 1984; 246:H267–273.
11. Iqbal K, Ottaway JH. Glutamine synthetase in muscle and kidney. Biochem J 1970; 119:145–156.
12. Smirnov VN, Asafov GB, Cherpachenko NM, Chernousova GB, Mozzhechkov VT, Krivov VI. Ammonia neutralization and urea synthesis in cardiac muscle. Circ Res 1974; 34(suppl III):58–69.
13. Henze E, Schelbert HR, Barrio JR, et al. Evaluation of myocardial metabolism with N-13 and C-11 labeled amino acids and positron computed tomography. J Nucl Med 1982; 23:671–681.
14. Safer B. The metabolic significance of the malate aspartate cycle in heart. Circ Res 1975; 37:527–533.
15. Williamson JR, Cooper RN. Regulation of the citric acid cycle in mammalian systems. FEBS Lett 1980; 177(suppl):K73-K85.

16. Mudge GH, Mills RM, Taegtmeyer H, Gorlin R, Lesch M. Alterations of myocardial amino acid metabolism in chronic ischemic heart disease. J Clin Inves 1976; 58:1185–1192.

17. Thomassen AR, Nielsen TT, Bagger JP, Henningsen P. Myocardial exchanges of glutamate, alanine, and citrate in controls and patients with coronary artery disease. Clinical Science 1983; 64:33–40.

18. Pisarenko OI, Baranov AV, Aleshin OI, et al. Features of myocardial metabolism of some amino acids and ammonia in patients with coronary artery disease. Eur Heart J 1989; 10:209–217.

19. Taegtmeyer H, Peterson MB, Ragavan VV, Ferguson AG, Lesch M. De novo alanine synthesis in isolated oxygen deprived rabbit myocardium. J Biol Chem 1977; 252:5010–5018.

20. Taegtmeyer H. Metabolic responses to cardiac hypoxia. Increased production of succinate by rabbit papillary muscles. Circ Res 1978; 43:808–815.

21. Sanborn T, Gavin W, Berkowitz S, Perille T, Lesch M. Augmented conversion of aspartate and glutamate to succinate during anoxia in rabbit heart. Am J Physiol 1979; 237:H535–541.

22. Rau EE, Shine KI, Gervais A, Douglas AM, Amos ECIII. Enhanced mechanical recovery of anoxic and ischemic myocardium by amino acid perfusion. Am J Physiol 1979; 236:H873–879.

23. Bittl JA, Shine KI. Protection of ischemic rabbit myocardium by glutamic acid. Am J Physiol 1983; 245:H406–412.

24. Choong YS, Gavin JB, Armiger LC. Effects of glutamic acid on cardiac function and energy metabolism of rat heart during ischemia and reperfusion. J Mol Cell Cardiol 1988; 20:1043–1051.

25. Pisarenko OI, Solomatina ES, Studneva IM, Ivanov VE, Kapelko VI, Smirnov VN. Protective effect of glutamic acid on cardiac function and metabolism during cardioplegia and reperfusion. Basic Res Cardiol 1983; 78:534–543.

26. Lazar HL, Buckberg GD, Manganaro AJ, Becker H, Maloney JV. Reversal of ischemic damage with amino acid substrate enhancement during reperfusion. Surgery 1980; 88:702–709.

27. Rosenkranz ER, Okamoto F, Buckberg GC, Vinten-Johansen J, Robertson JM, Bugyi H. Safety of prolonged aortic clamping with blood cardioplegia. II. Glutamate enrichment in energy-depleted hearts. J Thorac Cardiovasc Surg 1984; 88:402–410.

28. Gelbard AS, Benua RS, Reiman RE, McDonald JM, Vomero JJ, Laughlin JS. Imaging of the human heart after administration of L-[^{13}NH$_3$]glutamate. J Nucl Med 1980; 21:988–991.

29. Gelbard AS, Clarke LP, McDonald JM, Monahan WG, Tilbury RS, Kuo TYT, Laughlin JS. Enzymatic synthesis and organ distribution studies with ^{13}N-labeled L-glutamine and L-glutamic acid. Radiology 1975; 116:127–132.

30. Krivokapich J, Keen RE, Phelps ME, Shine KI, Barrio JR. Effects of anoxia of kinetics of [^{13}N]glutamate and ^{13}NH$_3$ metabolism in rabbit myocardium. Circ Res 1987; 60:505–516.

31. Knapp WH, Helus F, Ostertag H, Tillmanns H, Kubler W. Uptake and turnover of l-[^{13}N]glutamate in the normal human heart and in patients with coronary artery disease. Eur J Nucl Med 1982; 7:211–215.

32. Zimmermann R, Tillmanns H, Knapp WH, et al. Regional myocardial nitrogen-13 glutamate uptake in patients with coronary artery disease: inverse post-stress relation to thallium-201 uptake in ischemia. J Am Coll Cardiol 1988; 11:549–556.

33. Krivokapich J, Barrio JR, Huang S-C, Schelbert HR. Dynamic positron tomographic imaging with N-13 glutamate in patients with coronary artery disease: comparison with N-13 ammonia and F-18 fluorodeoxyglucose imaging. J Am Coll Cardiol 1990; 16:1158–1167.

34. Baumgartner F, Barrio JR, Henze E, et al. ^{13}N-labeled L-amino acids for in vivo assessment of local myocardial metabolism. J Med Chem 1981; 24:764–766.

35. Barrio JR, Egbert JE, Henze E, Schelbert HR, Baumgartner FJ. L-[4-^{11}C]aspartic

acid: Enzymatic synthesis, myocardial uptake and metabolism. J Med Chem 1982; 25:93–96.

36. Chua B, Siehl DL, Morgan HE. Effect of leucine and metabolites of branched-chain amino acids on protein turnover in heart. J Biol Chem 1979; 254:8358–8362.

37. Barrio JR, Baumgartner FJ, Henze E, et al. Synthesis and myocardial kinetics of N-13 and C-11 labeled branched-chain L-amino acids. J Nucl Med 1983; 24:937–944.

38. Gevers W. Protein metabolism of the heart. J Mol Cell Cardiol 1984; 16:30–32.

39. Mortimore GE, Poso AR. Intracellular protein catabolism and its control during nutrient deprivation and supply. Annu Rev Nutr 1987; 7:539–564.

40. Schreiber SS, Evans CD, Oratz M. Protein synthesis degradation in cardiac stress. Circ Res 1981; 48:601–611.

41. Schimke R. Protein degradation in vivo and its regulation. Circ Res 1976; 38(suppl II):I-131-I-134.

42. Moalic JM, Swynghedauw B. Regulation of gene expression in the normal and overloaded heart. In: Legato MJ, ed. The Stressed Heart. Boston: Martinus Nijhoff Publishing, 1987: 1–19.

43. Morgan HE, Gordon EE, Kira Y, et al. Biochemical mechanisms of cardiac hypertrophy. Annu Rev Physiol 1987; 49:533–543.

44. Gordon EE, Kira Y, Morgan HE. Aortic perfusion pressure, protein synthesis, and protein degradation. Circulation 1987; 75(suppl I):I-78-I-80.

45. Peterson MB, Lesch M. Protein synthesis and amino acid transport in the isolated rabbit right ventricular papillary muscle. Effect of isometric tension development. Circ Res 1972; 31:317–327.

46. Leffert HL, Koch KS. Growth regulation by sodium ion influxes. In: Boynton A, Leffert HL, eds. Control of Animal Cell Proliferation. New York: Academic Press, 1985; 367–413.

47. Kent RL, Hoober JK, Cooper G. Load responsiveness of protein synthesis in adult mammalian myocardium: Role of cardiac deformation linked to sodium influx. Circ Res 1989; 64:74–85.

48. Morgan HE. The newborn pig heart, a superior animal model of cardiac hypertrophy. In: Anand IS, Wahi PL, Dhalla NS, eds. Pathophysiology and Pharmacology of Heart Disease. Boston: Kluwer Academic Publishers, 1989; 1–7.

49. Parmacek MS, Magid NM, Lesch M, Decker RS, Samerel AM. Cardiac protein synthesis and degradation during thyroxine-induced left ventricular hypertrophy. Am J Physiol 1986; 251:C727–736.

50. Hjalmarson AC, Rannels DE, Kao R, Morgan HE. Effects of hypophysectomy, growth hormone and thyroxine on protein turnover in the heart. J Biol Chem 1975; 250:4556–4561.

51. Klein I, Hong C. Role of thyroid hormone in the regulation of cardiac hypertrophy. In: Dhalla N, Singal PK, Beamish RE, eds. Pathophysiology of Heart Disease. Boston: Martinus Nijhoff Publishing, 1987; 73–81.

52. Morgan HE, Hefferson LS, Wolpert EB, Rannels DE. Regulation of protein synthesis in heart muscle. II. Effect of amino acid levels and insulin on ribosomal aggregation. J Biol Chem 1971; 246:2163–2170.

53. McKee EE, Cheung JY, Rannels DE, Morgan HE. Measurement of the rates of protein synthesis and compartmentation of heart phenylalanine. J Biol Chem 1978; 253:1030–1040.

54. Chua BHL, Watkins CA, Siehl CL, Morgan HE. Effect of epinephrine and glucagon on protein turnover in perfused rat heart. Fed Proc 1978; 37:1333 (abstract).

55. Clark AF, DeMartino GN, Wildenthal K. Effects of glucocorticoid treatment on cardiac protein synthesis and degradation. Am J Physiol 1986; 250:C821–827.

56. Czerwinski SM, Kurowski TT, McKee EE, Zak R, Hickson RC. Myosin heavy chain turnover during cardiac mass changes by glucocorticoids. J Appl Physiol 1991; 70:300–305.

57. Samarel AM, Parmacek MS, Magid NM, Decker RS, Lesch M. Protein synthesis and degradation during starvation-induced cardiac atrophy in rabbits. Circ Res 1987; 60:933–941.

58. Preedy VR, Sugen PH. The effects of fasting or hypoxia on rates of protein synthesis in vivo in subcellular fractions of rat heart and gastrocnemium muscle. Biochem J 1989; 257:519–527.

59. Clark AF, Wildenthal K. Disproportionate reduction of actin synthesis in hearts of starved rats. J Biol Chem 1986; 261:13163–13172.

60. Jefferson LS, Wolpert EB, Giger KE, Morgan HE. Regulation of protein synthesis in heart muscle. III. Effect of anoxia on protein synthesis. J Biol Chem 1971; 246:2171–2178.

61. Lesch M, Taegtmeyer H, Peterson MB, Vernick R. Mechanism of the inhibition of myocardial protein synthesis during oxygen deprivation. Am J Physiol 1976; 230:120–126.

62. Chua B, Kao RL, Rannels DE, Morgan HE. Inhibition of protein degradation by anoxia and ischemia in perfused rat hearts. J Biol Chem 1979; 254:6617–6623.

63. Schreiber SS, Hearse DJ, Oratz M, Rothschild MA. Protein synthesis in prolonged cardiac arrest. J Mol Cell Cardiol 1977; 9:87–100.

64. Schreiber SS, Rothschild MA, Oratz M. Investigation into the causes of increased protein synthesis in acute hemodynamic overload. In: Kobayashi T, Ito Y, Rona G, eds. *Cardiac Adaptation*. Baltimore: University Park Press, 1978; 49–59.

65. Sparrow MP, Earl CA, Laurent GL, Everett AW. Turnover rates of muscle proteins in cardiac, skeletal, and smooth muscle: turnover rate related to muscle function. In: Kobayashi T, Ito Y, Rona G, eds. *Cardiac Adaptation*. Baltimore: University Park Press, 1978; 29–34.

66. Pritzl N, Zak R. Molecular biology of myocardial proteins. Circulation 1987; (suppl I)75:I-85-I-91.

67. Gupta MP, Gupta M, Stewart A, Zak R. Activation of alpha-myosin heavy chain gene expression by cAMP in cultured fetal rat heart myocytes. Biochem Biophys Res Com 1991; 174:1196–1203.

68. Everett AW, Sinha AM, Umeda PK, Jakovcic S, Rabinowitz M, Zak R. Regulation of myosin synthesis by thyroid hormone: relative change in the α- and β-myosin heavy chain mRNA levels in rabbit hearts. Biochemistry 1984; 23:1596–1599.

69. Korecky B, Zak R, Schwartz K, Aschenbrenner V. Role of thyroid hormone in regulation of isomyosin composition, contractility, and size of heterotopically isotransplanted rat heart. Circ Res 1987; 60:824–830.

70. Umeda PK, Darling DS, Kennedy JM, Jakovcic S, Zak R. Control of myosin heavy chain expression in cardiac hypertrophy. Am J Cardiol 1987; 59:49A-55A.

71. Phelps ME, Barrio JR, Huang S-C, Keen RE, Chugani H, Mazziotta JC. Criteria for the tracer kinetic measurement of cerebral protein synthesis in humans with positron emission tomography. Ann Neurol 1984; 15(suppl):S192-S202.

72. Keen RE, Barrio JR, Huang S-C, Hawkins RA, Phelps ME. In vivo cerebral protein synthesis rates with leucyl-transfer RNA used as a precursor pool: Determination of biochemical parameters to structure tracer kinetic models for positron emission tomography. J Cerebr Blood Flow Metab 1989; 9:432–448.

73. Hawkins RA, Huang S-C, Barrio JR, et al. Estimation of local cerebral protein synthesis rates with L-[1-^{11}C]leucine and PET: methods, model and results in animals and humans. J Cerebr Blood Flow Metab 1989; 9:446–460.

74. Barrio JR, Keen RE, Chugani H, Ackerman R, Chugani DC, Phelps ME. L-[1-^{11}C]Phenylalanine for the determination of cerebral protein synthesis rates in man with positron emission tomography. J Nucl Med 1983; 24:70 (abstract).

75. Revkin JH, Bukowski TR, Schwartz LM, Bassingthwaighte JB. Amino acid tracer transport in the heart. Circulation 1988; 78(suppl II):II-57 (abstract).

Chapter 9

Quantification of Regional Myocardial Oxidative Utilization with Positron Emission Tomography

Steven R. Bergmann, M.D., Ph.D. and Burton E. Sobel, M.D.

A salient thread in the history of cardiac physiology is the quest to elucidate determinants of myocardial oxygen requirements (demand) and of myocardial perfusion (supply). The pioneering work of Tennant and Wiggers demonstrated that cardiac contractions ceased virtually instantaneously when oxygen supply was interrupted.[1] Sarnoff et al elegantly delineated the major factors accounting for oxygen demand (and hence regional myocardial oxygen consumption per minute or $M\dot{V}O_2$) including heart rate, contractile state, wall stress, and shortening.[2] Braunwald formulated the seminal concept that the evolution of infarction is a dynamic process influenced by the imbalance between oxygen supply and demand.[3] Furthermore, he hypothesized that the imbalance could be redressed by therapeutic interventions and that the result would be salvage of jeopardized myocardium.

An elusive goal of cardiovascular research has been the noninvasive quantification of regional $M\dot{V}O_2$. Measurement of regional $M\dot{V}O_2$ is needed for investigations designed to define the relative efficacy of therapeutic interventions implemented to reduce myocardial oxygen requirements, increase supply, or both. It is needed to identify pathophysiologic factors in conditions such as angina with angiographically normal coronary arteries, and to improve the diagnosis of conditions as diverse as atherosclerotic coronary artery disease and microvascular coronary disease associated with connective tissue disorders, vasculitis, and diabetes mellitus among other etiologies. It is also needed to detect consequences of impaired perfusion such as limitation of coronary flow reserve and its effects on regional $M\dot{V}O_2$ in cardiac allografts with occult graft

From *Positron Emission Tomography of the Heart* edited by Steven R. Bergmann, MD, PhD and Burton E. Sobel, MD © 1992, Futura Publishing Inc., Mount Kisco, NY.

$H_2^{15}O$ by carbonic anhydrase in the lung and in blood). With the use of a mathematical formulation to correct the data obtained after administration of $O^{15}O$ for conversion to labeled water and to correct for spillover and partial volume effects, these investigators obtained close correlations between PET estimates of $M\dot{V}O_2$ and $M\dot{V}O_2$ measured directly.[21–23] However, oxygen extraction estimated with the constant inhalation approach was lower in absolute terms than that measured directly with invasive methods.

Results from Clinical Studies

Although it seems clear that estimation of regional $M\dot{V}O_2$ with $O^{15}O$ would be cumbersome for general clinical use, Iida and coworkers have extended their approach to human subjects.[24,25] In 5 normal volunteers, oxygen extraction ranged from 0.61 to 0.67 and a calculated average $M\dot{V}O_2$ ranged from 0.094 to 0.109 ml/min/g.[24,25] In 3 subjects, oxygen extraction declined by approximately 50% after infusion of dipyridamole (anticipated to increase perfusion without markedly altering $M\dot{V}O_2$).[24] In other normal volunteers studied at rest and again while dobutamine was being infused (to increase $M\dot{V}O_2$ by increasing oxygen demand secondary to augmentation of heart rate and contractility), estimated $M\dot{V}O_2$ increased.[25]

Although these preliminary results suggest that estimates of $M\dot{V}O_2$ and of oxygen extraction are possible with the use of the $O^{15}O$ inhalation technique, the approach may be limited by the imaging intervals required. The scanning procedure requires steady-state administration of $O^{15}O$; $C^{15}O_2$, which is converted to $H_2^{15}O$; and $C^{15}O$ for labeling the blood pool as well as acquisition of a transmission scan. Maintenance of a hemodynamic steady-state throughout, necessary for accurate estimates, is difficult and more complex if interventions are to be assessed. Corrections for spillover from lung to heart and corrections for conversion of $O^{15}O$ to $H_2^{15}O$ require rigorous acquisition of data and complex analysis. Nevertheless, the results are important and demonstrate that tomographic assessment of regional $M\dot{V}O_2$ directly with $O^{15}O$ is feasible.

^{11}Carbon-Acetate

Rationale for the use of ^{11}C-acetate

Because of the limitations encountered in the use of $O^{15}O$, we developed a method for estimation of regional myocardial $M\dot{V}O_2$ with ^{11}C-acetate, a short-chain acid that is metabolized virtually exclusively by mitochondrial oxidative metabolism.[26,27] Because of the close coupling between the rate of oxidation of acetate and the overall rate of oxidative phosphorylation, we hypothesized that oxidation of acetate could provide an indirect estimate of overall, regional tricarboxylic acid cycle flux and consequently of overall, regional oxygen utilization despite the possibility that some acetate could be metabolized through alternative pathways. Also, under some conditions, the rate of oxidative phosphorylation might not remain closely coupled to the rate of metabolism of ^{11}C-acetate.[26]

Metabolism of many diverse substrates by mitochondria involves their conversion to acetyl coenzyme A (CoA) and subsequent entry into the tricarboxylic acid cycle[4-6](also see Chapter 3). Acetate is converted directly to acetyl CoA by acetyl CoA synthase. Even though acetate can be oxidized readily by myocardium, the concentration of acetate in plasma is so low under physiologic conditions (30 to 400 µM) that oxidation of acetate contributes only negligibly to overall production of adenosine triphosphate (ATP) and to energy production in the heart.

Extraction of acetate by human myocardium under steady-state conditions averages 40% to 50%.[28] Myocardial oxygen consumption of acetate has been estimated to be approximately 90 nmol/g/min. In rat myocardium, the turnover rate of acetyl CoA averages 80 to 400 nmol/g/min, a much higher value than the steady-state content of acetyl CoA (0.05 to 0.15 nmol/g).[29] Although variations in the pattern of substrate utilization can alter the ratio of tricarboxylic acid cycle flux to oxygen consumption, the magnitude of the change is minute. For example, if the heart used exclusively glucose, lactate, or palmitate as the sole substrate for oxidative metabolism, it would consume 3.0, 3.0, and 2.9 mol of oxygen per mole of acetyl CoA consumed, respectively. Accordingly, if oxidative metabolism shifted from exclusive oxidation of palmitate to exclusive oxidation of glucose, the maximal error in the estimate of oxygen consumption based on assessment of the overall tricarboxylic acid flux would be 4%. Because of the admixture of substrates normally utilized by the heart, the error in the estimates of oxidative metabolism based on assessment of tricarboxylic acid cycle flux with ^{11}C-acetate would actually be less.

Hypothetically, the rate of oxidation of radiolabeled acetate should not be affected by a change in the particular substrate that serves as the precursor of acetyl CoA as long as the size of the precursor pool is small compared with the amount of the pool utilized in a given interval, and as long as the pool size remains relatively constant. As judged from results of numerous studies, these assumptions appear valid. Acetyl CoA can be incorporated into fatty acid by de novo synthesis or chain elongation. However, the extent of such incorporation is less than 1% of that in normoxic hearts.[30] Even though the rate can increase up to 12-fold with hypoxia,[31] the fraction of incorporation of acetyl CoA into lipid with respect to the total intracellular pool of acetyl CoA is small. Although acetate can be incorporated into amino acids and ketones as well,[32,33] we and others have shown that the magnitude of acetate flux through these synthetic pathways is so modest under diverse conditions that use of ^{11}C-acetate for estimation of $M\dot{V}O_2$ is not likely to be compromised.[26,34] Furthermore, despite the fact that the acetyl CoA pool size can change under certain conditions (e.g., perfusion of isolated hearts with supraphysiologic concentrations of acetate, ethanol intoxication in intact animals or human subjects, or dialysis with media containing high concentrations of acetate), changes of pool size encountered under physiologic and most pathophysiologic conditions does not markedly influence the turnover rate of labeled acetyl CoA.

Results in Studies in Experimental Animal Preparations

In 1980, investigators at Hammersmith Hospital in the United Kingdom demonstrated that the clearance of labeled acetate from the heart appeared to be monoexponential and to be decreased in ischemic myocardium.[35] Our laboratory demonstrated in isolated perfused rabbit hearts [26] and in hearts of intact dogs [27] that the clearance of ^{11}C from the heart after administration of ^{11}C-acetate was attributable virtually entirely to the myocardial production of ^{11}C-carbon dioxide and directly proportional to the rate of oxidative metabolism over a wide range of flow and diverse conditions of metabolism. In the hearts of laboratory animals, clearance of ^{11}C-radioactivity from the heart after administration of ^{11}C-acetate was shown to be biexponential.[26,27] Results in laboratory studies have shown that the rapid phase of clearance (k_1) represents oxidation of ^{11}C-acetate to $^{11}CO_2$ and that the slower phase (k_2) represents incorporation of tracer into amino acids (predominantly glutamate and aspartate) through transamination of tricarboxylic acid cycle intermediates and their metabolism (see Chapter 3).

In isolated perfused rabbit hearts, the steady-state extraction fraction of acetate averaged $62 \pm 4\%$.[26] Oxidation of radiolabeled acetate, assessed from the rate of efflux of radiolabeled CO_2 in venous effluents, correlated closely with $M\dot{V}O_2$ under conditions of normoxia, ischemia, hypoxia, and reperfusion ($r = 0.97$). Under conditions of ischemia, greater than 80% of the efflux of label is attributable to labeled CO_2 despite a slight increase in the production of non-CO_2 labeled metabolites. The efflux of total radioactivity correlates very closely with $M\dot{V}O_2$ even under these circumstances. With ischemia or hypoxia, the rate of clearance decreases reflecting diminished oxidative metabolism independent of changes in flow. With ischemia, modest backdiffusion of labeled acetate occurs. Radiolabel liberated from acetate appears in the aqueous rather than the organic phase of extraction media indicating that incorporation of the acetate into lipid is minimal despite increased production of triglycerides with ischemia.

We have characterized uptake and clearance of radioactivity from the heart in intact, anesthetized dogs after intravenous administration of ^{11}C-acetate under physiologic conditions, in response to high workloads (induced with beta-agonists), and in response to low workloads (induced with beta-blockade).[27] Uptake of radioactivity after intravenous bolus administration of ^{11}C-acetate was avid. Clearance of radioactivity from the blood was rapid. As a result, images of myocardium were of high quality (Color Figure 4).

In dog hearts, the steady-state extraction of unlabeled acetate averaged 33%. The unidirectional extraction fraction of labeled acetate is likely to be even greater. As with isolated hearts, the clearance of ^{11}C-radioactivity from myocardium was biexponential (Figure 9-1A,B). The rate of the rapid phase of clearance correlated with oxidation of acetate to $^{11}CO_2$ measured directly and with $M\dot{V}O_2$ measured directly over a wide range of flow and under diverse metabolic states (Figure 9-2).[26,27,36,37] Under normoxic conditions, approximately 81% of the label was cleared rapidly from the heart. This percentage remained constant despite increased cardiac work.

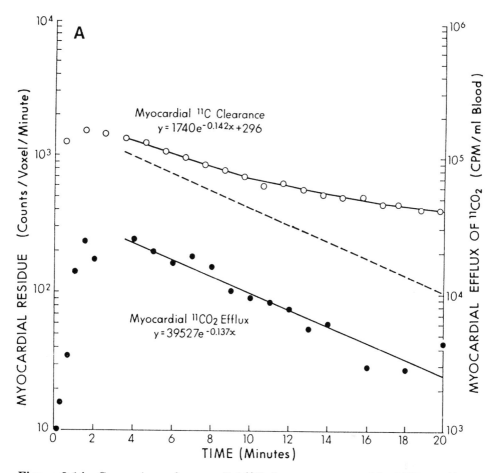

Figure 9-1A. *Comparison of myocardial ^{11}C clearance measured by PET and $^{11}CO_2$ efflux measured from direct coronary sinus sampling. A biexponential solution was closely fitted to the PET data. The dashed line represents clearance due to the rapid phase (k_1) and is similar to the rate constant of directly measured $^{11}CO_2$ efflux (0.142 and 0.137 min^{-1}, respectively). Thus, tomographically detectable clearance from myocardium represents oxidation of extracted tracer by the mitochondria. CPM represents counts per minute.*

In dogs given infusions of glucose, insulin, and potassium, or infusions of fatty acids to modify substrate supply and the pattern of myocardial substrate use, the relationship between clearance of ^{11}C-acetate and $M\dot{V}O_2$ measured directly was unaltered (after adjustment of estimated $M\dot{V}O_2$ for the changes in hemodynamics induced by the interventions) (Figure 9-2).[36] Recently, Buck et al. suggested that mathematical modeling to account for recirculation of tracer may improve estimates of $M\dot{V}O_2$ with ^{11}C-acetate.[38] However, under most circumstances this appears to be unnecessary.

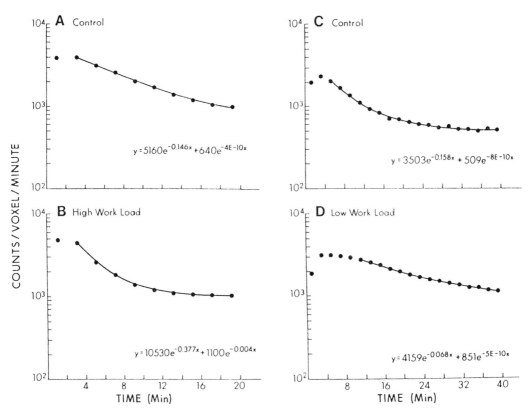

Figure 9-1B. *Myocardial time-activity curves obtained from serial, 2 minute tomographic scans from a dog studied under control conditions (A) and again after induction of a high workload with norepinephrine (B). Time-activity curves are shown in C and D for a dog studied under control conditions and again after a low workload was induced with the administration of propranolol and sodium nitroprusside. Biexponential solutions, shown by the solid lines, have been fitted from the PET data. The rate constant of the rapid phase varies directly with workload. (Reproduced with permission from Brown et al.[27])*

Physiologic Implications

The recovery of $M\dot{V}O_2$ after either brief or prolonged ischemia followed by reperfusion and its relationship to functional recovery was soon evident. Short intervals of ischemia preceding reperfusion resulted in prompt recovery of $M\dot{V}O_2$.[26,37,39] Recovery of oxidative metabolism was delayed after longer intervals of ischemia followed by reperfusion. Recovery of $M\dot{V}O_2$ detectable with ^{11}C-acetate was a prerequisite for recovery of contractile function.

After reperfusion following a brief, 15 minute coronary occlusion, both $M\dot{V}O_2$ and contractile performance were diminished. However, both could be augmented by paired pacing.[40] These results suggest that the early diminution of ventricular performance induced by ischemia and the early reduction of $M\dot{V}O_2$ are not attributable exclusively to defects in the contractile apparatus or

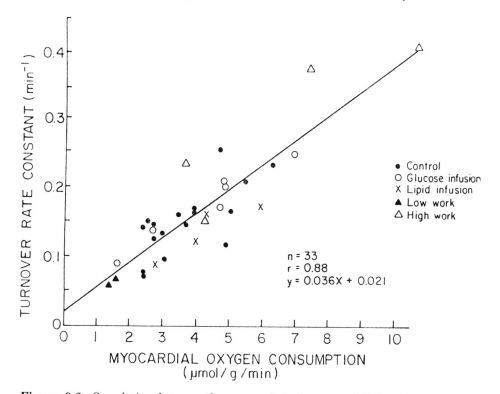

Figure 9-2. *Correlation between the myocardial clearance of* [11]*C-radioactivity from analysis of dynamic myocardial PET data, and directly measured MV̇O₂ obtained in dogs under baseline conditions and again after myocardial work had either been increased or decreased, or after the pattern of myocardial substrate utilization had been altered by infusion of glucose or lipid. The correlation is close over a wide range of metabolic states and workloads, and indicates the validity of estimates of myocardial oxygen consumption using* [11]*C-acetate. The results shown in this graph summarize data from our group.*[27,36] *(Reproduced with permission from Bergmann.*[57]*)*

the cellular biochemical systems responsible for oxidative metabolism. Instead, they are consistent with a defect in excitation-contraction coupling, perhaps induced by increased intracellular concentrations of calcium.

Results of Studies in Patients

After intravenous administration of ^{11}C-acetate, extraction of the tracer by human myocardium is avid and clearance from the blood pool is rapid.[41] Accordingly, images of myocardium are of high quality (Color Figure 5). In most subjects studied at rest, clearance from myocardium appears to be mo-noexponential (Figure 9-3) in contrast to the case in hearts of laboratory animals, probably because of the lower workload of the human myocardium compared with that of myocardium of anesthetized laboratory animals. Under some circumstances, biexponential clearance is observed. In fact, clearance is proba-

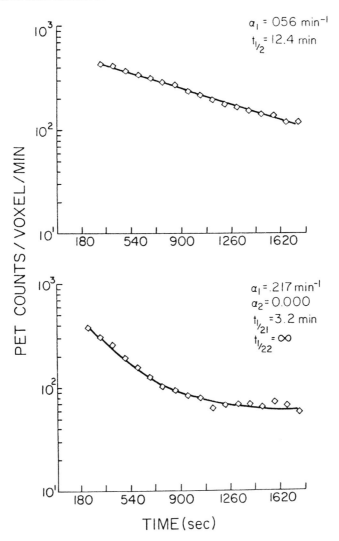

Figure 9-3. *Time-activity curves representing clearance of *^{11}*C-radioactivity from the left ventricular myocardium of a healthy human subject studied at rest (upper panel) and again during the infusion of dobutamine (bottom panel). At rest, clearance appears monoexponential whereas the overall shape conforms to a biexponential clearance during infusion of dobutamine which raises MV̇O*$_2$*. The rate of clearance of radioactivity of the early phase of clearance is increased during infusion of dobutamine. A*$_1$* and A*$_2$* represent the Y intercept of the fast (k*$_1$*) and slow (k*$_2$*) component of the time-activity curve. (Reproduced with permission from Henes et al.[41])*

bly truly biexponential in all subjects at rest, with the second component obscured by the relatively slow rate of disappearance attributable to the first component and by statistical noise. In some subjects for whom it was possible to perform a biexponential fit of data obtained at rest, the magnitude of the second component averaged only 4% of that of the first and the second component clearance rate, k_2, averaged less than 0.1% of k_1.[41] Clearance of radioactivity from myocardium after administration of 0.4 mCi/kg of ^{11}C-acetate intravenously was homogeneous and apparently monoexponential in subjects at rest.[41] The average rate of clearance was 0.054 ± 0.014 min[-1], corresponding to a biological half-time of approximately 13 minutes. Use of the relationship between k and $M\dot{V}O_2$ established in canine hearts enabled us to calculate an $M\dot{V}O_2$ of 0.97 μmol/g/min in human hearts (a value close to that previously obtained directly in measurements with invasive procedures). The modest difference between results with the two methods may reflect an interspecies difference in the relationship between k and $M\dot{V}O_2$. Use of the relationship enabled generation of functional, three-dimensional images of regional $M\dot{V}O_2$ (Color Figure 6). In addition, correlations between k and the rate-pressure product (an indirect index of oxygen demand) are similar in humans and dogs (Figure 9-4).

When dobutamine (15 to 20 μg/kg/min) was used as a pharmacologic stressor to augment regional myocardial metabolism (under conditions suitable for imaging with steady-state conditions throughout a 30 minute interval, in contrast to the case with exercise) the rate-pressure product increased by an

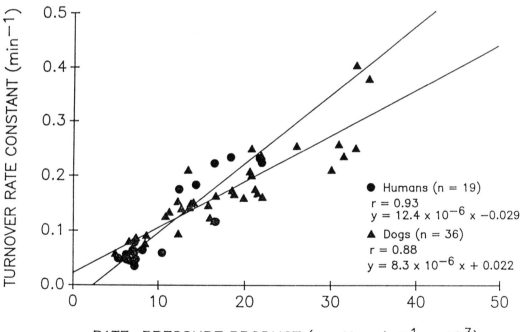

Figure 9-4. *Correlation between the myocardial turnover rate constant (k_1) and the rate-pressure product for data acquired in human subjects and those acquired in experimental animals under a variety of conditions. The regression lines are not statistically different. These data suggest that results with ^{11}C-acetate are an accurate reflection of myocardial oxygen demand. (Reproduced with permission from Henes et al.[41])*

average of 141%. Under these conditions, clearance of ^{11}C-acetate was clearly biexponential (Figure 9-3) and homogeneous throughout the myocardium. The second component of clearance is essentially infinite. The slope of the rapid phase and the rate-pressure product correlated closely. Of interest, in another study providing additional confirmation of the specificity of ^{11}C-acetate clearance for estimation of MV̇O₂, Bol et al. demonstrated that changes in clearance of ^{11}C-acetate paralleled changes observed with the use of O^{15}O in normal subjects studied at rest and again after infusion of dobutamine.[25] These findings suggested that performance of cardiac PET with ^{11}C-acetate and dobutamine stress will permit quantification of regional myocardial oxidative metabolic reserve in patients with cardiac diseases of diverse etiologies and assessment of the efficacy of interventions designed to enhance the recovery of metabolically compromised myocardium.

To determine whether acute myocardial infarction is accompanied by changes in regional MV̇O₂, Walsh et al. studied patients treated conservatively, i.e., without thrombolytic drugs.[42] In the central infarct region, myocardial oxidative metabolism was markedly depressed to approximately 6% of levels in remote, presumably normal tissue (Color Figure 6 and Figure 9-5). The depression persisted unchanged and was still evident in follow-up studies performed immediately before hospital discharge (Figure 9-5). Subsequently, we characterized the extent of restoration of oxidative metabolism induced by thrombolytic drugs administered early after the onset of ischemia.[43] At the time of initial PET study, soon after coronary thrombolysis, nutritive perfusion was nearly normal (Figure 9-6; also see Chapter 11, Figure 11-2). Nevertheless, regional oxidative metabolism in the infarct zone assessed with ^{11}C-acetate was only 45% of that in remote, normal regions. Within the first 24 hours, it increased to 59% of normal. By the time of hospital discharge, it had increased further, to 68% of normal (Figure 9-7; also see Chapter 11, Figure 11-6). Recovery of regional wall motion was observed only in those segments that exhibited early restoration of both nutritive perfusion and oxidative metabolism.

The utility of PET with ^{11}C-acetate and its specificity for delineation of regional MV̇O₂ were confirmed soon thereafter in studies performed in patients an average of 6 days after their admission for acute myocardial infarction. Myocardial perfusion was assessed with ^{15}O-water, utilization of glucose with ^{18}F-fluorodeoxyglucose, and oxidative metabolism with ^{11}C-acetate. Recovery of function after revascularization was documented by wall motion analysis.[44] Maintenance of clearance of ^{11}C-acetate at a rate equivalent to 74% or greater of that in normal myocardium was the best predictor of recovery of function after revascularization. In contrast, regional utilization of glucose, (even when normalized to regional perfusion) was markedly variable, and its maintenance was less predictive of recovery of function. Thus, preservation of oxidative metabolism was confirmed to be a necessary prerequisite for recovery of regional function after coronary recanalization, and estimation of regional MV̇O₂ with ^{11}C-acetate was documented to provide a reliable descriptor of viability of myocardium and its capacity for functional recovery.

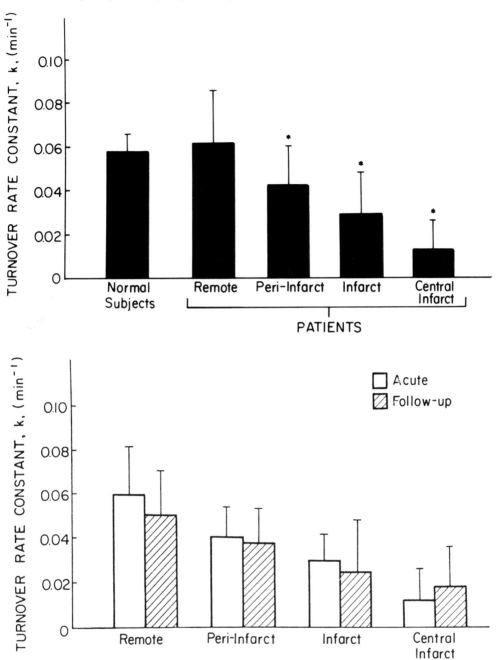

Figure 9-5. *(Top) Histogram depicting the regional myocardial rate constant (k_1) from normal subjects, and from patients with acute myocardial infarction treated conservatively (without recanalization therapy). The data from the patients reflects the turnover of ^{11}C-radioactivity from remote, presumably normal regions, and in peri-infarct, infarct, and central infarct regions of interest. Regional myocardial oxygen consumption was severely diminished in the zone of infarction. The asterisks represents $P < 0.05$ compared with k_1 in remote regions. (Bottom) Histogram displaying the myocardial turnover rate constant, k_1, from patients studied during the acute phase of infarction and again before hospital discharge. In these patients managed conservatively, there was no change in regional k_1 with time. (Reproduced with permission from Walsh et al.[42])*

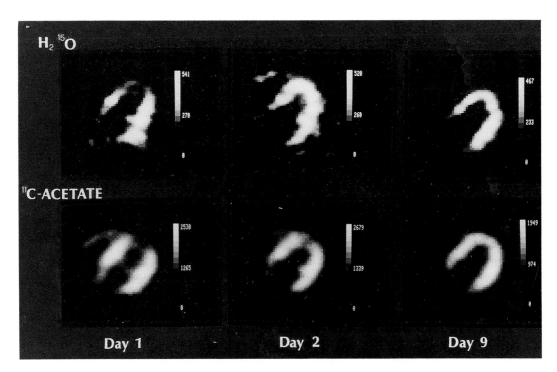

Figure 9-6. *Sequential tomograms obtained on days 1, 2, and 9 from a patient with myocardial infarction treated with thrombolytic therapy. As depicted in the midventricular tomograms on the top, myocardial perfusion (estimated with $H_2{}^{15}O$) is initially diminished in the anterior myocardium but recovered by day 2. The accumulation of ^{11}C-acetate (Bottom) is delayed compared with recovery of perfusion indicating the delayed recovery of myocardial oxygen consumption compared with perfusion. By day 9, both perfusion and metabolism have recovered to near normal levels, indicating substantial myocardial salvage. Recovery of oxidative metabolism presages recovery of function. (Reproduced with permission from Henes et al.[43])*

^{18}F-Fluoromisonidazole

Delineation of jeopardized but still viable, hypoxic myocardium with a tracer that provides a positive image of the compromised tissue is another approach to improved detection and assessment of the severity of spontaneous or inducible myocardial ischemia and accordingly of coronary artery disease and its pathophysiologic significance in individual patients. ^{18}F-fluorodeoxyglucose has been used for this purpose. However, uptake of this tracer is dependent on the metabolic state of the myocyte, on flow, and on the pattern of substrate use.[4–6,10–12] Accordingly, uptake is only modestly predictive of recovery of function when the tracer is administered under conditions of acute myocardial ischemia.[44–48] An alternative under active exploration is a class of compounds with high electron affinity, the nitroimidazoles.[49–51] Misonidazole is known to accumulate in regions of hypoxia but not in regions of necrosis in tumors. Accordingly, we recently characterized its behavior in myocardium.

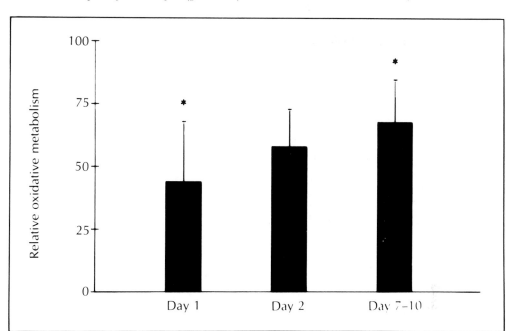

Figure 9-7. *The mean rate of oxidative metabolism (estimated with* ^{11}*C-acetate) in jeopardized zones from patients with acute myocardial infarction treated with thrombolytic therapy, expressed as a fraction of that in remote, normal zones calculated as a percentage. Progressive improvement of relative oxidative metabolism occurs in the region at risk studied acutely and again before hospital discharge (P < 0.05). Thus, PET with* ^{11}*C-acetate can be used to define the extent and magnitude of therapeutic interventions. (Reproduced with permission from Henes et al.*[43]*)*

Misonidazole diffuses across cell membranes and undergoes reduction in the cytoplasm to form a radical.[49–51] When oxygen is abundant in the cell, it reacts with the radical anion formed to yield superoxide and noncharged misonidazole that diffuses out of the cell (Figure 9-8). When intracellular hypoxia is present, the misonidazole radical anion is reduced further to form nitrous compounds including hydroxyl and other amides that combine covalently with intracellular macromolecules and are thereby trapped intracellularly. Necrotic myocardium exhibits less binding because its capacity for enzymatic nitroreduction is diminished and intracellular trapping of macromolecules is offset by loss of integrity of the sarcolemma.

Results in Studies in Laboratory Animal Preparations and in Patients

In both isolated myocytes[52] and isolated perfused hearts,[53] ^{18}F-fluoromisonidazole accumulated in proportion to the severity of intracellular depletion of oxygen. Uptake and binding of ^{18}F-fluoromisonidazole in isolated hearts was

Proposed Metabolism of ^{18}F-Fluoromisonidazole

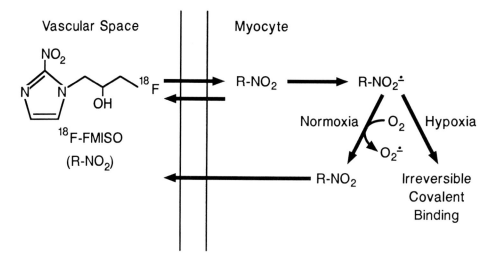

Figure 9-8. *Schematic diagram of the proposed metabolism of ^{18}F-fluoromisonidazole (^{18}F-FMISO) in the heart. R-NO$_2$ represents reduced nitrate (see text). (Reproduced with permission from Shelton et al.[54])*

characterized under control conditions, with ischemia, with hypoxia without low flow, and with reperfusion after ischemia.[53] Myocardial retention of tracer averaged 18% in normal tissue and increased to 46% in hearts subjected to either ischemia or hypoxia. When tracer was administered during the course of reperfusion after a period of ischemia, uptake in myocardium was again normal (Figure 9-9). The biological half-life of tracer that had been retained was greater than 40 hours, indicative of irreversible binding of extracted tracer.

In hearts of intact dogs, retention of tracer in normal myocardium averaged 2%.[54] It increased to 23% in myocardium subjected to 3 hours of ischemia, an interval still brief enough to permit substantial salvage of myocardium with reperfusion. When ischemia was present for more prolonged intervals before administration of the tracer, retention of the tracer was much less. In addition, perfusion of less than 40% of normal appeared necessary to increase extraction of tracer, suggesting that this level of ischemia is necessary to create tissue hypoxia.

^{18}F-fluoromisonidazole persists in the blood pool for prolonged intervals. With delayed imaging ($>$ 4 hours), positive images of ischemic myocardium can be obtained.[55] Alternatively, subtraction of blood pool related activity can be employed with a second tracer such as C^{15}O (Color Figure 7) enabling identification of hypoxic myocardium within 30 to 45 minutes of tracer administration.[54] Recently, increased uptake has been demonstrated in patients with chronic stable angina.[56] Accordingly, use of this tracer is promising for the

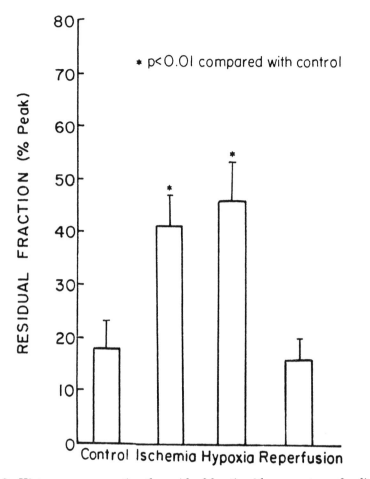

Figure 9-9. *Histogram representing the residual fraction (the percentage of radioactivity retained at the end of the washout period compared with peak radioactivity just before washout) for isolated perfused rabbit hearts studied under control conditions, during ischemia, during hypoxia and during reperfusion after ischemia. Hearts subjected to ischemia or hypoxia retain significantly more tracer than that retained in hearts subjected to control perfusion. The enhanced retention was not due simply to bulk flow since hearts subjected to hypoxia were perfused at normal flow rates but with hypoxic media. After transient ischemia (i.e., during reperfusion), the kinetics of tracer extraction returned to normal. (Reproduced with permission from Shelton et al.[53])*

noninvasive identification of jeopardized but still salvageable ischemic myocardium by positive imaging.

Conclusions

Cardiac PET has played a pivotal role in a fundamental quest in cardiovascular research. It has provided the means, for the first time, to noninvasively quantify regional myocardial oxygen consumption in hearts of human subjects under specific physiologic and pathophysiologic conditions. Its use will undoubtedly help to answer persistent questions that have confronted clinicians and investigators for decades such as the extent to which, if any, the hypertrophied ventricle can outgrow its blood supply; the extent to which the syndrome of angina with angiographically normal coronary arteries is attributable to microvascular coronary disease; the extent to which specific, potentially therapeutic interventions restore or preserve regional oxidative metabolism and consequently permit recovery of regional function in jeopardized ischemic myocardium; and the extent to which modulation of myocardial oxygen requirements with pharmacologic regimens such as beta-adrenergic blockers in patients with dilated cardiomyopathy can retard deterioration of cardiac function and improve prognosis. Development of the approach has been difficult due to the complex multiple pathways that contribute to $M\dot{V}O_2$ and the need for novel mathematical and tracer approaches. Nevertheless, cardiac PET now provides a powerful tool for noninvasive quantification of regional $M\dot{V}O_2$

Acknowledgments

The authors thank Sue Furey for secretarial assistance and Beth Engeszer for editorial review. Work from the authors' laboratory was supported in part by the National Institutes of Health Grant HL 17646-Specialized Center of Research in Coronary and Vascular Disease.

References

1. Tennant R, Wiggers CJ: The effect of coronary occlusion on myocardial contraction. Am J Physiol 1935; 112:351–361.
2. Sarnoff SJ, Braunwald E, Welch GH Jr, Case RB, Stainsby WN, Macruz R: Hemodynamic determinants of oxygen consumption of heart with special reference to tension-time index. Am J Physiol 1958; 192:148–156.
3. Braunwald, E: Regulation of the circulation. N Engl J Med 1974; 290:1420–1425.
4. Bing RJ: Cardiac metabolism. Physiol Rev 1965; 45:171–213.
5. Neely JR, Morgan HE: Relationship between carbohydrate and lipid metabolism and the energy balance of heart muscle. Annu Rev Physiol 1974; 36:413–459.
6. Liedtke AJ: Alterations of carbohydrate and lipid metabolism in the acutely ischemic heart. Prog Cardiovasc Dis 1981; 23:321–336.
7. Schelbert HR, Henze E, Schon HR, Keen R, Hansen H, Selin C, Huang S-C, Barrio JR, Phelps ME: C-11 palmitate for the noninvasive evaluation of regional myocardial fatty acid metabolism with positron computed tomography. III. In vivo demonstration of the effects of substrate availability on myocardial metabolism. Am Heart J 1983; 105:492–504.
8. Schelbert HR, Henze E, Sochor H, Grossman RG, Huang S-C, Barrio JR, Schwaiger M, Phelps ME: Effects of substrate availability on myocardial C-11 palmitate kinetics by positron emission tomography in normal subjects and patients with ventricular dysfunction. Am Heart J 1986; 111:1055–1064.
9. Fox, KAA, Abendschein D, Ambos HD, Sobel BE, Bergmann SR: Efflux of metabolized and nonmetabolized fatty acid from canine myocardium. Implications for quantifying myocardial metabolism tomographically. Circ Res 1985; 57:232–243.

10. Phelps ME, Hoffman EJ, Selin C, Huang SC, Robinson G, MacDonald N, Schelbert H, Kuhl DE: Investigation of [^{18}F]2-fluoro-2-deoxyglucose for the measure of myocardial glucose metabolism. J Nucl Med 1978; 19:1311–1319.

11. Gropler RJ, Siegel BA, Lee KJ, Moerlein SM, Perry DJ, Bergmann SR, Geltman EM: Nonuniformity in myocardial accumulation of fluorine-18-fluorodeoxyglucose in normal fasted humans. J Nucl Med 1990; 31:1749–1756.

12. Myears DW, Sobel BE, Bergmann SR: Substrate use in ischemic and reperfused canine myocardium: quantitative considerations. Am J Physiol: Heart Circ Physiol 1987; 253:H107-H114.

13. Parker JA, Beller GA, Hoop B, Holman BL, Smith TW: Assessment of regional myocardial blood flow and regional fractional oxygen extraction in dogs, using ^{15}O-water and ^{15}O-hemoglobin. Circulation 1978; 42:511–518.

14. Metzger JM: Myocardial blood flow and oxygen consumption using $H_2{}^{15}O$ and ^{15}O-hemoglobin. Ph.D. Thesis, Washington University, St. Louis, Mo.1972.

15. Fox KAA, Bergmann SR, Rand AL, Ambos HD, and Sobel BE: External measurement of myocardial oxygen extraction with 0-15-labeled oxygen. J Nucl Med 1983; 24:P20 (abstract).

16. Fox KAA, Ambos HD, Bergmann SR, Sobel BE: External measurement of myocardial oxygen utilization with O-15 labeled oxygen. Circulation 1983; 68:III-82 (abstract).

17. Bergmann SR, Fox KAA, Geltman EM, Sobel BE: Positron emission tomography of the heart. Prog Cardiovasc Dis 1985; 28:165–194.

18. Jones T: The continuous inhalation of Oxygen-15 for assessing regional oxygen extraction in the brain of man. Br J Radiol 1976; 49:339–343.

19. Mintun MA, Raichle ME, Martin WRW, Herscovitch P: Brain oxygen utilization measured with O-15 radiotracers and positron emission tomography. J Nucl Med 1984; 25:177–187.

20. Kanno I, Uemura K, Higano S, Murakami M, Iida H, Miura S, Shishido F, Inugami A, Sayama I: Oxygen extraction fraction at maximally vasodilated tissue in the ischemic brain estimated from the regional CO_2 responsiveness measured by positron emission tomography. J Cereb Blood Flow Metab 1988; 8:227–235.

21. Iida H, Rhodes CG, Araujo LI, Taylor CJV, Jones T, Tochon-Danguy H, Maseri A, Kanno I, Ono Y: Measurement of myocardial metabolic rate of oxygen (MMRO2) using $^{15}O_2$ and PET. J Nucl Med 1991; 31:736 (abstract).

22. Yamamoto Y, de Silva R, Rhodes CG, Iida Y, Taylor C, Jones T, Maseri A: Validation of quantification of myocardial oxygen consumption and oxygen extraction fraction using $^{15}O_2$ and positron emission tomography. Circulation 1991; 84(suppl II):II-47 (abstract).

23. Bol A, Melin JA, Essamri B, Vogelaers D, Iida H, Vanbutsele R, Heyndrickx GR, Wijns W: Assessment of myocardial oxidative reserve with PET: Comparison with Fick oxygen consumption. Circulation 1991; 84(suppl II):II-425 (abstract).

24. Iida H, Rhodes CG, Yamamoto Y, Jones T, de Silva R, Araujo LI: Quantitative measurement of myocardial metabolic rate of oxygen (MMRO2) in man using $^{15}O_2$ and positron emission tomography. Circulation 1990; 82(suppl III): III-614 (abstract).

25. Bol A, Iida H, Essamri B, Vanbutsele R, Labar D, Grandin C, Wijn W, Melin JA: Assessment of myocardial oxidative reserve with PET: Comparison of C-11 acetate kinetics with quantitation of metabolic rate of oxygen (MRO2) using 0–15 02. J Nucl Med 1991; 32:988–989 (abstract).

26. Brown MA, Marshall DR, Sobel BE, Bergmann SR: Delineation of myocardial oxygen utilization with carbon-11 labeled acetate. Circulation 1987; 76:687–696.

27. Brown MA, Myears DW, Bergmann SR: Noninvasive assessment of canine myocardial oxidative metabolism with carbon-11 acetate and positron emission tomography. J Am Coll Cardiol 1988; 12:1054–1063.

28. Lindeneg O, Mellemgaard K, Fabricius J, Lundquist F: Myocardial utilization of acetate, lactate and free fatty acids after injection of ethanol. Clin Sci 1964; 27:427–435.

29. Randle PJ, Tubbs PK: Carbohydrate and fatty acid metabolism. In: RM Berne, N Sperelakis, SR Geiger, Eds.*Handbook of Physiology, The Cardiovascular System. Volume I, The Heart.* American Physiological Society, Bethesda, Maryland, 1979; 805–844.

30. Randle PJ, England PJ, Denton RM: Control of the tricarboxylate cycle and its interactions with glycolysis during acetate utilization in rat heart. Biochem J 1970; 117:677–695.

31. Harris P, Gloster J: The effects of acute hypoxia on lipid synthesis in the rat heart. Cardiology 1971/1972; 56:43–47.

32. Bailey IA, Gadian DG, Matthews RM, Radda GK, Seeley PJ: Studies of metabolism in the isolated, perfused rat heart using ^{13}C NMR. FEBS Lett 1981; 123:315–318.

33. Neurohr KH, Barrett EJ, Shulman RG: In vivo carbon-13 nuclear magnetic resonance studies of heart metabolism. Proc Natl Acad Sci USA 1983; 80:1603–1607.

34. Buxton DB, Schwaiger M, Nguyen A, Phelps ME, Schelbert HR: Radiolabeled acetate as a tracer of myocardial tricarboxylic acid cycle flux. Circ Res 1988; 63:628–634.

35. Allan RM, Selwyn AP, Pike VW, Eakins MN, Maseri A: In vivo experimental and clinical studies of normal and ischemic myocardium using ^{11}C-acetate. Circulation 1980; 62(suppl III): III-74 (abstract).

36. Brown MA, Myears DW, Bergmann SR: Validity of estimates of myocardial oxidative metabolism with carbon-11 acetate and positron emission tomography despite altered patterns of substrate utilization. J Nucl Med 1989; 30:187–193.

37. Armbrecht JJ, Buxton DB, Schelbert HR: Validation of [1-^{11}C] acetate as a tracer for noninvasive assessment of oxidative metabolism with positron emission tomography in normal, ischemic, postischemic, and hyperemic canine myocardium. Circulation 1990; 81:1594–1605.

38. Buck A, Wolpers HG, Hutchins GD, Savas V, Mangner TJ, Nguyen N, Schwaiger M: Effect of carbon-11-acetate recirculation on estimates of myocardial oxygen consumption by PET. J Nucl Med 1991; 32:1950–1957.

39. Brown MA, Nohara R, Vered Z, Perez JE, Bergmann SR: The dependence of recovery of stunned myocardium on restoration of oxidative metabolism. Circulation 1988; 78(suppl II):II-467 (abstract).

40. Bergmann SR, Shelton ME, Weinheimer CJ, Sobel BE, Perez JE: Persistence of perfusion, metabolic, and functional reserve capacity in stunned myocardium. J Nucl Med 1990; 31:794 (abstract).

41. Henes CG, Bergmann SR, Walsh MN, Sobel BE, Geltman EM: Assessment of myocardial oxidative metabolic reserve with positron emission tomography and carbon-11 acetate. J Nucl Med 1989; 30:1489–1499.

42. Walsh MN, Geltman EM, Brown MA, Henes CG, Weinheimer CJ, Sobel BE, Bergmann SR: Noninvasive estimation of regional myocardial oxygen consumption by positron emission tomography with carbon-11 acetate in patients with myocardial infarction. J Nucl Med 1989; 30:1798–1808.

43. Henes CG, Bergmann SR, Perez JE, Sobel BE, Geltman EM: The time course of restoration of nutritive perfusion, myocardial oxygen consumption, and regional function after coronary thrombolysis. Coronary Artery Dis 1990; 1:687–696.

44. Gropler RJ, Siegel BA, Sampathkumaran K, Perez JE, Sobel BE, Bergmann SR, and Geltman EM: Dependence of recovery of contractile function on maintenance of oxidative metabolism after myocardial infarction. J Am Coll Cardiol, 1992; 989–997.

45. Schwaiger M, Brunken R, Grover-McKay M, Krivokapich J, Child J, Tillisch JH, Phelps ME, Schelbert HR: Regional myocardial metabolism in patients with acute myocardial infarction assessed by positron emission tomography. J Am Coll Cardiol 1986; 8:800–880.

46. Pierard LA, De Landsheere CM, Berthe C, Rigo P, Kulbertus HE: Identification of viable myocardium by echocardiography during dobutamine infusion in patients with myocardial infraction after thrombolytic therapy: Comparison with positron emission tomography. J Am Coll Cardiol 1990; 15:1021–1031.

47. Buxton DB, Vaghaiwalla MF, Krivokapich J, Phelps ME, Schelbert H: Quantitative measurement of sustained metabolic abnormalities in reperfused canine myocardium. J Nucl Med 1990; 31:795 (abstract).

48. Sebree L, Bianco JA, Subramanian R, Wilson MA, Swanson D, Hegge J, Tschudy J, Pyzalski R: Discordance between accumulation of C-14 deoxyglucose and Tl-201 in reperfused myocardium. J Mol Cell Cardiol 1991; 23:603–616.

49. Chapman JD: Hypoxic sensitizers: implications for radiation therapy. N Engl J Med 1979; 301:1429–1432.

50. Frank AJ, Chapman JD, Doch CJ: Binding of misonidazole to EMT6 and V79 spheroids. Int J Radiat Oncol Biol Phys 1982; 8:737–739.

51. Miller GG, Ngan-Lee J, Chapman JD: Intracellular localization of radioactivity labeled misonidazole in EMT-6 tumor cells in vitro. Int J Radiat Oncol Biol Phys 1982; 8:741–744.

52. Martin GV, Cerqueira MD, Caldwell JH, Rasey JS, Embree L, Krohn KA: Fluoromisonidazole: A metabolic marker of myocyte hypoxia. Circulation 1990; 67:240–244.

53. Shelton ME, Dence CS, Hwang D-R, Welch MJ, Bergmann SR: Myocardial kinetics of fluorine-18 misonidazole: A marker of hypoxic myocardium. J Nucl Med 1989; 30:351–358.

54. Shelton ME, Dence CS, Hwang D-R, Herrero P, Welch MJ, Bergmann SR: In vivo delineation of myocardial hypoxia during coronary occlusion using fluorine-18 fluoromisonidazole and positron emission tomography: A potential approach for identification of jeopardized myocardium. J Am Coll Cardiol 1990; 16:477–485.

55. Martin GV, Caldwell JH, Rasey JS, Grunbaum Z, Cerqueira M, Krohn KA: Enhanced binding of the hypoxic cell marker [³H] fluoromisonidazole in ischemic myocardium. J Nucl Med 1989; 30:194–201.

56. Revenaugh JR, Caldwell JH, Martin GV, Grierson JL, Krohn KA: Positron emission tomography (PET) imaging of myocardial hypoxia with ¹⁸F-fluoromisonidazole (FMISO) in post myocardial infarction patients. Circulation 1991; 84 (suppl II):II-424 (abstract).

57. Bergmann SR: Clinical applications of assessments of myocardial substrate utilization with positron emission tomography. Mol Cell Biochem 1989; 88:201–209.

58. Bergmann, SR: Positron emission tomography of the heart. In: Gerson, M, Ed. *Cardiac Nuclear Medicine*. New York: McGraw-Hill, 1990; 299–335.

59. Miller TR, Wallis JW, Geltman EM, and Bergmann SR: Three-dimensional functional images of myocardial oxygen consumption from positron tomography. J Nucl Med 1990; 31:2064–2068.

Chapter 10

Noninvasive Evaluation of the Cardiac Sympathetic Nervous System with Positron Emission Tomography

Markus Schwaiger, M.D., Gary D. Hutchins, Ph.D., and Donald M. Wieland, Ph.D.

The autonomic nervous system plays an important role in the regulation of cardiovascular performance under various physiologic and pathophysiologic conditions. The sympathetic and parasympathetic innervation of the heart facilitates its electrophysiologic and hemodynamic adaptation to changing cardiovascular demands. Both sympathetic and parasympathetic tone control the rate of electrophysiologic stimulation, whereas the heart's contractile performance is primarily modulated by sympathetic neurotransmission.

Almost 70 years ago Loewi et al. reported that stimulation of cardiac sympathetic nerves results in increased heart rate and force of ventricular contraction.[1] About 25 years later, norepinephrine was described as the primary neurotransmitter of the sympathetic nervous system.[2,3] Technologic advances (e.g., the development of fluorometric assay methods) allowed definition of the differential role of norepinephrine as a neurotransmitter synthesized in sympathetic nerve terminals and of epinephrine as a hormonal neurotransmitter secreted by the adrenal gland.[4] With the further refinement of assays of neurotransmitter concentrations in plasma and tissue, the kinetics of neuronal uptake and secretion of norepinephrine could be studied. Based on these breakthroughs, the characterization of cardiac neurophysiology has become possible by the use of radiotracer approaches to measure plasma levels of norepinephrine and its metabolites in arterial and coronary sinus blood.[5] In addition to these sophisti-

This work was done during the tenure of an established investigatorship from the American Heart Association (M. Schwaiger), and supported in part by the National Institutes of Health, Bethesda, MD, RO1 HL41047-01 and R01 HL27555-06, and the American Heart Association of Michigan #88-0699-J1.

From *Positron Emission Tomography of the Heart* edited by Steven R. Bergmann, MD, PhD and Burton E. Sobel, MD © 1992, Futura Publishing Inc., Mount Kisco, NY.

cated measurements of cardiac sympathetic function in animals and in patients undergoing catheterization, radiolabeled pharmaceuticals have been recently introduced for the noninvasive assessment of the sympathetic nervous system by the use of nuclear medicine imaging approaches.[6] The recent improvements in radiochemistry and imaging technology allow the specific visualization of sympathetic nerve terminals and adrenergic receptors of the living heart.

This chapter addresses the emerging role of positron emission tomography (PET) in the noninvasive characterization of the cardiac sympathetic nervous system. It provides a review of the physiology of the sympathetic nervous system and covers radiochemical approaches to trace sympathetic neurotransmission and methods for the quantification of neuronal function with the use of tracer kinetic modeling. A description of initial experimental and clinical experience with radiopharmaceuticals developed at the University of Michigan for the imaging of the sympathetic nervous system is included.

Physiology of the Sympathetic Nervous System

The heart is innervated by both sympathetic and parasympathetic nerve fibers. The atria of the heart, the sinus, and the atrioventricular node are regulated by both the sympathetic and parasympathetic nervous system, but the neuronal structures in the ventricular myocardium and vascular tree represent primarily sympathetic nerve fibers. However, since the atrium and conduction system of the heart cannot be imaged by current techniques, this discussion is limited to the sympathetic innervation of the ventricular myocardium.

Sympathetic Nerve Terminal

The postganglionic sympathetic fibers travel along vascular structures on the surface of the heart. On entering the myocardial wall, the fibers branch into multiple plexi referred to as sympathetic nerve terminals. These terminals include vesicles, which represent a storage pool for neurotransmitters, enzymes, and other proteins.

Norepinephrine, the dominant neurotransmitter in the cardiac sympathetic nerve terminals, is synthesized from the amino acid tyrosine in several enzymatic steps (Figure 10-1). Synthesis occurs in the postganglionic sympathetic neurons. The conversion from tyrosine to dopa, and from dopa to dopamine, takes place in the cytoplasm of the neuron. The synthesis of dopa from tyrosine is the rate-limiting step in the biosynthesis of catecholamines.[7] After the conversion from dopa to dopamine by dopa decarboxylase, dopamine is transported into storage vesicles by an active mechanism and norepinephrine is synthesized by the dopamine beta hydroxylase (DBH) within the storage vesicles.[8,9]

Upon nerve stimulation, norepinephrine is released from nerve terminals. This occurs as the vesicles approach the neuronal membrane, where they re-

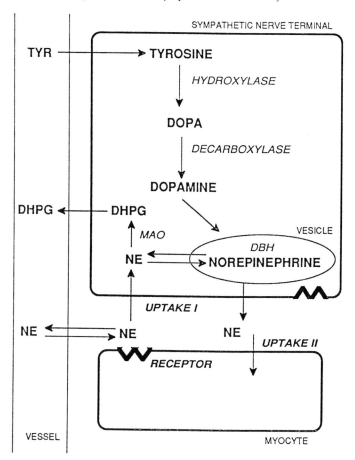

Figure 10-1. *Schematic display of sympathetic nerve terminal. NE = norepinephrine; DBH = dopamine-β-hydroxylase; MAO = monoamine oxidase; DHPG = dihydroxyphenylglycol; Tyr = tyrosine.*

lease their contents by exocytosis. A single nerve stimulation leads to the exocytosis of norepinephrine from only a fraction of the many thousands of storage vesicles in the sympathetic nerve terminals. Therefore, it is thought that although most norepinephrine is released by exocytosis, nonvesicular release also occurs. After exocytosis the retained membranes of the empty vesicles are taken up into the cytoplasm and reloaded, and the cycle of exocytosis is repeated.

The regulation of neuronal norepinephrine release is complex. Activation of the α_2-receptors on the membrane of the presynaptic nerve terminal [10] by norepinephrine leads to a negative feedback of the exocytotic process. In addition to the presynaptic α_2-adrenergic receptor, the presence of other inhibitory presynaptic receptors suggests that multiple control mechanisms modulate norepinephrine release from sympathetic nerve terminals. For example, muscarinic receptors and adenosine receptors play an important role, especially in the heart.[11] As recently shown, histamine and 5-hydroxytryptamine may also inhibit norepinephrine release in peripheral sympathetic nervous systems.[12]

The fate of released norepinephrine varies: only a small amount is available in the synaptic cleft to activate receptors on the surface of the myocyte, or to enter the cardiac cell directly (i.e., the uptake$_2$ mechanism). A fraction diffuses into the vascular space, where it can be measured as "norepinephrine spillover" in the coronary sinus venous blood, but the majority of extraneuronal norepinephrine is removed by the nerve terminal itself. The reuptake of norepinephrine from the synaptic cleft is an important and efficient mechanism for the regulation of extraneuronal stores;[13] as much as 70% of that released from the nerve terminal is taken up via this mechanism (i.e., uptake$_1$ mechanism).[14] After reuptake, norepinephrine "recycles" into the storage vesicles by active transport.[15] Other amines structurally related to norepinephrine, including epinephrine, dopamine, and metaraminol, are also taken up by the nerve terminal. The uptake$_1$ mechanism can be blocked by drugs such as cocaine, amphetamine, and desipramine,[16] whereas the storage of norepinephrine and analogs in the neuronal vesicles is inhibited by reserpine.[15]

Norepinephrine undergoes rapid metabolism in neuronal and extraneuronal tissue; it is metabolized in the neuronal cytosol by monoamine oxidase to dihydroxyphenylglycol, which clears into the vascular space, or by catechol-o-methyltransferase (COMT), which appears predominantly to be concentrated in non-neuronal tissue.

Adrenergic Receptors

The postsynaptic adrenergic receptors are classified as α or β, based on pharmacologic studies describing specific functional responses of each receptor system. Knowledge of receptor systems has rapidly expanded with the recent introduction of radioligand binding techniques to directly identify receptors.[17-19]

Cardiac adrenergic receptors are currently classified as α_1-, α_2-, β_1-, and β_2-receptor subtypes,[20] and are coupled to distinct effect pathways. Both β_1- and β_2-receptors stimulate the enzyme adenylate cyclase leading to the production of cyclic adenosine monophosphate (AMP), a biochemical response regulated by guanine nucleotide regulatory proteins (Gs).[21] In contrast, α_2-receptors inhibit adenylate cyclase via the G-protein (G$_i$). The α_1-adrenergic receptors activate the enzyme phospholipase C, but the involved G-protein is not defined.

The positive inotropic response of catecholamine stimulation is primarily mediated by β-receptors. In the normal left and right ventricular myocardium, β_1-receptors average about 80% of the total pool of β-receptors.[22] It has been speculated that β_2-receptors are more prevalent in the atria, and that β_2-selective agonists elicit a more chronotropic response than do β_1-selective drugs.[23] β_1-Receptors are targets of both epinephrine and norepinephrine, while β_2-receptors have a higher affinity for epinephrine than for norepinephrine. Recent investigations indicate that, in the heart, β-receptors may exist on the external surface of cell membranes as well as on the intracellular site of the membrane. Such internalization may correspond to the upward and downward regulation of β-receptors observed under various physiologic and pathophysiologic conditions.[24]

Radiopharmaceuticals

Based on this brief description of the sympathetic nervous system, it becomes apparent that the assessment of neuronal function with a single tracer may be difficult. The dual role of the sympathetic nerve terminal consists of synthesis and release of norepinephrine as well as its reuptake and metabolism. The characterization of this complex physiologic system with radiopharmaceuticals requires an in-depth understanding of their physiologic behavior. Competition with endogenously released neurotransmitters, intraneuronal metabolism by monoamine oxidase, and pharmacologic effects are only a few of the possible factors confounding the interpretation of clinical scintigraphic data. Thus, tracers of various designs have been examined for use in the evaluation of the sympathetic nervous system, including norepinephrine analogs, norepinephrine precursors, and receptor binding ligands.

Norepinephrine Analogs

Radiopharmaceutical research efforts have focused initially on the design of radiotracers that serve as markers for the presynaptic neuron. Radiolabeled norepinephrine is an obvious tracer for the delineation of adrenergic nerve endings. Imaging of the heart in vivo based on adrenergic nerve accumulation of a radiotracer was first accomplished with carbon-11 (^{11}C)-norepinephrine in 1976.[25] This radiotracer, labeled on the α-carbon by synthetic incorporation of ^{11}C-cyanide, provided planar images of the dog heart with the use of a standard gamma camera. Because PET imaging systems were in their infancy at this time, tomographic neuronal imaging of the heart was delayed for another decade.

In the early 1980s, iodine-123 (^{123}I)-metaiodobenzyl-guanidine (MIBG) was developed at the University of Michigan for selective mapping of the heart's sympathetic nerve endings with the use of single-photon emission computed tomographic (SPECT) instrumentation.[26] MIBG, an analog of the antihypertensive drug guanethidine, is a false adrenergic neurotransmitter that is taken up and stored by the neuron and is most likely released along with endogenous norepinephrine upon stimulation of the nerve. Unlike norepinephrine however, MIBG has a low affinity for postsynaptic adrenergic receptors, so that the message it transmits, if not "false," is at least greatly attenuated.

The subsequent development of PET neuronal radiopharmaceuticals was influenced by the University of Michigan's earlier experience with iodinated false neurotransmitters. The false transmitter metaraminol, a phenolamine

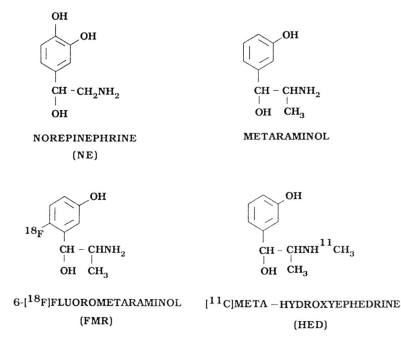

Figure 10-2. *Chemical structures of norepinephrine, metaraminol, ^{18}F-fluorometaraminol, and ^{11}C-HED.*

that is a close structural analog of norepinephrine (Figure 10-2), was chosen for detailed study. Metaraminol has been used extensively for the study of the transport characteristics of the neuronal uptake$_1$ carrier.[27] It appears to be an ideal adrenergic tracer because it has a high affinity for the amine pump (uptake$_1$) and its retention in tissue is uncomplicated by neuronal metabolism. The metabolic refractoriness of the drug relative to norepinephrine is due to the presence of the alpha methyl group, which effectively blocks the action of monoamine oxidase, and to the absence of a catechol group, which confers resistance to COMT. Once in the neuronal cytoplasm, metaraminol is co-sequestered with norepinephrine in the storage vesicles. Upon nerve impulse both norepinephrine and metaraminol are released by exocytosis. There has been controversy regarding the time course, extent, and mechanism by which metaraminol is sequestered in the intraneuronal storage vesicles.[28] However, based on the work of Shore and coworkers[29] and on our recent studies, it is evident that metaraminol labeled in vivo accumulates in the storage vesicle via the energy-requiring and reserpine-sensitive vesicular transport carrier, the same carrier that sequesters norepinephrine in the vesicles. Metaraminol's appeal is also enhanced by its structural similarity to norepinephrine. MIBG, with its highly lipophilic iodophenyl head, may display considerable non-neuronal binding in heart tissue shortly after injection. In contrast, the highly polar phenolic head of metaraminol provides high neuronal selectivity with little non-neuronal binding in the heart.[30]

After the initial validation of hydrogen-3 (^{3}H)-metaraminol as a suitable presynaptic tracer in the rat heart, 6-fluorine-18 (^{18}F)-fluorometaraminol was synthesized by the electrophilic fluorination method. The 6-position was chosen for the site of ^{18}F incorporation based on studies with fluorodopa and other catecholamines that demonstrated that fluorine in this position minimally alters the biochemistry of the native tracer. The specific activity of ^{18}F-metaraminol achievable with this synthetic method, however, averages about 1 to 15 Ci/mmol. The mass of unlabeled fluorometaraminol in projected clinical doses is thus too close to a pharmacologic level to allow safe use in human subjects.

Three N-methyl sympathomimetics (i.e., epinephrine, phenylephrine, and meta-hydroxyephedrine [HED]) were tritiated and evaluated in rats[31] as possible alternatives to fluorometaraminol. Epinephrine and HED were both superior to phenylephrine in their potential for neuronal imaging of the heart, but ^{3}H-HED was found to have the same characteristics in vivo as ^{3}H-metaraminol and fluorometaraminol. It should be noted that HED is identical in structure to metaraminol except for the presence of the N-methyl group in the former (Figure 10-2). It is not surprising that HED and metaraminol display similar dispositions in vivo since norepinephrine and epinephrine, which share the same structural homology, also have similar distributions in vivo. Thus, HED was chosen for ^{11}C labeling and for more extensive studies as an alternative to fluorometaraminol.

^{11}C-HED was synthesized by direct reaction of the free base form of metaraminol with ^{11}C-CH$_3$-I in dimethylformamide and was purified by radio high-pressure liquid chromatography (HPLC).[32] Radiochemical yields approached 40% and the specific activity ranged from 500 to 2000 Ci/mmol (i.e., over 500 times higher than that achieved with fluorometaraminol). Metabolic studies with ^{11}C-HED in guinea pigs showed that only unchanged tracer was present in heart tissue,[32] in accord with results of earlier metabolic studies with fluorometaraminol.[33] However, metabolites of ^{11}C-HED and fluorometaraminol have been observed in blood. Based on studies of metaraminol by Fuller and coworkers,[34] the two blood metabolites derived from HED are most likely α-methylepinephrine and its 3-O-methyl ether.

Norepinephrine Precursors

The rate of endogenous norepinephrine synthesis is a biochemical variable that might be used to assess sympathetic tone. 6-^{18}F-Fluorodopamine has been used for neuronal imaging of the canine heart.[35] Studies in vivo have demonstrated that this agent is partially converted to 6-^{18}F-fluoronorepinephrine in the rat heart.[36] It is difficult, however, to estimate the rate at which dopamine-β-hydroxylase metabolizes 6-^{18}F-fluorodopamine since both tracers, substrate as well as product, are retained in the adrenergic storage vesicles. A tracer approach aimed at measuring tyrosine hydroxylase activity in the heart may be a valuable tool because this enzyme is the rate-limiting step in norepinephrine synthesis. Unfortunately tyrosine and radiolabeled analogs such as L-2-^{18}F-fluorotyrosine[37] are incorporated mainly (>90%) into myocyte protein, and thus lack specificity for catecholamine synthesis. Tyrosine hydroxylase displays a high degree of substrate specificity so that there are limitations on the structural changes that can be made with the basic tyrosine structure. Meta-tyrosine is known to concentrate in sympathetic neurons but, unlike tyrosine, does not undergo protein incorporation. Meta-tyrosine has been labeled with ^{18}F in the 6-position and has been shown to accumulate in central dopaminergic neurons, mainly as the metabolite 6-^{18}F-fluoro-meta-hydroxyphenylacetic acid.[38] The behavior of 6-^{18}F-fluoro-meta-tyrosine in the peripheral adrenergic neuron has not been reported, but it will likely circumvent the rate-limiting tyrosine hydroxylase pathway and act as an immediate substrate for aromatic amino acid decarboxylase.

Adrenergic Receptor Ligands

Presynaptic Receptors

A number of receptor sites or uptake carriers in the adrenergic neuron could be targeted with positron-labeled ligands. Antidepressants such as desipramine and drugs that are abused, such as cocaine, bind to the uptake$_1$ carrier on the plasma membrane; reserpine and tetrabenazine bind to the vesicular carrier on the norepinephrine storage vesicles. The autoreceptor control of the release of norepinephrine is mediated by presynaptic α_2-adrenoceptors and such drugs as clonidine and idazoxan might be candidates for positron labeling. Although ^{11}C-prazosin has been proposed as an imaging agent for neuronal α_1-receptors, its high nonspecific binding may limit its use.[39]

Postsynaptic receptors

Numerous reports exist on the subject of radiolabeled adrenergic receptor antagonists. Both ^{11}C-propanolol and ^{11}C-practolol have been synthesized and evaluated for PET imaging.[40] As in the case of the presynaptic blockers of uptake site, most of these radioligands are highly lipophilic and exhibit considerable nonspecific binding. Also, many of the ligands bind to the adrenergic receptors with near picomolar affinity, and thus, their tissue uptake is highly dependent on blood flow. Receptor/ligand internalization and "hibernating" receptors may further complicate the interpretation of the tissue kinetics. Delforge and coworkers[41] have recently introduced butyl amino-2-hydroxypropoxy-benzimidazol (CGP12177) as a receptor ligand. This hydrophilic β-receptor antagonist binds to cell surface binding sites and therefore delineates functionally active receptors. The compound has been labeled with ^{11}C with ^{11}C-phosgene as precursor.

Quantitative Assessment of Tracer Kinetics

The fact that PET radionuclide distribution images can yield information about the functional status of both the pre- and postsynaptic components of the nervous system of the myocardium is well established.[42] The primary goal of quantitative PET studies of the nervous system of the heart is to evaluate the functional integrity of the system in the presence of disease or to evaluate the physiologic response to pharmacologic intervention. As described earlier, the physiologic and biochemical mechanisms of the cardiac nervous system are complex. Therefore, the development of quantitative PET procedures requires radiopharmaceuticals that isolate specific components of the system (e.g., tracers that selectively bind to specific receptor sites, or compounds that mimic the uptake and storage mechanisms of catecholamines in the presynaptic nerve terminal).

In PET, mathematical models are developed to define the kinetic behavior of radiopharmaceuticals as a function of the physiologic or biochemical processes of interest. Parameters describing these processes include those reflecting the delivery and removal of the radiopharmaceutical from the tissue by the vasculature, the rate at which the radiolabeled substance is accumulated or bound by the process of interest, and release of the substance from the accumulation sites. In addition, terms are often added to this parameter set to describe biochemical interactions of the radiopharmaceutical in the tissue that are not associated with the physiologic system under examination (nonspecific binding). The regulation of many of these transport systems is accomplished through the regulation of a small number of rate-limiting steps. Therefore, the determination of all values in these multiparameter sets cannot be accomplished in a single experiment, but rather multiple experiments must be performed in which some of the transport processes are interfered with via interventions such as pharmacologic blocking or displacement.[9,39,43] Since many of these pharmacologic interventions cannot be safely performed in human subjects, they are not available for use in conjunction with PET. Therefore, the complex mathematical description of radiopharmaceutical kinetics must be simplified such that the model parameters reflect combinations of processes, and the parameter magnitudes are determined primarily by the rate-limiting step of each combination.

Figure 10-3 illustrates a four-compartment model frequently used for the assessment of neuronal function in PET.[44] In this model, the compartments represent 1) the concentration of the radiopharmaceutical in the arterial blood available for transport into the tissue (Ca), 2) the free fraction of the radiopharmaceutical in the tissue available to interact with either specific or nonspecific biochemical mechanisms (Ce), 3) the specifically bound or trapped radiopharmaceutical (Cb), and 4) the nonspecifically bound tracer (Cns). The rate constants (K_1-K_6) of the model represent the unknown parameters that are estimated from the PET data.

Imaging procedures for the estimation of the kinetic model parameters generally fall into two distinct categories: dynamic and equilibrium methods. With the dynamic method, statistically based algorithms for estimation of parameters are applied to a set of tissue concentration time-activity curves acquired after the administration of the radiopharmaceutical.[40,45–47] Since the concentration of the radiopharmaceutical in the blood perfusing the tissue as a function of time is an essential component of the mathematical model, it must be measured along with the tissue data. Typically, nonlinear regression, which

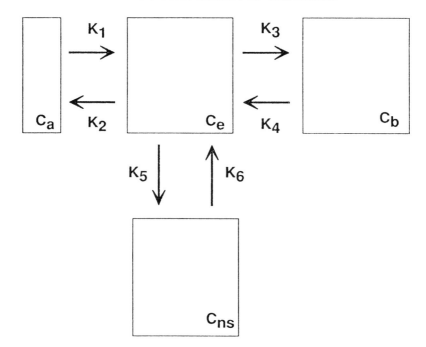

Figure 10-3. *Generalized compartmental model used for PET measurements of presynaptic and postsynaptic function of the sympathetic nervous system. The compartments of this model represent the arterial blood (Ca), the extracellular space (Ce), and the specifically bound and nonspecifically bound label (Cb and Cns, respectively). The rate of transport of the label between compartments is defined by the model parameter (K_1-K_6).*

minimizes the sum of squared residuals between the model estimate and the measured data, is used in the dynamic approach.

The second method, the equilibrium approach, is applicable to labeled pharmaceuticals that have rapid release rates from the bound state so that equilibrium can be achieved.[22] By this approach, a series of equilibrium studies are performed at various concentrations of radiopharmaceutical, and semigraphic analysis procedures are used to produce estimates of the density of binding sites in the tissue and the equilibrium dissociation constant of the radiopharmaceutical-binding site complex.

Presynaptic Sympathetic Function

The above description of the physiology of the cardiac sympathetic nervous system indicates the complex mechanisms involved in the uptake and release of catecholamines from presynaptic varicosities. A mathematical model that describes the processes of delivery and removal of the radiopharmaceutical to and from the tissue by the vascular system, the neuronal and vesicular accumulation of the tracer, and release via exocytosis on nerve stimulation would be extremely complex. In addition, terms should be included in the model to describe biochemical interactions involving the radiopharmaceutical that are not associated with the physiologic processes of interest (nonspecific interactions). Fortunately, many of these transport systems are regulated by a small number of rate-limiting steps so that the mathematical description of the radiopharmaceutical kinetics can be simplified to a subset of the four-compartment model previously described. Preliminary studies of 6-^{18}F-fluorometaraminol and ^{11}C-HED have demonstrated the suitability of this model (with the nonspecific compartment eliminated) for the description of observed kinetics.[48] An example of ^{11}C-HED kinetics in the open-chest dog after intracoronary injection of radiopharmaceutical as a bolus is shown in Figure 10-4. The biexponential behavior of the detected photon efflux from the tissue can clearly be delineated, which corresponds with the described model configuration. The overlayed curve in the Figure represents the observed kinetic behavior of ^{11}C-HED after the administration of a dose of 5 mg/kg desipramine to block the cellular uptake of the tracer. The rapid efflux of the tracer from the tissue in this study demonstrates the low nonspecific component of tracer accumulation in the tissue. In this model (Figure 10-3), the rate constants K_1 and K_2 represent the delivery and removal of the radiopharmaceutical via the vascular system of the heart. The rate constants K_3 and K_4 represent the combination of cellular and vesicular uptake mechanisms via diffusion or active transport mechanisms and the catecholamine release from the presynaptic nerve terminals by both exocytosis and cellular transport mechanisms, respectively. Preliminary kinetic studies in human

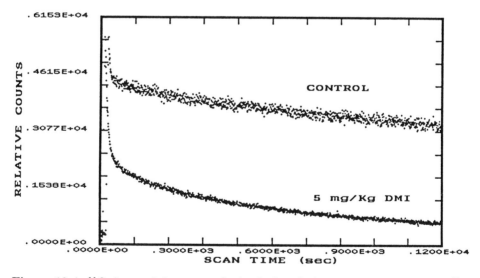

Figure 10-4. *[11]C time-activity curves obtained after the intracoronary injection of ^{11}C-HED in the open-chest dog (bolus injection). The control curve (top) shows high extraction of ^{11}C-HED by myocardium, with only slow clearance of the activity from tissue. The time-activity curve on the bottom was obtained after pretreatment with 5 mg/kg desipramine (DMI). [11]C activity cleared rapidly from tissue, resulting in markedly decreased tissue retention of the tracer, which indicates very little nonspecific binding of the tracer in myocardial tissue.*

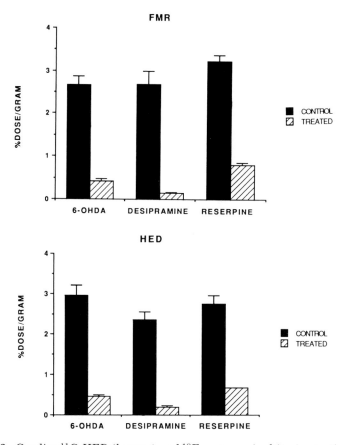

Figure 10-6. *Cardiac* ^{11}C*-HED (bottom) and* ^{18}F*-metaraminol (top) retention in the rat under control conditions and after pretreatment with 6-hydroxydopamine (6-OHDA), desipramine, and reserpine. Retention of tracer in cardiac tissue is expressed as percent injected dose per gram and was determined 30 minutes after intravenous injection of tracer.*

PET was used in closed-chest dogs to evaluate ^{18}F-metaraminol and ^{11}C-HED for the noninvasive assessment of the distribution of the sympathetic nerve terminals by imaging techniques. Images were acquired after intravenous injection of the tracer. Regional blood flow was assessed in this experiment by use of ^{13}N-ammonia and the results were correlated with the regional retention of the catecholamine analog. Uptake kinetics in normal and denervated myocardium were determined in a chronic dog model in which regional denervation was achieved by epicardial application of phenol. Figure 10-7 shows a representative example of an ^{18}F-metaraminol study in an animal 5 days after epicardial application of phenol. The blood flow studies on the right show homogeneous blood flow distribution throughout the left ventricle. The corresponding ^{18}F-metaraminol images on the left indicate markedly decreased uptake of the tracer in the area of previous phenol application. The myocardium is well visualized in contrast to the ventricular chamber and surrounding lung tissue.

Correlation of the retention of tracer in vivo with tissue content of norepineph-rine showed a close linear relationship between the measurements (Figure 10-8). These data indicate that ^{18}F-metaraminol and ^{11}C-HED provide images of excellent quality and allow specific delineation of normal and denervated myocardium in the dog. Application of a kinetic model for both tracers provided quantitative assessment of regional tracer distribution volume. The volume of distribution for ^{18}F-metaraminol derived from PET data correlated closely with tissue content of norepinephrine.[48]

An animal preparation of brief regional ischemia and subsequent reperfu-sion was used to demonstrate the sensitivity of sympathetic neurons to is-chemia.[49] In the open-chest dog, ^{18}F-metaraminol was injected after a 30 min-ute occlusion of the left anterior descending artery and tissue activity was

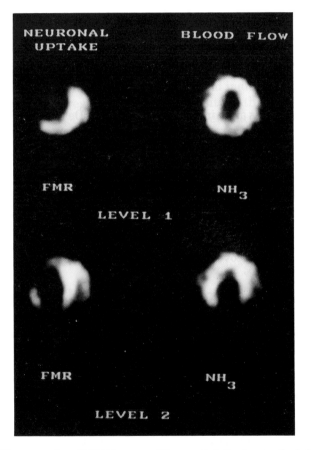

Figure 10-7. *Cross-sectional PET images of tracer distribution in the left ventricle after the injection of ^{13}N-ammonia (blood flow tracer; right) and ^{18}F-metaraminol (left). Myo-cardial blood flow is homogeneous throughout the left ventricle. The fluorometaraminol images on the left show regional reduction of tissue retention of ^{18}F-metaraminol. In this animal, regional sympathetic denervation was performed by the epicardial application of phenol 5 days before the PET study.*

of presynaptic nerve terminals in these patients. Color Figure 11 shows cross-sectional images obtained after the intravenous injection of ^{11}C-HED from a patient with congestive cardiomyopathy. In contrast to the relative homogeneous myocardial perfusion as assessed with [82]Rb, ^{11}C-HED retention is markedly reduced, especially in the more distal aspects of the left ventricle. This heterogeneous pattern of ^{11}C-HED uptake has been confirmed in the majority of patients with congestive cardiomyopathy studied.[56] With the use of the described kinetic model for ^{11}C-HED described above, myocardial tracer retention has been quantified as tracer volume of distribution and compared in healthy volunteers, patients with recent cardiac transplantation, and patients with congestive cardiomyopathy (Figure 10-11). This index of neuronal catecholamine storage capacity was markedly reduced in patients with cardiomyopathy, in whom values approached those in the denervated transplanted heart, although the relatively large standard deviation of the measurements indicates a large variability in the findings. These quantitative data indicate that the presynaptic uptake of catecholamines is severely altered in patients with cardiomyopathy, which may affect the reuptake of extraneuronal norepinephrine by sympathetic nerve terminals, and hence results in an overexposure of myocytes to norepinephrine. This hypothesis is supported by recent findings indicating a beneficial effect of β-receptor blockade in patients with congestive

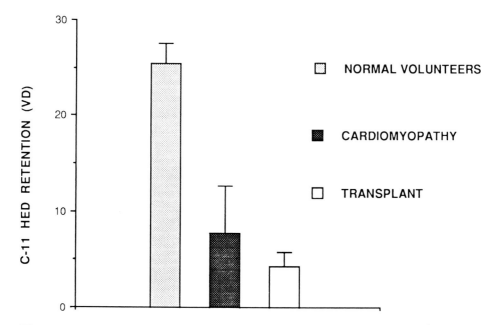

Figure 10-11. *Quantitative assessment of myocardial retention of ^{11}C-HED by use of a tracer kinetic model (Figure 10–3). The volume of distribution (VD) of tracer was averaged in 5 healthy volunteers, 4 patients with congestive cardiomyopathy, and 5 patients with recent cardiac transplants. VD was significantly reduced in both latter groups. VD in the patients with cardiomyopathy approached that in transplant patients, but demonstrated considerable variability.*

heart failure.[45] Thus, the quantitative delineation of sympathetic nervous function in such patients by PET may aid in the selection of individuals for therapy with β-receptor blockers, and enhance understanding of the cardiac sympathetic nervous system in patients with congestive cardiomyopathy.

Conclusion

PET appears to permit accurate regional delineation of tissue concentration of tracer. With the use of this modality with new radiopharmaceuticals, the presynaptic sympathetic nerve terminal and β-receptor distribution can be noninvasively evaluated.

The approaches being developed represent a start in efforts to describe quantitatively the cardiac integrity of function of the sympathetic nervous system. Radiolabeled analogs and precursors of norepinephrine may allow the specific evaluation of amine uptake and norepinephrine synthesis. The qualitative evaluation of regional tracer distribution will allow identification of global and regional denervation but appears to be limited in assessing functional abnormalities of the sympathetic nervous system. Quantitative data analysis by use of a tracer kinetic model appears to be feasible for ^{11}C-HED and CGP12177 but requires further validation. Thus, not only detailed knowledge about uptake and binding characteristics of the radiopharmaceuticals but also the definition of metabolic fate of the compounds is necessary for accurate measurement of tracer kinetics.

A multidisciplinary approach that involves neurocardiologists, radiochemists, and physicists is needed to maximize the full potential of PET for the noninvasive assessment of regional neuronal function. The clinical application of such imaging approaches in patients with various cardiac diseases should provide important insights regarding the involvement of the sympathetic nervous system in specific pathophysiologic conditions. Undoubtedly, neuronal imaging will have major value as a research tool. Its future clinical role is difficult to predict presently but clearly merits further definition.

References

1. Loewi O. Uber humorale ubertragbarkeit der herznervenwirkung. Pfluegers Arch 1921; 189:239.
2. von Euler U. A specific sympathomimetic ergone in adrenergic nerve fibers (sympathin) and its relation to adrenaline and noradrenaline. Acta Physiol Scand 1946; 12:73.
3. Peart W. The nature of splenic sympathin. J Physiol 1949; 108:491.
4. Lund A. Simultaneous fluorometric determinations of adrenaline and noradrenaline in blood. Acta Pharmacol Toxicol 1950; 6:137.
5. Goldstein D. Plasma norepinephrine as an indicator of sympathetic neural activity in clinical cardiology. Am J Cardiol 1981; 48:1147.
6. Wieland D, Brown L, Rogers W, Worthington K, Wu J, Clinthorne N, Otto C,

Swanson D, Beierwaltes W. Myocardial imaging with a radioiodinated norepinephrine storage analog. J Nucl Med 1983; 24:1127–1134.

7. Levitt M, Spector S, Sjoerdsma A, Udenfriend S. Elucidation of the rate-limiting step in norepinephrine biosynthesis in the perfused guinea-pig heart. J Pharmacol Exp Ther 1965; 148:1.

8. Bareis D, Slotkin T. Synaptic vesicles isolated from rat heart: L-(H3) norepinephrine uptake properties. J Neurochem 1979; 32:345.

9. Toll L, Howard B. Role of MG_{2+}-ATPase and a pH gradient in the storage of catecholamines in synaptic vesicles. Biochemistry 1978; 17:2517.

10. Langer S. Presynaptic receptors and modulation of neurotransmission: pharmacological implications and therapeutic relevance. Trends Neurosci 1980; 3:110–112.

11. Muscholl E, Ritzel H, Rossler K. Presynaptic muscarinic control of neuronal adrenaline release. In: Langer S, Stark K, Dubocovich M, eds. Presynaptic Receptors. Oxford: Pergamon, 1979; 287–291.

12. Francis G. Modulation of peripheral sympathetic nerve transmission. J Am Coll Cardiol 1988; 12:250–254.

13. Goldstein D, Brush J Jr, Eisenhofer G, Stull R, Esler M. In vivo measurement of neuronal uptake of norepinephrine in the human heart. Circulation 1988; 78:41–48.

14. Axelrod J. The fate of adrenaline and noradrenaline. In: Vane J, Wolstenholme G, O'Connor M, Eds. Adrenergic Mechanisms.Boston: Little, Brown & Co., 1960; 28–39.

15. Njus D, Kelley P, Harnadek G. Bioenergetics of secretory vesicles. Biochim et Biophys Acta 1986; 853:237–265.

16. Hertting G, Axelrod J, Kopin J, Whitby L. Effect of drugs on the uptake and metabolism of H3-norepinephrine. J Pharmacol Exp Ther 1961; 134:146–153.

17. Lefkowitz R, Mukherjee C, Coverstone M, Caron M. Stereospecific [3H](-)- alprenolol binding sites, beta-adrenergic receptors and adenylate cyclase. Biochem Biophys Res Commun 1974; 60:703–709.

18. Aurbach G, Fedak S, Woodard C, Palmer JS, Hauser D, Troxler F. Beta-adrenergic receptor: Stereospecific interaction of iodinated beta-blocking agent with high affinity site. Science 1974; 186:1223–1224.

19. Levitzki A, Atlas D, Steer M. The binding characteristics and number of beta-adrenergic receptors on the turkey erythrocyte. Proc Natl Acad Sci USA 1974; 71:2773–2776.

20. Lefkowitz R, Caron M. Adrenergic receptors. J Biol Chem 1988; 263:4993–4996.

21. Casey P, Gilman A. G protein involvement in receptor-effector coupling. J Biol Chem 1988; 263:2577–2580.

22. Stiles G, Taylor S, Lefkowitz R. Human cardiac beta-adrenergic receptors: Subtype heterogeneity delineated by direct radioligand binding. Life Sci 1983; 33:467–473.

23. Carlsson E, Dahlof C, Hedberg A, Persson H, Tangstrand B. Differentiation of cardiac chronotropic and inotropic effects of beta-adreno-ceptor agonists. Naunyn-Schmiedebergs Arch Pharmacol 1977; 300:101–106.

24. Bristow MR, Ginsburg R, Minobe W, Cubicciotti RS, Sageman WS, Lurie K, Bullingham ME, Harrison DC, Stinson EB. Decreased catecholamine sensitivity and beta-adrenergic receptor density in failing human hearts. N Engl J Med 1982; 307:205–211.

25. Fowler J, Wolf A, Cristman R, MacGregor R, Ansari A, Atkins H. Carrier-free ^{11}C-labeled catecholamines. In: Subramanian G, Rhodes B, Cooper J, Sodd V, Eds. Radiopharmaceuticals. New York: Society of Nuclear Medicine, 1975; 196–204.

26. Wieland D, Brown L, Rogers W, Worthington K, Wu J-L, Clinthorn N, Otto C, Swanson D, Beierwaltes W. Myocardial imaging with a radioiodinated norepinephrine storage analog. J Nucl Med 1981; 22:22–31.

27. Ross S. Structural requirements for uptake into catecholamine neurons. In: Paton, Ed. The Mechanism of Neuronal and Extraneuronal Transport of Catecholamines. New York: Raven Press, 1976; 67–93.

28. Anton A, Berk A. Distribution of metaraminol and its relation to norepinephrine. Eur J Pharmacol 1977; 44:161–167.

29. Crout J, Alpers H, Tatum E, Shore P. Release of metaraminol (Aramine) from the heart by sympathetic nerve stimulations. Science 1964; 145:828–830.

30. Wieland D, Rosenspire K, Hutchins G, Van Dort M, Rothley J, Mislankar S, Lee H, Massin C, Gildersleeve D, Sherman P, Schwaiger M. Neuronal mapping of the heart with 6-[^{18}F]fluorometaraminol. J Med Chem 1990; 33:956–964.

31. Van Dort M, Gildersleeve D, Wieland D. Synthesis of ^{3}H-labeled sympathomimetic amines for neuronal mapping. J Label Compounds Radiopharm 1990; 28:831–840.

32. Rosenspire K, Kaka M, Jewett D, Van Dort M, Gildersleeve D, Schwaiger M, Wieland D. Synthesis and preliminary evaluation of [^{11}C]meta-hydroxyephedrine: A false transmitter agent for heart neuronal imaging. J Nucl Med 1990; 31:163–167.

33. Rosenspire K, Gildersleeve D, Massin C, Mislankar S, Wieland D. Metabolic fate of the heart agent [^{18}F]6-fluorometaraminol. Nucl Med Biol 1989; 16:735–739.

34. Fuller R, Snoddy H, Perry K, Bernstein J, Murphy P. Formation of alpha-methyl-norepinephrine as a metabolite of metaraminol in guinea pigs. Biochem Pharmacol 1981; 30:2831–2836.

35. Goldstein D, Chang P, Eisenhofer G, Miletich R, Finn R, Bacher J, Kirk K, Bacharach S, Kopin I. Positron emission tomographic imaging of cardiac sympathetic innervation and function. Circulation 1990; 81:1606–1621.

36. Eisenhofer G, Hovevey-Sion D, Kopin I, Miletich R, Kirk K, Finn R, Goldstein D. Neuronal uptake and metabolism of 2- and 6-fluorodopamine: False neurotransmitters for positron emission tomographic imaging of sympathetically innervated tissues. J Pharmacol Exp Ther 1989; 248:419–427.

37. Coenen H, Kling P, Stocklin G. Cerebral metabolism of L-[2- ^{18}F]fluorotyrosine, a new PET tracer for protein synthesis. J Nucl Med 1989; 30:1367–1372.

38. Firnau G, Chirakal R, Nahmias C, Garnett E. [F-18]fluorometa-L-tyrosine is a better PET tracer than [F-18]fluoro-L-DOPA for the delineation of dopaminergic structures in the human brain. Proc 8th Inter Sympos Radiopharm Chem, Princeton University, Princeton, NJ, June 24–29, 1990; 272–273.

39. Syrota A. Positron emission tomography: Evaluation of cardiac receptors. In: Marcus ML, Skorton DJ, Schelbert HR, Wolf GL, Eds. (Braunwald E, Consulting Ed). *Cardiac Imaging—Principles and Practice: A Companion of Braunwald's Heart Disease.* Philadelphia: W.B. Saunders 1991; 1256–1270.

40. Syrota A, Marty J, Seto M, Fournier D, Crouzel C, Vallois J, Crouzel M, Maze M. Halothane-induced decrease of ^{11}C-CGP 12177 binding to myocardial beta adrenergic receptor demonstrated by PET in the dog. J Nucl Med 1988; 29:940.

41. Delforge J, Syrota A, Lancon J-P, Nakajima K, Lock C, Janier M, Valloise J-M, Cayla J, Crouzel C. Cardiac beta-adrenergic receptor density measured in vivo using PET, CGP 12177 and a new graphical method. J Nucl Med 1991; 32:739–748.

42. Dormont D, Syrota A, Berger G, Maxiere M, Prenant C, Sastre J, Davy J, Aumont M, Motte G, Gourgon R. C-11 ligand binding to adrenergic and muscarinic receptors in the human heart studied in vivo by PET. J Nucl Med 1983; 24:P20.

43. Kopin I, Gordon E. Metabolism of norepinephrine-3H by tyramine and reserpine. J Pharmacol Exp Ther 1962; 138:351–358.

44. Farde L, Hakan H, Ehrin E, Sedvall G. Quantitative analysis of D2 dopamine receptor binding in the living human brain by PET. Science 1986; 231:258–261.

45. Waagstein F, Caidahl K, Wallentin I, Bergh C-H, Hjalmarson A. Long-term β-blockade in dilated cardiomyopathy: Effects of short- and long-term metoprolol treatment followed by withdrawal and readministration of metoprolol. Circulation 1989; 80:551–563.

46. Sole M, Helke C, Jacobowitz D. Increased dopamine in the failing hamster heart: Transvesicular transport of dopamine limits the rate of norepinephrine synthesis. Am J Cardiol 1982; 49:1682.

47. Syrota A, Comar D, Paillotin G, Davy J, Aumont M, Stulzaft O, Maziere B. Muscarinic cholinergic receptor in the human heart evidenced under physiological conditions by positron emission tomography. Proc Natl Acad Sci (USA) 1985; 82:584–588.

48. Hutchins G, Schwaiger M, Haka M, Rosenspire K, Wieland D. Compartmental analysis of the behavior of catecholamine analogs in myocardial tissue. J Nucl Med 1989; 30:767.
49. Schwaiger M, Guibourg H, Rosenspire K, McClanahan T, Gallagher K, Hutchins G, Wieland D. Effect of regional myocardial ischemia on sympathetic nervous system as assessed by F-18 metaraminol. J Nucl Med 1990; 31:1352–1357.
50. Chiueh C, Zukowska-Grojec Z, Kirk K, Kopin I. Fluoro-catecholamines as false adrenergic neurotransmitters. J Pharmacol Exp Ther 1983; 225:529–533.
51. Pascal O, Syrota A, Berger G, Sastre J, Collard P, Huchon G, Chretien J. Lung uptake of ^{11}C-imipramine and ^{11}C-propranolol in patients with sarcoidosis evaluated by positron emission tomography. In: Marsac, Chretien, eds. *Sarcoidosis and Other Granulomatous Disorders*. Paris: Pergamon Press, 1981; 404–408.
52. Boullais C, Crouzal C, Syrota A. Synthesis of 4-(3-t-butylamino-2-hydroxypropoxy)-benzimidazole-2(^{11}C)-one (CGP 12177). J Label Compounds Radiopharm 1986; 5:565–567.
53. Schwaiger M, Kalff V, Rosenspire K, Haka M, Molina E, Hutchins G, Deeb M, Wolfe E Jr., Wieland D. The noninvasive evaluation of the sympathetic nervous system in the human heart by PET. Circulation 1990; 82:457–464.
54. Schwaiger M, Hutchins G, Kalff V, Molina E, Rosenspire K, Haka M, Deeb M, Wieland D. Evidence of regional catecholamine uptake and storage sites in the transplanted human heart by positron emission tomography. J Clin Invest 1991; 87:1681–1690.
55. Wolpers H, Nguyen N, Rosenspire K, Haka M, Wieland D, Schwaiger M. Comparison of C-11 HED and I-131 MIBG for the assessment of ischemic neuronal injury in the canine heart. J Nucl Med 1990; 31:725 (abstract.)
56. Schwaiger M, Hutchins G, Rosenspire K, Haka M, Wieland D. Quantitative evaluation of the sympathetic nervous system by PET in patients with cardiomyopathy. J Nucl Med 1990; 31:792 (abstract).

Chapter 11

Clinical Applications of Cardiac Positron Emission Tomography

Robert J. Gropler, M.D.,
Edward M. Geltman, M.D.,
and Burton E. Sobel, M.D.

Positron emission tomography (PET) is an established and powerful tool for characterizing cardiac cellular physiology and pathophysiology, quantifying regional myocardial perfusion and oxygen consumption, and delineating myocardial biochemical manifestations of cardiomyopathy of diverse etiologies.[1–3]

Regardless of the imaging modality used, cardiac imaging is undertaken either to provide observations in well-defined subsets that elucidate novel diagnostic and therapeutic advances or to obtain information needed for management of individual patients. PET's value in the first category is unequivocal; for example, it has demonstrated normalization of myocardial perfusion reserve after angioplasty and documented salutary effects of coronary thrombolysis on myocardial oxidative metabolism.[4,5] Its value in the second category, management, is becoming increasingly well appreciated.

Regional Myocardial Perfusion, Metabolism, and Function

Characterization of coronary blood flow at the level of macroscopic vessels requires angiography or digital subtraction angiography; estimates at the level of tissue perfusion generally entail single-photon scintigraphy with agents such as thallium 201 (^{201}Tl); and the impact of limited flow is often assessed indirectly by exercise radionuclide ventriculography or stress echocardiography. PET can yield estimates of regional myocardial perfusion per se, in absolute terms.[6] With respect to quantifying regional myocardial metabolism, im-

From *Positron Emission Tomography of the Heart* edited by Steven R. Bergmann, MD, PhD and Burton E. Sobel, MD © 1992, Futura Publishing Inc., Mount Kisco, NY.

aging modalities other than PET, such as scintigraphy with iodinated fatty acids, exhibit marked limitations.[7] In contrast, PET can delineate fluxes through specific metabolic pathways underlying normal or abnormal cardiac function.

Several imaging approaches have been developed to assess regional contractile function: two-dimensional echocardiography, radionuclide ventriculography, and nuclear magnetic resonance imaging, to name but a few. PET can delineate changes in ventricular geometry and wall motion but its limited spatial resolution detracts from its utility for definitive characterization of regional and ventricular performance.

The following material summarizes major contributions of PET in clinical research that requires delineation of regional myocardial perfusion and myocardial metabolism as well as its contributions to diagnosis and management of individual patients.

General Principles

Localization of emitted positrons, tomographic instrumentation, image reconstruction, and production of radiopharmaceuticals will be reviewed only briefly here. As discussed in Chapter 2, positron-emitting radionuclides decay with generation of two 511 keV photons that are dispersed at an angle of approximately 180°. Coincidence counting, the detection of 2 photons by opposing detectors within a pre-established interval typically 5 to 20 nsec), can therefore localize the emission event within a collinear field of view. Coincidence detection can compensate for attenuation regardless of the locus of the emitter with respect to either of the 2 detectors in each pair. Within the limits of spatial resolution of the tomograph used, the kinetic energy of the positron-emitting radionuclide used, which predominately determines the path length of positrons in the tissue before annihilation, and the degradation of data attributable to cardiac and respiratory motion, coincidence detection permits absolute quantification of the amount of radioactivity within a given field of view.

A major attribute of PET is its applicability to tracers of physiologic compounds. Positron-emitting radionuclides of carbon (^{11}C), nitrogen (^{13}N), and oxygen (^{15}O) can be incorporated into diverse metabolic substrates (and with fluorine [^{18}F] into substrate-analogues) that participate in diverse biochemical pathways without distorting the biochemical properties of the substrate of interest (Table 11-1). Accurate interpretation of the kinetics of a particular radiopharmaceutical requires knowledge of the metabolic pathways involved, of the fates of specific pools of the radiopharmaceutical, and the fate of the tracer as it is incorporated in numerous products of metabolism. The short physical half-life exhibited by most positron-emitting radionuclides is well suited to performance of brief and sequential studies with limited radiation burdens to the subject. However, this property (except for ^{18}F, $t_{1/2} = 110$ min) generally mandates on-site production with an on-site cyclotron. Nevertheless, generator-produced positron-emitting radionuclides such as copper-62 ([62]Cu), gallium-68 (^{68}Ga), and rubidium-82 ([82]Rb), and cyclotron-produced ^{18}F can be used by centers without isotope production capabilities.

Table 11-1
Positron-emitting Compounds Currently Used with PET for Cardiac Studies

Radionuclide	Half Life	Compound	Present Use
Cyclotron Produced			
Oxygen 15	2.04 min	H_2O	Blood flow
		CO	Blood volume
		CO_2	Blood flow
Nitrogen 13	10.0 min	NH_3	Blood flow
		Various amino acids	Amino acid metabolism
Carbon 11	20.4 min	Acetate	Oxidative metabolism
		Pyruvate	Intermediary metabolism
		Palmitate	Fatty acid metabolism
		Glucose	Glucose metabolism
		HED	Norepinephrine distribution
		Microspheres	Blood flow
		Butanol	Blood flow
Fluorine 18	110 min	Deoxyglucose	Glucose metabolism
		Misonidazole	Marker of hypoxia
		Metaraminol	Norepinephrine distribution
Generator Produced			
Rubidium 82	1.25 min	RbCl	Blood flow
Copper 62	9.73 min	Cu-PTSM	Blood flow
Gallium 68	68.0 min	Microspheres	Blood flow

Abbreviations: HED = hydroxyephedrine; PTSM = bis-4-N-methylthiosemicarbazone.

Measurement of Perfusion

Clinically important abnormalities of perfusion are often regional. In some instances (e.g., cardiac allograft rejection, left ventricular hypertrophy, or cardiomyopathy attributable to small-vessel coronary disease) they may be homogeneous. Definitive assessment of both global and regional myocardial perfusion at rest and after vasodilator (or exercise) stress or after a therapeutic intervention designed to improve nutritive perfusion is of intense interest.

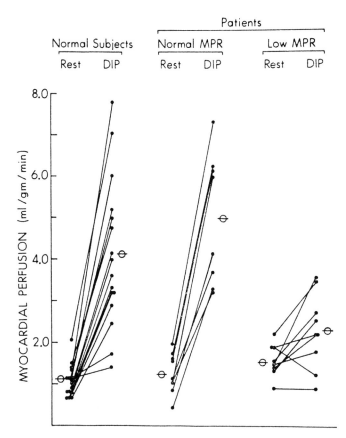

Figure 11-1. *Estimates of myocardial perfusion determined by PET with $H_2{}^{15}O$ and dynamic analysis in normal subjects and patients with chest pain and angiographically normal coronary arteries. Myocardial perfusion reserve (MPR) was reduced (< 2.5) in response to dipyridamole (DIP) in 9 of 17 patients and 2 of 16 normal subjects. (Reproduced with permission from Geltman et al.[16])*

coronary arteries and the response of the syndrome to potentially therapeutic interventions.[16]

Detection of Late Rejection of Cardiac Allografts

Survival after cardiac transplantation within 1 year is limited primarily by complications such as infection and rejection of the allograft. Long-term survival is frequently limited by development of "coronary artery disease" in the allograft.[17] It is unclear whether the cause of this type of coronary disease is the same as that in patients with typical atherosclerotic, coronary artery disease or whether it is mediated by late, immunologic rejection of the donor heart's vasculature. Presently, its detection requires annual or more frequent coronary angiography in recipients, in part because of the absence of pain with ischemia in a denervated heart. Despite aggressive angiographic surveillance, coronary arterial compromise is frequently difficult to detect because of the diffuse nature of the process.[17] Several studies using intracoronary Doppler flow probes have demonstrated reduced perfusion reserve in patients with either early or late rejection.[18,19] Recently, we have shown that PET with $H_2^{15}O$ detects reduced perfusion reserve in response to intravenous dipyridamole in recipients of cardiac transplants.[20] The reduction is attributable to an increase in perfusion at rest, approximately 80% greater than that in normal subjects, rather than a reduction in the maximal hyperemic flow response.[21] These results indicate that cardiac PET may be useful not only in detecting coronary artery disease in transplanted hearts, hence facilitating selection of patients requiring invasive procedures such as angiography and myocardial biopsy, but also in elucidating the pathogenesis of the insult, thereby facilitating development and evaluation of prophylactic measures.

Assessment of Patients with Left Ventricular Hypertrophy

Angina pectoris is a frequent symptom in patients with left ventricular hypertrophy even in patients without macrovascular coronary artery disease. These symptoms most likely reflect abnormalities in the coronary microcirculation resulting in an impairment in myocardial perfusion reserve. Marcus and coworkers demonstrated that perfusion reserve, derived from Doppler flow velocity measurements of the left anterior descending artery, was decreased in patients with left ventricular hypertrophy.[22] Goldstein and Haynie, using PET and ^{82}Rb in 9 patients with left ventricular hypertrophy and 16 control subjects, measured myocardial perfusion under resting conditions and after the combination dipyridamole and handgrip-induced stress. Using a semiquantitative approach of myocardial perfusion reserve (based on the ratio of myocardial activity after dipyridamole and handgrip stress divided by myocardial activity under resting conditions), they demonstrated that myocardial perfusion reserve was limited in the patients with left ventricular hypertrophy and that the impairment in perfusion reserve was global, not regional.[23] More recently, Camici et al., using ^{13}N-ammonia and PET, demonstrated impaired perfusion reserve in patients with asymmetric left ventricular hypertrophy. They found impaired perfusion reserve in these patients, even in nonhypertrophied regions. Patients with hypertrophy and a history of chest pain had more pronounced reductions in perfusion reserve than did those without chest pain.[24] Thus, evaluation of perfusion reserve in patients with hypertrophy should better quantify the degree of impairment in perfusion reserve and help delineate whether the impairment reflects primarily an elevation in myocardial perfusion under resting conditions, a reduced response to pharmacologic or exercise-induced stress, or both.

Characterization of Potentially Therapeutic Interventions

Restoration of nutritive myocardial perfusion is the cornerstone of modern treatment of disorders such as acute myocardial infarction. Salutary effects on myocardial metabolism and function follow if ischemia is interrupted promptly and if the restoration of perfusion is sustained.

Revascularization

Available methods for documentation of restoration of perfusion and perfusion reserve after coronary revascularization by any means are limited. Coronary angiography delineates graft patency and the extent of residual stenosis in native vessels. It provides no information defining the impact of an intervention on myocardial perfusion per se. Intracoronary Doppler flow probes can document normalization of perfusion velocity reserve after interventions such as angioplasty, but the approach is invasive, and the accuracy of results is critically dependent on the expertise of the individual operator. No estimate of actual volume of flow, as opposed to flow velocity, is provided. Scintigraphy can document reversible defects in myocardial uptake of ^{201}Tl for intervals as long as 1 month after successful coronary angioplasty,[25] but it is not clear whether such defects represent physiologically significant abnormalities of perfusion as opposed to correlates of myocardial stunning (with altered intra- or extracellular transport of ^{201}Tl). Nevertheless, restoration of perfusion after coronary artery bypass surgery detected scintigraphically is paralleled by improved regional contractile function. Thus, in 23 patients studied after surgery, 19 of 23 segments with abnormal contractile function before surgery exhibited improved perfusion reserve with exercise after surgery in segments supplied by a patent bypass graft. Improvement in contractile function was seen as well. In contrast, in 9 of 10 segments with persistent abnormalities of regional contractility perfusion deficits were induced by exercise, and the coronary bypass graft was either occluded or markedly compromised.[26]

Cine-computed tomography (fast CT) with its high temporal and spatial resolution provides sensitivity, specificity, and diagnostic accuracy of greater than 90% in determining graft patency.[27,28] Nevertheless, ^{201}Tl scintigraphy remains the most commonly used method for identifying restenosis after angioplasty or surgery. Sensitivity, specificity, and diagnostic accuracy have been reported to be in the range of 80% each.[29–31]

Results of clinical studies with positron-emitting perfusion tracers have documented the efficacy of revascularization procedures in augmenting nutritive perfusion. For example, in 100% of a small group of patients undergoing successful angioplasty, PET with ^{82}Rb delineated improvement in perfusion reserve. Although results were limited by the underestimation of absolute levels in perfusion reserve (because of underestimation of hyperemic flow attributable to altered extraction fraction when end points are images), augmentation of myocardial perfusion reserve after coronary angioplasty[32] was delineated as well. More recently, we used $H_2{}^{15}O$ and a mathematical approach to measure regional perfusion in absolute terms and showed that myocardial perfusion normalized after angiographically successful coronary angioplasty (Color Figure 12).[4] Even in zones supplied by arteries with high-grade residual stenoses, regional perfusion was restored.

Cardiac PET has clarified the status of regional perfusion after coronary artery bypass surgery. Thus, in 67% of patients with preoperative electrocardiographic and tomographic criteria of ischemia, coronary bypass surgery relieved ischemia entirely. However, in approximately 30% of patients, exercise-induced perfusion abnormalities were demonstrable with [82]Rb despite angiographically demonstrable patent grafts. These results imply impairment in nutritive perfusion and may be attributable to lesions distal to the site of implantation of the bypass grafts into epicardial vessels.[33]

Treatment of Acute Myocardial Infarction

A mainstay of modern treatment of acute myocardial infarction is prompt restoration of nutritive perfusion, usually implemented pharmacologically with thrombolytic drugs.[34–36] If reperfusion is prompt enough, myocardium can be salvaged, left ventricular contractility preserved, and mortality reduced substantially.[37–39] Much investigation during the past decade has focused on coronary thrombolysis, and particularly, quantification of the extent of reperfusion and subsequent myocardial salvage elicited by specific regimens. Initial studies relied on serial coronary angiography as a sole or primary end point. Their results documented patency with various thrombolytic agents given by various modes of administration.[40,41] However, patency (defined as an open vessel at a specific interval after treatment without reference to previous angiographic documentation of thrombotic occlusion) of the infarct-related artery is not necessarily indicative of the extent of reperfusion. The patent vessel may never have been occluded, collateral flow may have been virtually as great as flow through a truly recanalized vessel, or myocardium supplied may be irreversibly injured and therefore be incapable of being salvaged.[42] In addition, microvascular occlusion, compression, or plugging may impair perfusion despite recanalization of macroscopic vessels. Accordingly, approaches have been defined to assess nutritive perfusion per se. Granato and coworkers measured ^{201}Tl myocardial kinetics in dogs at selected intervals after coronary occlusion and reperfusion. When ^{201}Tl was administered after 1 hour of occlusion followed by rapid reperfusion, the extent of redistribution correlated with the extent of myocardial salvage. However, when ^{201}Tl was given immediately after a 1 hour occlusion, ^{201}Tl myocardial uptake overestimated the amount of myocardial salvage because of excess ^{201}Tl uptake by necrotic myocytes exposed to hyperemia with early reperfusion. The clearance of ^{201}Tl was faster from the necrotic than from the normal myocardium. Even though the extent of necrosis was similar, myocardial defects were significantly smaller in dogs when ^{201}Tl was given after the onset of reperfusion after 1 hour of occlusion than they were in dogs when ^{201}Tl was given while the vessel was occluded before reperfusion.[43] No significant redistribution was observed when ^{201}Tl was given after 3 hours of occlusion without reperfusion. Thus, ^{201}Tl uptake and clearance are significantly influenced by the timing of administration of the tracer relative to the time of onset of reperfusion. Nevertheless, resolution of ^{201}Tl myocardial perfusion defects with time is frequently associated with improvement in regional contractility in patients with angiographically successful coronary thrombolysis.[44]

of involvement of specific coronary arteries, particularly when coupled with quantitative image analysis.[51]

Thallium-201 scintigraphy has advantages compared with PET in that standard gamma camera detection systems can be used and experience is extensive. Some information is acquired regarding tissue viability. However, suboptimal imaging characteristics, the long physical half-life of the tracer, and a relative lack of instantaneous and universal availability of the radionuclide detract from its attributes.

The imaging characteristics of Tc-MIBI are more favorable than those of ^{201}Tl. Its relatively short physical half-life and ready availability (by synthesis with ^{99m}Tc) are advantages. It exhibits little or no redistribution in nonreperfused tissue and is being evaluated extensively for detection of coronary artery disease. Kahn and coworkers demonstrated that pre- and postexercise Tc-MIBI myocardial imaging was only slightly more sensitive than SPECT ^{201}Tl scintigraphy for detection of coronary artery disease documented angiographically. However, Tc-MIBI imaging was superior to SPECT with ^{201}Tl in localizing involvement of specific coronary arteries of supply.[52]

Exercise radionuclide ventriculography, like electrocardiography, detects consequences of ischemia rather than diminished perfusion per se. It has been used widely for detection of coronary artery disease. Despite its high sensitivity (greater than 90%), its specificity is unacceptably low.[53] An analogous approach involves echocardiography. However, stress or exercise echocardiography is limited by several technical constraints, including the ability to image in only one plane at one time. In addition, wide variability has been encountered in image quality. Accordingly, the role of stress echocardiography for general application has not yet been fully elucidated.[54]

From first principles, PET with tracers of perfusion is a particularly attractive approach for detecting and quantifying regional myocardial ischemia (Table 2). For detection of coronary artery disease with PET, ^{82}Rb has been used enthusiastically. Its appeal reflects in part its short physical half-life and its production by generator systems that obviate the need for an on-site cyclotron. Gould and coworkers studied a total of 50 patients with PET, 27 with ^{82}Rb, and 23 with ^{13}N-ammonia. Images were acquired before and after intravenous administration of dipyridamole followed by isometric handgrip exercise to induce vasodilator stress (Color Figure 13). Visual interpretation of the ^{82}Rb and ^{13}N-ammonia images detected coronary artery disease with a sensitivity of 95% and a specificity of 100% in patients with angiographically calculated coronary flow reserve of less than 3.0.[55] In a direct comparison of ^{82}Rb imaging with ^{201}Tl SPECT imaging, Stewart and coworkers showed that sensitivities were similar (84% for ^{82}Rb and 84% for thallium-SPECT), but that specificity was superior with ^{82}Rb (88%) compared with ^{201}Tl (53%),[56] probably because of superior correction for photon attenuation in tissues available with PET as opposed to SPECT.

^{13}N-ammonia has been evaluated extensively as a flow tracer for detection of coronary artery disease by PET. It provides excellent image quality. Its 10 min half-life permits pre- and postexercise perfusion imaging (Figure 11-3). Disadvantages include a relatively long half-life, which limits frequent sequen-

Table 11-2
Positron Tomographic Myocardial Perfusion Studies for the Detection of CAD

	Number of Subjects	Sensitivity	Specificity	Comments
^{82}Rb				
Gould et al.[55]	27*	95	100	Visual interpretation of perfusion images compared with angiographic measures of CFR. Sensitivity 31% in patients with mild CAD (CFR 3-4).
Stewart et al.[56]	60	87	82	Sensitivity of PET and ^{201}Tl SPECT similar but specificity of PET higher than ^{201}Tl SPECT (57%).
Demer et al.[67]	82	NP	NP	Visual interpretation of perfusion images correlated with quantitative angiographic measures of stenosis severity.
Go et al.[120]	202	93	78	Sensitivity of PET higher than ^{201}Tl SPECT (76%); however, study design may have been biased against ^{201}Tl SPECT.
^{13}N-ammonia				
Schelbert et al.[57]	45	97	100	Patients with angiographic documentation of CAD. ^{13}N-ammonia PET correctly localized 90% of stenoses.
Gould et al.[55]	23*	95	100	Same as for ^{82}Rb.
Yonekura et al.[121]	60	97	99	Patients with angiographic documentation of CAD. Circumferential profiles used to analyze perfusion images.
Tamaki et al.[58]	51	88	90	Similar sensitivity and specificity as ^{201}Tl SPECT (81% and 94%).
Demer et al.[67]	111*	NP	NP	Same as ^{82}Rb.
^{15}O-water				
Iida et al.[14]	15	NP	NP	Measurements of regional perfusion in absolute terms demonstrated diffuse reductions in regional perfusion in patients with 3-vessel CAD.
Walsh et al.[59]	33	93%	NP	Estimates of relative regional perfusion compared with quantitative angiographic measures of stenosis severity.

* = Separate estimates of sensitivity and specificity for ^{82}Rb and [^{13}N]ammonia not provided.
CAD = Coronary artery disease.
CFR = Coronary flow reserve.
NP = Not provided.

tial imaging, the need for an on-site cyclotron, and increased lung activity in patients who smoke. In a study that included 13 normal subjects and 32 patients with known coronary artery disease, ^{13}N-ammonia perfusion imaging was 97% sensitive and 100% specific in detecting myocardium supplied by coronary arteries with stenosis of 50% or more.[57] In a direct comparison with

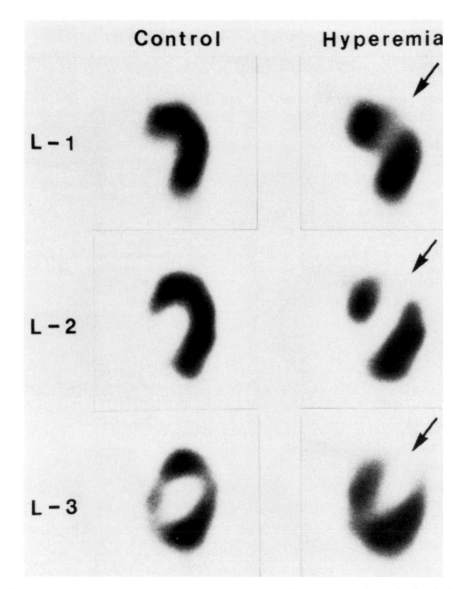

Figure 11-3. *Transaxial positron emission tomographic reconstructions obtained after the intravenous administration of $^{13}NH_3$ before (left), and after (right) administration of dipyridamole to a patient with a 100% stenosis of the proximal left anterior descending artery that filled via collaterals from the right coronary artery. The distribution of radioactivity is homogeneous at rest, but defects in the anterior wall are evident with vasodilator stress, as shown by the arrows. (Reproduced with permission from Schelbert et al.[57])*

[201]Tl SPECT imaging in patients with angiographically documented coronary disease, ^{13}N-ammonia exhibited similar sensitivity (98% for ^{13}N-ammonia and 96% for thallium SPECT) and specificity (90% for ^{13}N-ammonia compared with 94% for ^{201}Tl SPECT).[58]

Results of recent studies by our group[59] and others demonstrate the utility of $H_2^{15}O$ compared with [82]Rb and ^{13}N-ammonia for quantification of perfusion as opposed to simply imaging with PET. In contrast with ^{13}N-ammonia, $H_2^{15}O$ is metabolically inert. Because of its virtually free diffusibility in myocardium, $H_2^{15}O$ permits measurement of myocardial blood flow in absolute terms. Because extraction fraction does not vary with flow, as it does with [82]Rb and ^{13}N-ammonia, use of $H_2^{15}O$ permits quantitative assessment of perfusion.

Quantification of regional perfusion is of inestimable value for investigational purposes, but it is not yet clear whether quantitative assessment of perfusion is necessary for routine diagnosis of coronary artery disease. When severe three-vessel disease is present, however, reductions in perfusion may be global rather than regional either under baseline conditions or with pharmacologic or physiologic stress. Under such circumstances, quantification of perfusion may be helpful or necessary for objective, noninvasive detection of coronary artery disease.

To define regional perfusion by PET with $H_2^{15}O$, a correction for $H_2^{15}O$ radioactivity in the blood pool has been applied with the use of ^{15}O-carbon monoxide and calculation of the ratio of $H_2^{15}O$ to ^{15}O-carbon monoxide in the blood pool image (Color Figure 14). We have found that PET with $H_2^{15}O$ delineates regional ischemia reflecting coronary artery disease in patients at rest and after intravenous dipyridamole.[59] When absolute quantification of perfusion is needed, multiparameter estimation can be performed with acquisition of data dynamically and without correction for blood pool [15]O activity after the intravenous bolus injection of $H_2^{15}O$.[6]

Assessment of Severity of Coronary Artery Disease

In patients with effort-induced angina that is clinically stable, the extent of coronary artery disease is a major determinant of long-term survival, as is the extent of left ventricular dysfunction.[60,61] Although coronary angiography can define the extent of epicardial coronary artery involvement, it does not delineate the physiologic significance of lesions with respect to limitation of perfusion at rest or with stress in an individual patient. Exercise electrocardiography can identify subgroups of patients who are at particularly high risk, but its sensitivity and specificity are limited.[62-64] Thallium-201 scintigraphy can stratify patients into low- and high-risk groups, with risk defined in terms of likelihood of future cardiac events, as shown by Gill et al. with ^{201}Tl scintigraphy combined with exercise electrocardiography. These investigators demonstrated that uptake of ^{201}Tl by the lungs after exercise is the most powerful predictor of future cardiac events when compared with clinical or electrocardiographic predictors such as a history of angina, previous myocardial infarction, or ST segment depression with exercise.[65] Similar criteria with ^{201}Tl scintigraphy plus low-level exercise testing have been useful in identifying low-risk patients early after myocardial infarction.[66]

Preliminary results in studies with PET indicate that this modality will be helpful in delineating the severity of coronary artery disease. With tracers of perfusion (^{82}Rb and ^{13}N-ammonia) reductions of regional perfusion in relative terms have been shown by Demer et al. to correlate with severity of disease delineated by quantitative angiography, although scatter was considerable.[67] Iida and coworkers measured regional myocardial blood flow in absolute terms with PET with $H_2{}^{15}O$ and have demonstrated reductions of myocardial blood flow in all three vascular territories of supply in patients with trivessel coronary artery disease (Color Figure 15).[14] Their results underscore the potential importance of quantitative estimates of regional perfusion in patients in whom no disparities would be evident in imaging estimates of relative perfusion in which comparisons were made on a region-to-region basis, but who are nevertheless at high risk with severe coronary artery disease. In patients studied early after myocardial infarction, reductions in myocardial blood flow assessed with ^{13}N-ammonia were significantly greater in regions with extensive irreversible injury than in those with large proportions of still viable myocardium.[68] Thus, in this setting as well, assessment of perfusion with PET appears to provide prognostically useful information. In a recent report, a low risk of angiographically severe lesions but maintained nutritive perfusion has been demonstrated.[69]

Myocardial Metabolism

Abnormalities in cardiac pump function such as impaired regional contractile performance generally reflect underlying derangements in myocardial metabolism—either secondary to ischemia or to a primary myopathic process. Even when the heart fails because of increased afterload secondary to prolonged severe hypertension, severe aortic stenosis, or increased preload secondary to severe mitral or aortic regurgitation, the proximate cause of failure is likely to be impaired myocardial metabolism. Consequently, characterization of changes in myocardial metabolism with specific disease processes is needed to delineate pathogenetic mechanisms, define diagnostic criteria in terms of metabolic "fingerprints," and identify promising targets for therapeutic intervention.

Under physiologic conditions, myocardial metabolism is virtually exclusively aerobic.[70] The heart meets its energy demands largely by oxidizing fatty acid and glucose. Even under fasting conditions, nonesterified fatty acids are the preferred energy source. With ischemia, nonesterified fatty acids can no longer be oxidized. Anaerobic metabolism supervenes. Extraction of glucose increases as glycolytic flux (anaerobic) accelerates. As much as 70% of glucose extracted is metabolized. Glucose becomes the primary substrate not only for increased anaerobic glycolysis with consequent lactate production but also for overall, albeit diminished oxidative metabolism.[71] When ischemic myocardium is reperfused, utilization of both glucose and free fatty acid increases initially. Thus, relative contribution to overall oxidative metabolism by glucose decreases. With time, myocardial glucose utilization declines.[72] Consequently, even though oxidative metabolism may persist to some extent throughout the time course of induction and relief of reversible ischemia, the relative contribution of glucose utilization to overall oxidative metabolism is variable.

Because of the importance of free fatty acids in myocardial energetics, we studied ^{11}C-palmitate metabolism extensively, first in isolated perfused hearts, subsequently in intact animals, and ultimately in hearts of patients with coronary artery disease and other cardiac disorders.[73–75] Carbon-11 palmitate is extracted rapidly by normoxic myocardium.[73,76] After an initial vascular transit phase, clearance of tracer is biexponential with an initial rate largely reflecting β-oxidation and a slower rate largely reflecting turnover of triglyceride pools into which the administered tracer had been incorporated.[77] With ischemia, both extraction and initial clearance of tracer are decreased, reflecting decreased β-oxidation.[76] Nevertheless, quantitation of regional myocardial oxidative metabolism with ^{11}C-palmitate alone is difficult because of contributions to overall oxidative metabolism from oxidation of glucose and ketone bodies as well as fatty acid.[71] In addition, backdiffusion of tracer from myocardium into the vascular compartment, increased with ischemia, may complicate interpretation of results of dynamic tomographic studies.[78] Despite these limitations, PET with ^{11}C-palmitate has proven useful for qualitative recognition of metabolic changes accompanying ischemia.

Because glucose metabolism (anaerobic and aerobic) predominates in ischemic myocardium, ^{18}F-fluorodeoxyglucose (FDG) has been used in PET studies of patients with coronary artery disease.[79] FDG is a glucose analog that traces initial components of metabolic flux of glucose, including transmembranous transport and hexokinase-mediated phosphorylation. Phosphorylated FDG is trapped effectively within myocytes because the sarcolemma is relatively impermeable to it and because it is a poor substrate for further metabolism by either glycolytic or glycogen-synthetic pathways. Dephosphorylation of glucose-6-phosphate and presumably FDG-6-phosphate appears to be quite slow.[80] The regional distribution of FDG radioactivity assessed 40 to 60 minutes after administration of FDG, an interval sufficient for uptake and phosphorylation of tracer, is thought by many to reflect overall anaerobic and aerobic regional glycolytic flux.[81] As is the case with ^{11}C-palmitate, the extent of myocardial uptake of FDG is dependent on not only the metabolic state of the tissue with respect to normoxia or ischemia, but also on the pattern of substrates presented to myocardium. Increases in FDG uptake occur under conditions of relative glucose, and thus insulin, excess. Recently, we have demonstrated[82] that the regional distribution of FDG within normal human myocardium is dependent critically on prevailing metabolic conditions (Color Figure 16). Thus, under fasting conditions, FDG uptake is significantly lower in anteroseptal than posterolateral myocardium, even though regional oxidative metabolism and flow remain homogenous. After glucose loading, the regional disparities in FDG uptake are attenuated.[82] Such variability in FDG accumulation may confound interpretation of PET studies with this tracer.

Because metabolism of ^{11}C-palmitate or of FDG can provide an index of oxidative metabolism attributable to only a subset of metabolic pathways involved in overall myocardial oxygen utilization, we hypothesized that ^{11}C-acetate would be a particularly useful tracer. Because acetate is metabolized virtually exclusively within mitochondria, and coupling between acetate oxidation and oxidative phosphorylation is likely to be tight, we hypothesized that ^{11}C-acetate turnover would provide an index of overall regional oxidative metabolism definable by cardiac PET. Results of studies in isolated perfused hearts and hearts in situ in experimental animals demonstrated close correlations between myocardial clearance of ^{11}C-acetate and myocardial oxygen consumption over a wide range of flow, with marked changes in cardiac work, and in normoxic, ischemic, and reperfused myocardium.[83,84] The kinetics of clearance of ^{11}C-acetate from myocardium were shown to be remarkably insensitive to changes in patterns of substrate presented to the heart as well.[85] These results were shown to apply to patients as well,[86] and have been confirmed by others.[87]

Research Applications

Present approaches, other than PET, with promise for characterization of regional myocardial metabolism in human subjects are quite limited. Applications of nuclear magnetic resonance spectroscopy in vivo are still in their infancy and are profoundly limited with respect to accurate spatial localization and the need for large sample volumes.[88] Scintigraphic delineation of accumulation of iodinated fatty acids has shown some promise for qualitative assessment of regional fatty acid metabolism but suffers from the same limitations as those applicable to PET with ^{11}C-palmitate plus those associated with use of single-photon radionuclides in general.[7] Thallium-201 scintigraphy has been used to delineate viable myocardium, but the kinetics of accumulation and clearance of this tracer from myocardium are influenced by myocardial blood flow, myocyte cell membrane function, and changes in extraction fraction unrelated to metabolic processes themselves.

Because PET can interrogate tissue with respect to biologically specific metabolic processes, it is a particularly promising modality for detection of specific metabolic derangements underlying particular cardiac disorders and manifestations.

Results of Studies in Patients with Clinically Stable Coronary Artery Disease

In patients with angiographically documented coronary artery disease and normal left ventricular function at rest, myocardial uptake and clearance of ^{11}C-palmitate are similar in regions of myocardium supplied by an artery with significant stenosis compared to uptake and clearance in myocardium supplied by normal coronary arteries, as shown by Grover-McKay and coworkers. With rapid atrial pacing, however, zones supplied by stenotic arteries exhibited decreased uptake and clearance of ^{11}C-palmitate consistent with decreased β-oxidation compared with uptake and clearance in zones supplied by angiographically normal coronary arteries. None of the patients studied experienced angina or manifested electrocardiographic signs of ischemia. More than 50% developed subtle wall motion abnormalities.[89] These observations demonstrate the sensitivity of metabolic imaging with PET for detection of metabolic derangements secondary to myocardial ischemia.

Additional abnormalities of metabolism have been recognized by Camici et al., who showed that FDG uptake remained elevated in zones with exercise-induced perfusion defects detected by PET with [82]Rb even after the perfusion abnormalities had resolved in patients with angiographically documented coronary artery disease (Figure 11-4).[90] The persistence of abnormalities in glucose metabolism even after resolution of ischemia suggests that recovery of normal cellular metabolism is quite delayed. However, it is not clear whether the increased FDG uptake is indicative of augmented aerobic or anaerobic glycolytic flux or both, replenishment of glycogen stores, or altered metabolism associated with the stunned myocardium.[2]

Results of Studies in Patients with Unstable Coronary Artery Disease

Araujo and coworkers demonstrated augmented global and regional myocardial metabolism of glucose with PET in patients with unstable angina. The augmentation of accumulation of FDG occurred in the absence of other objective criteria of ischemia. Furthermore, augmented accumulation of FDG was reduced by nifedipine in parallel with a reduction of chest pain and episodic ST depression documented by Holter monitoring.[91] These results indicate that metabolic abnormalities induced by ischemia in patients are remarkably persistent and that treatment designed to improve the balance between myocardial oxygen supply and demand may exert salutary effects on myocardial metabolism in addition to ameliorating symptoms.

We have shown that PET can accurately identify, localize, and quantify the extent of myocardial infarction by delineating the distribution of impaired myocardial fatty acid oxidation. Initially we showed that infarct size reflected by PET with ^{11}C-palmitate correlated closely with morphologic and enzymatic estimates of infarction in dogs.[92] These observations suggested that irreversible injury evolved rapidly since the tomographic estimates, made virtually immediately, presaged enzymatic and morphologic estimates that only could be made later. In patients with remote myocardial infarction we showed that the locus of infarction could be identified readily with ^{11}C-palmitate and PET and that the extent of infarction in human subjects studied with PET and ^{11}C-palmitate correlated closely with enzymatic estimates of infarct size available only later.[75,93,94] Furthermore, we found that Q wave infarction could be differentiated from non-Q wave infarction tomographically based on the appearance of the metabolic defect in PET images obtained with ^{11}C-palmitate.[94] The PET approach developed elucidated the nature of electrocardiographically reciprocal ST segment depression in patients with Q wave infarction. PET with ^{11}C-palmitate showed that such changes were truly electrophysiologically reciprocal in approximately 50% of patients, but indicative of ischemia at a distance in a substantial minority.[95]

In subsequent studies we used PET with ^{11}C-palmitate to determine whether coronary artery thrombolysis improved the heart itself in patients with acute myocardial infarction. In patients in whom thrombolysis was angio-

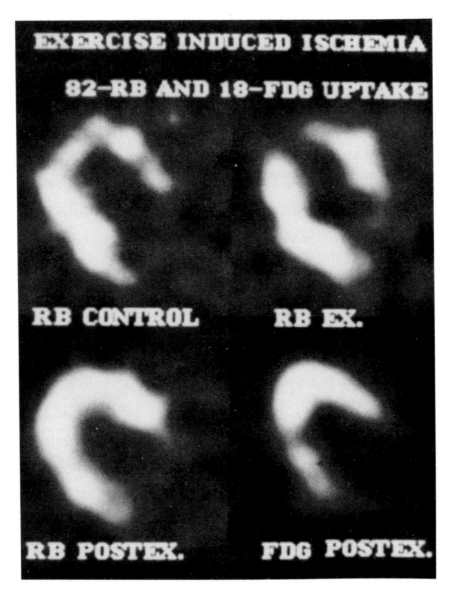

Figure 11-4. *Positron emission tomographic reconstructions at the midventricular level acquired after the intravenous administration of ^{82}Rb and ^{18}FDG in a patient with exercise-induced ischemia. The top of each image is anterior and the left represents the patient's left. The distribution of rubidium was homogenous at rest, but an anterior defect was seen with exercise. The distribution of rubidium normalized within 6 minutes after exercise (bottom left). ^{18}FDG was injected 8 minutes after the completion of exercise, and data collection commenced 60 minutes thereafter. Accumulation of ^{18}FDG was greatest in the anterior wall that had exhibited a perfusion abnormality with exercise. (Reproduced with permission from Camici et al.[90])*

graphically successful, the severity of metabolic defects representing zones of jeopardized tissue on myocardial ^{11}C-palmitate PET images declined by 29%—a decline documenting salvage of myocardium by the intervention (Color Figure 17).[96] Transient reductions in the severity of metabolic compromise assessed with PET and ^{11}C-palmitate have been noted in some patients treated with nifedipine[97] even though, as judged from several large, multicenter trials,this intervention does not diminish the overall extent of infarction in general.[70]

To define the relationship between compromise of perfusion and the presence or absence of irreversible injury and hence the potential for salvage of jeopardized, ischemic myocardium, PET has been performed with FDG and with ^{13}N-ammonia in which changes in regional myocardial accumulation of FDG have been referenced to changes in regional perfusion. Normal myocardium, with the patient in the postprandial state, typically exhibits nearly homogenous accumulation of FDG and homogenous regional perfusion reflected by uptake of ^{13}N-ammonia. Zones in which infarction is present typically exhibit concordant reduction of uptake of both tracers, indicative of concomitant reduction of perfusion and viability. Such concordance has been referred to as "matched" defects. In zones of myocardium rendered ischemic in which viable, metabolically active tissue persists, accumulation of FDG is increased relative to uptake of NH_3, indicative of perfusion yielding what has been called a "flow-metabolism mismatch" (Figure 11-5).[98] Frequently, such zones will exhibit improved regional wall motion. The mismatch pattern has been considered to reflect the persistence of jeopardized but still viable myocardium that is amenable to salvage by prompt and effective coronary recanalization.

In studies of patients with remote Q wave myocardial infarction, Brunken and coworkers showed that only 32% of zones with Q waves exhibited concordant decreases in flow and metabolism assessed by PET with ^{13}N-ammonia and FDG. Mismatches between flow and metabolism or the presence of apparently normal perfusion and FDG uptake were evident in the other 68% of zones despite Q waves.[99] Thus, regions of myocardium typically manifesting conventional, electrocardiographic signs of necrosis contained some metabolically active and presumably still viable tissue in most instances. However, consistent with the clinical impression that zones of infarction not generating Q waves typically contain more viable tissue than zones reflected by Q wave infarction, Hashimoto et al. documented augmented accumulation of FDG in 91% of patients with non-Q wave and only 36% of those with Q wave insults.[100]

Results of studies from our group with ^{11}C-acetate have characterized changes in regional myocardial oxygen consumption associated with acute myocardial infarction. In patients with recent (< 48 hours) Q wave infarction treated without thrombolysis or immediate angioplasty myocardial oxygen consumption in central zones of infarction was less than 6% of that in normal zones. Myocardial oxygen consumption in peri-infarct zones was reduced to only approximately 50% of that of normal zones. Sequential studies demonstrated persistence of these changes for at least 7 days after the onset of infarction.[86] In addition, we demonstrated with combined PET studies with $H_2^{15}O$ and ^{11}C-acetate that perfusion returns to nearly normal levels within 24 hours

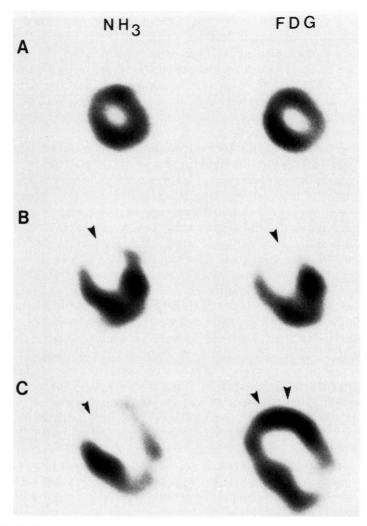

Figure 11-5. *Positron emission tomographic images from hearts of three subjects after the intravenous injection of $^{13}NH_3$ (left) and ^{18}FDG (right): a) from a normal volunteer exhibiting homogeneous accumulation of $^{13}NH_3$ (perfusion) and ^{18}FDG (glucose utilization); b) from a patient with remote anterior myocardial infarction exhibiting concordantly decreased accumulation of $^{13}NH_3$ and ^{18}FDG; and c) from a patient with three-vessel coronary artery disease with a "mismatch" pattern of decreased perfusion in the anteroseptal wall but preserved or increased accumulation of ^{18}FDG relative to blood flow, indicative of preserved metabolic activity. (Reproduced with permission from Schelbert et al.[122])*

after coronary thrombolysis and persists at normal levels for at least 7 days after the onset of reperfusion. In contrast, however, myocardial oxidative metabolism is depressed within the first 24 hours after reperfusion and increases only slowly over the subsequent 7 days (Figure 11-6). The recovery of oxidative metabolism presages recovery of function.[5]

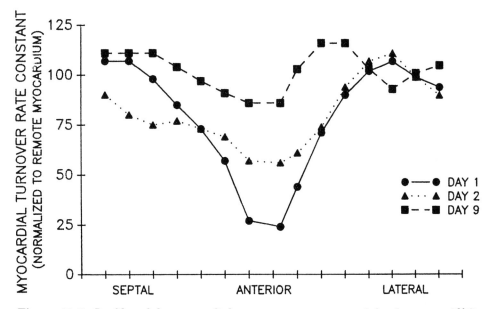

Figure 11-6. *Profiles of the myocardial turnover rate constant of the clearance of* [11]*C-acetate from a patient with anterior myocardial infarction in whom thrombolysis led to recanalization (see Chapter 9, Figure 9-6). Initially, clearance was markedly slowed in the central infarct zone with lesser degrees of slowing in the border between the infarct and normal zones. It increased modestly on the second day after thrombolysis and was nearly normal 9 days after thrombolysis. (Reproduced with permission from Henes et al.[5])*

These results have clinically important implications. They indicate that myocardium that is initially depressed both functionally and metabolically may retain striking potential for recovery with reperfusion. In addition, they imply that exclusion of invasive intervention should not be predicated solely on attenuation of function or oxidative metabolism at one point in time. They suggest that differentiation between stunned and irreversibly injured myocardium cannot be made unequivocally with static measurements alone, even sophisticated ones, and raise the possibility that sequential assessments are needed for definitive differentiation. Because recovery of function occurs only in zones with previous recovery of oxidative metabolism, the results show that restoration of regional oxidative metabolism is a necessary although not a sufficient condition for recovery of contractile performance as well as salvage of myocardium—in keeping with concepts derived from results of laboratory studies of hearts of experimental animals.[101]

In concert, results of metabolic assessments by PET in patients with unstable coronary artery disease are promising. Such assessments appear to be capable of delineating the presence of still viable myocardium in jeopardized zones and may therefore improve selection of patients suitable for angioplasty or coronary surgery. They may be particularly useful in evaluating putative therapeutic interventions designed to salvage jeopardized myocardium and in elucidating the pathophysiology of stunning of myocardium, i.e., protracted depression of regional ventricular function after resolution of ischemia.

Clinical Applications

Tomographic Assessments of Myocardial Metabolism after Myocardial Infarction

Coronary revascularization early after myocardial infarction is predicated on the concept that viable but dysfunctional tissue that has been rendered ischemic can be salvaged by restoration of nutritive perfusion. Patient selection is therefore difficult but critical. Dysfunctional but still viable myocardium may be "hibernating" or "stunned."[102,103] "Hibernating" refers to consequences of myocardial ischemia such as impaired regional wall motion that are immediately reversed by restoration of adequate perfusion. Such impairment may be protective in that decreased metabolic demands are matched to decreased perfusion. "Stunned" refers to postischemic regional dysfunction that persists long after perfusion has been restored, for hours to weeks. Both phenomena, "hibernation" and "stunning," may share some underlying metabolic common denominators.

To identify "stunned" or "hibernating" myocardium, regional ventricular function has been assessed under conditions at rest and after cardiac stimulation. However, difficulties in controlling influences on global and regional ventricular performance of variations in loading conditions, the neurohumoral milieu, and altered physical properties of myocardium rendered ischemic have obscured interpretation. Changes in ^{201}Tl perfusion defects with respect to those present initially after exercise can identify myocardium that remains viable after transient ischemia, but limitations associated with single-photon scintigraphy in general and variations in kinetics of accumulation and clearance of ^{201}Tl from myocardium limit discrimination. Repeated administration of ^{201}Tl may unmask viable myocardium in zones with apparently fixed ^{201}Tl perfusion defects.[104] The need for definitive localization of viable yet dysfunctional myocardium that is recovering from an ischemic insult has not yet been met optimally. PET offers a particularly promising approach.

Assessment of Clinically Stable Coronary Artery Disease

Considerable progress has been made in detection with PET of still viable myocardium in patients with stable coronary artery disease. In studies by Tillisch and coworkers of patients with left ventricular dysfunction at rest secondary to coronary artery disease with PET, ^{13}N-ammonia, and FDG before coronary artery bypass surgery, 73 ventricular segments were identified in which contractile function was abnormal. Among these, 67 were believed to have been revascularized adequately by subsequent surgery. Three patterns of flow and FDG uptake were observed: normal flow and normal uptake of FDG (25 segments), increased uptake of FDG relative to flow (16 segments), and decreased uptake of FDG with decreased flow (27 segments). Functional improvement was evident in 85% of the segments that exhibited preservation of uptake of FDG. In contrast, 92% of the segments with reduced FDG uptake failed to exhibit functional improvement after surgery.[79] Tamaki et al. acquired analogous results in a study in which flow and uptake of FDG were characterized before and after coronary bypass surgery. With preservation of FDG accumulation evident preoperatively, contractile function was evident in 78% of zones characterized after surgery. However, somewhat surprisingly, 22% of zones with reduced FDG accumulation exhibited improved function after surgery as well. In all segments with decreased accumulation of FDG after surgery, regional function improved. Thus, restoration of nutritive perfusion exerted salutary effects not only on regional contractile function but also on regional metabolism.[105]

In comparing FDG PET imaging with either planar or SPECT ^{201}Tl myocardial scintigraphy for detection of viable myocardium, numerous investigators have shown that approximately 50% of dysfunctional segments with fixed ^{201}Tl perfusion defects contain myocardium that retains the capacity to accumulate FDG.[106] Hypothetically, such segments are likely to contain viable myocardium that can benefit from revascularization. However, because of the lack of serial assessments of regional function after revascularization, it is not yet clear whether all segments in which FDG accumulation is preserved can exhibit functional improvement with restoration of perfusion.

In a recent study, we have shown that maintenance of oxidative metabolism is a major determinant of the potential for recovery of regional contractile function after revascularization. In patients with resting left ventricular dysfunction secondary to coronary artery disease, regional perfusion, accumulation of FDG, and the rate of oxidative metabolism were delineated by PET with H_2^{15}O, FDG, and ^{11}C-acetate, respectively. Studies were performed before myocardial revascularization, and results were correlated with improvements in regional function after revascularization with respect to initial regional ventricular performance. Regional perfusion was reduced similarly in segments destined to exhibit improved function and those in which no functional improvement occurred (to 79% and 74% of normal). In segments destined to exhibit improved function, oxidative metabolism averaged 95% of that in normally functioning segments. Accumulation of FDG was greater relative to flow in these segments than in other segments. In dysfunctional segments that were not destined to improve, oxidative metabolism averaged only 66% of that in normally functioning segments, and accumulation of FDG was variable relative to flow. Some segments exhibited marked depression of oxidative metabolism but augmented accumulation of FDG. This phenomenon suggests that anaerobic glycolysis alone is not sufficient to maintain tissue viability, in keeping with results in studies of experimental animals.[107]

Detection of Viable Myocardium in Patients with Unstable Coronary Artery Disease

Schwaiger et al. used PET with ^{13}N-ammonia and FDG in patients with acute myocardial infarction within 72 hours of its onset to estimate perfusion and regional metabolism, which were correlated with functional improvement assessed 6 weeks later.[108] The patients studied were managed conservatively without thrombolytic drugs, angioplasty, or coronary bypass surgery. Among ventricular myocardial segments in which accumulation of FDG was preserved at the time of the initial PET study, 50% failed to exhibit improved mechanical function over time.[108] In virtually all segments in which accumulation of FDG was reduced initially, mechanical impairment persisted as well. However, because PET with FDG cannot differentiate aerobic from anaerobic metabolism of glucose and because glucose utilization varies with time after the onset of reperfusion, FDG may be of only limited value in detecting viable myocardium early after myocardial infarction. In contrast, maintenance of oxidative metabolism early after reperfusion detectable with PET with ^{11}C-acetate is a powerful descriptor of subsequent recovery of function.[107] To date, approximately 100 patients have been studied prospectively to determine the accuracy of assessment of metabolism with PET in predicting return of regional mechanical function (Table 3). Optimal criteria for identifying dysfunctional but still viable myocardium have not yet been elucidated rigorously. Nevertheless, cardiac PET is likely to provide definitive criteria for characterization of myocardial viability, reflected by the capacity for recovery of regional mechanical function with restoration of sustained perfusion, and to serve as a "gold standard" for comparison in development of more widely applicable indexes obtainable with more universally available procedures.

The Promise of PET for Elucidation and Detection of Cardiomyopathy

Most cardiomyopathy encountered clinically is of obscure cause and pathogenesis. Even conditions with clear genetic origins such as familial, hypertrophic cardiomyopathy are generally idiopathic. Because many primary and secondary cardiomyopathies are attributable to underlying derangements in metabolism, with altered rates of synthesis or degradation of myocardial proteins, cell membrane constituents, organelles, modulators of ion transport, or intracellular components such as the sarcoplasmic reticulum influencing electromechanical coupling, it is likely that their elucidation will require delineation of specific derangements in metabolism contributing to each. In view of the quantitative power of cardiac PET for delineation of fluxes through specific biochemical pathways in vivo, PET is particularly promising for elucidation of the cause and pathogenesis of cardiomyopathy. Most observations to date have been descriptive and have not defined primary metabolic derangements or microvascular abnormalities underlying the manifestations of cardiomyopathy. Nevertheless, such observations have been useful in improving the recognition of cardiomyopathic conditions and delineating differences between them.

In an early study of patients with dilated cardiomyopathy, we demonstrated that PET with ^{11}C-palmitate detected spatially heterogeneous accumulation of the tracer in hearts of patients with ischemic heart disease with striking segmental variation (Color Figure 18). Subsequently, we compared patients with idiopathic dilated cardiomyopathy with those with ischemia and found that spatial heterogeneity of accumulation was abnormal but in a more diffuse fashion.[109] Thus, PET detected abnormalities in both groups of patients and

Table 11-3

Correlation of PET Criteria of Myocardial Viability and Functional Recovery of Myocardium

	Number of Subjects	Predictive Value (viable)	Predictive Value (nonviable)	Comments
18F-fluorodeoxyglucose				
Brunken et al.[99]	5	83%*	100%*	PET criteria of viability compared with changes in wall motion after CABG. Only 2 regions defined as nonviable.
Tillisch et al.[79]	17	85%*	92%*	Patients with stable CAD studied prior to CABG. 54% of "PET-viable" regions demonstrated normal flow and metabolism, 46% demonstrated "flow-metabolic" mismatch.
Tamaki et al.[105]	28	78%*	80%*	PET and echocardiographic studies performed pre- and post-CABG. Functional recovery usually associated with resolution and perfusion and metabolic abnormalities.
Piérard et al.[68]	17	55%†	100%†	Patients studied 9 days post MI. Functional improvement occurred in 100% of patients with normal flow and metabolism but in only 17% of patients with "flow-metabolic" mismatch.
11C-acetate				
Henes et al.[5]	8	NP	NP	Sequential PET studies performed in patients early after thrombolysis. Functional recovery associated with improvement in oxidative metabolism.
Gropler et al.[107]	16	NP	NP	PET-11C-acetate and FDG studies performed in patients with stable CAD prior to CABG or PTCA. Functional recovery dependent upon maintenance of oxidative metabolism not glucose metabolism.

Predictive value $= \dfrac{\text{True positive}}{\text{True positive + False positive}}$

* = Predictive values based on numbers of regions analyzed.
† = Predictive values based on numbers of patients analyzed.
CABG = Coronary artery bypass grafting.
CAD = Coronary artery disease.
MI = Myocardial infarction.
FDG = 18F-fluorodeoxyglucose.
PTCA = Percutaneous transluminal coronary angioplasty.
NP = Not provided.

provided criteria distinguishing the two, despite the similarity of hemodynamic impairment, depressed ventricular performance, and radiographic and echocardiographic manifestations of cardiac failure.

Hypertrophic Cardiomyopathy

Because hypertrophic cardiomyopathy occurs in both a familial and a sporadic form and because recent observations have localized the genetic defect in at least some instances to a specific chromosome, it appears likely that cardiac PET will aid in the identification of derangements in specific metabolic pathways underlying expression of the disorder. One can envision the use of precursors of nucleic acids or proteins such as nucleosides and amino acids to detect accelerated or inhibited incorporation of specific intracellular components into macromolecules. To date, however, observations with PET in patients with hypertrophic cardiomyopathy have been only descriptive. Grover-McKay and coworkers demonstrated decreased septal accumulation of FDG compared with accumulation in the posterolateral wall in hearts of patients with hypertrophic cardiomyopathy. In contrast, accumulation of ^{13}N-ammonia and ^{11}C-palmitate was spatially homogeneous. The authors speculated that their results were indicative of a primary metabolic abnormality.[110] Such observations are provocative because of the known propensity of hypertrophic cardiomyopathy to be manifest early in its course or predominantly by septal hypertrophy. However, these results must be interpreted cautiously. As noted above, accumulation of FDG in the septum is markedly dependent on prevailing concentrations of glucose in plasma and the presence or absence of a fasting state when the patient is studied.[82] Furthermore, it appears unlikely that altered accumulation of FDG is indicative of a fundamental derangement in carbohydrate metabolism underlying hypertrophic cardiomyopathy because the disorder can affect the entire left and sometimes right ventricle, and because accumulation of FDG is dependent on overall glycolytic flux, aerobic and anaerobic, with one or the other component or both being vulnerable to a secondary alteration as a result of hypertrophy disproportionate to vascularization and blood flow.

PET in Patients with Duchenne's Muscular Dystrophy

Many forms of muscular dystrophy affect cardiac as well as skeletal muscle. Even though clinical manifestations of disease in skeletal muscle may dominate, death is sometimes attributable to subtle yet critical cardiac disease. Examples include myotonic dystrophy and the more common sex-linked muscular dystrophy, Duchenne's muscular dystrophy. The latter is associated with myocardial fibrosis and scarring often particularly prominent in the posterobasal and contiguous lateral wall of the left ventricle. Perloff and coworkers demonstrated decreased perfusion by cardiac PET with ^{13}N-ammonia in hearts of patients afflicted with Duchenne's muscular dystrophy. They observed augmented accumulation of FDG in those ventricular segments with apparently decreased perfusion. They concluded that the derangements detected were primary.[111] However, the relative diminution of FDG accumulation in the septum may have reflected an altered nutritional state associated, nonspecifically, with the debility of severe illness. In addition, replacement of myocardial cells with fibrous tissue, regardless of the cause, may give rise to disparities between perfusion and metabolism detectable by cardiac PET. Nevertheless, these observations underscore the potential utility of cardiac PET for improved detection and differentiation of cardiomyopathic states in vivo without the need for cardiac biopsy and provide an index that may be useful in characterizing responses of specific cardiomyopathic conditions, including ethanol abuse, viral infection, polyarteritis nodosa, scleroderma, severe and prolonged hypertension, or aortic valvular disease, to specific therapeutic interventions such as cessation of exposure to potential toxins, immunosuppression or use of cytokines, administration of afterload-reducing agents, or valvuloplasty, or surgery.

Miscellaneous Applications of Cardiac PET

Although infarct imaging by scintigraphy with ^{99m}Tc permits detection of regions of infarction, so-called hot spot imaging is used rarely because of the overwhelming diagnostic sensitivity and specificity of plasma enzyme determinations,[112] the electrocardiogram, and other universally applicable criteria of infarction. Nevertheless, when patients present relatively late after the onset of infarction, when the diagnosis is particularly obscure, when other causes of enzyme elevations or electrocardiographic abnormalities may mask signs of possible infarction, or when anatomic localization is particularly difficult and critical, infarct imaging may be helpful. Accumulation of ^{99m}Tc-pyrophosphate depends on binding of the tracer to free, presumably intracellular calcium as a result of damage to sarcolemma and flooding of intracellular calcium binding sites with extracellular calcium that would be excluded or extruded under physiologic conditions.[113] Myocardial accumulation of the tracer varies with time after the onset of infarction and is not evident for many hours after intravenous administration. These considerations detract somewhat from its utility.

An alternative approach to infarct imaging involves administration of radiolabeled monoclonal myosin-specific antibody. This agent accumulates in myocytes in which sarcolemmal integrity has been compromised as a result of severe and prolonged ischemia sufficient to induce necrosis.[114] Clinical utilization of radiolabeled monoclonal myosin-specific antibody is not yet widespread.

We have recently demonstrated that fluoromisonidazole labeled with ^{18}F diffuses readily into myocardium and is metabolized in normoxic tissue to the parent compound, which readily diffuses out of the cell. In contrast, in hypoxic myocardium the tracer is chemically reduced, rendered insoluble intracellularly, and thereby trapped. Necrotic cells cannot mediate the chemical reduction and, as a result, do not trap labeled material. Accordingly, accumulation of ^{18}F-fluoromisonidazole detects regions of reversible ischemia in which myocytes within the jeopardized zone remain viable. Accumulation of tracer in such zones differentiates them from zones of normal myocardium, which do not trap the material at all, and from zones of infarction, which cannot trap it because they cannot mediate the chemical reduction necessary for trapping.[115] Clinical utilization of such so-called hypoxic sensitizers may be helpful in detecting unstable angina and differentiating it from non-Q wave infarction or Q wave infarction early in its course before the electrocardiographic evolution of Q wave abnormalities could have occurred.

Because of the unavoidable spatial limitations of PET related in part to the path lengths of positrons in tissue before annihilation and the physical characteristics of instrumentation needed for detection and localization of emitters, the utility of cardiac PET for assessment of ventricular performance, regional wall motion, and contractility is limited. A priori, many other cardiac imaging modalities are superior because of their intrinsically greater spatial resolution despite their own limitations such as requirement for ionizing radiation, expense, and difficulty in acquiring optimal echocardiographic windows among others. Despite its limitations, cardiac PET can provide useful information regarding regional and global ventricular performance, particularly when electrocardiographic gating[116] or novel approaches to gating of the cardiac cycle are used.[117] With PET, regional perfusion, metabolism, and mechanical function can be assessed under conditions of the same geometry and virtually simultaneously. Thus, under particular conditions, cardiac PET may be particularly helpful in defining the extent to which transitory or persistent impairment of regional function is associated with impairment of perfusion or derangements in regional metabolism.

Anticipated Developments

In the near future, cardiac PET is likely to be most essential in clinical investigation. It should help to elucidate fundamental, biochemical, and physiologic derangements underlying the pathogenesis and manifestations of specific disease processes resulting ultimately in cardiac dysfunction. It should provide definitive criteria for assessment of specific interventions that can serve as reference criteria for accuracy, reliability, sensitivity, and specificity of more universally available and applicable end points.

The development of positron emission tomographs capable of very rapid data acquisition, high spatial and temporal resolution, large axial fields of view, and short processing intervals will permit generation and display of genuinely three-dimensional images of the heart. Images indicative of specific physiologic processes, such as regional oxygen consumption, can be constructed to provide investigators and clinicians with visually useful information that integrates phenomena presently integrated by inference based on results of off-line processing.

Development of novel tracers suitable for convenient, rapid, sequential, and specific delineation of regional myocardial perfusion and specific metabolic pathways in myocardium, development and validation of physiologically based mathematical models delineating kinetics of specific tracers required, and further elucidation of alterations in perfusion and metabolism responsible for specific cardiac disorders will undoubtedly expand the use of cardiac PET for diagnosis and for monitoring the efficacy of treatment. It appears likely that PET will soon permit delineation of the distribution of radiolabeled pharmacologic agents designed to interact with specific receptors, thereby facilitating noninvasive characterization of cardiac innervation under physiologic and pathologic conditions. In view of the obvious importance of adrenergic and parasympathetic stimulation of the heart in arrhythmogenecity and the impact of denervation on symptoms in recipients of cardiac allografts to name but two examples, elucidation of regional autonomic nervous system activity in the myocardium is likely to become increasingly important in clarification of pathogenesis and cardiac diagnosis.[118]

The extent to which cardiac PET will become generally used in diagnosis is difficult to predict. Its complexity and expense will remain disadvantages, but in view of its capacity to provide quantitative information delineating metabolism and perfusion sensitively and noninvasively, it may well play an increasing role in detection of disease and the assessment of its severity. One example is vascular disease in cardiac allograft recipients, thought to be a manifestation of late rejection, frequently asymptomatic because of cardiac denervation, and quantitatively the most important cause of ultimate failure of cardiac transplantation. Presently, assessment of allograft status requires invasive procedures, including repetitive endocardial biopsy and coronary arteriography. Noninvasive detection of occult vascular disease meriting evaluation angiographically may well prove to be cost effective and medically desirable.

Management of patients with coronary artery disease has been revolutionized by the demonstrable importance of early recanalization induced pharmacologically, by angioplasty, and by surgery. Assessments of regimens that may improve these approaches have generally required invasive procedures such as angiography to demonstrate recanalization and ventriculography to characterize regional wall motion abnormalities. Because of its quantitative power to quantify perfusion as well as the metabolic response to ischemia, cardiac PET may prove to be invaluable in comparing the relative merits of diverse interventions used to induce recanalization and protect jeopardized myocardium.[119]

Pioneering studies of cardiac positron tomography were undertaken approximately 20 years ago. During the past decade, opportunistic applications tended to dominate the field, as is the case with any technologic advance. Progress already made has set the stage, however, for more probing, mechanistic studies in which cardiac PET can fulfill its promise for elucidating cause and pathogenesis, detecting occult disease at a time when it is most amenable to favorable modification, and objectively assessing the efficacy of therapeutic interventions targeted against specific pathophysiologic mechanisms.

References

1. Bergmann SR, Fox KAA, Geltman EM, Sobel BE. Positron emission tomography of the heart. Prog Cardiovasc Dis 1985; 28:165–194.
2. Braunwald E, Sobel BE. Coronary blood flow and myocardial ischemia. In: Braunwald E, Ed. *Heart Disease, Third Edition*.Philadelphia: W. B. Saunders Company, 1988; 1191–1221.
3. Geltman EM, Bergmann SR, Sobel BE. Cardiac positron emission tomography.

In: Reivich M, Ed. *Positron Emission Tomography*. New York: Alan R. Liss, Inc., 1985; 345–385.

4. Walsh MN, Geltman EM, Steele RL, Kenzora JL, Ludbrook PA, Sobel BE, Bergmann SR. Augmented myocardial perfusion reserve after coronary angioplasty quantified by positron emission tomography with $H_2{}^{15}O$. J Am Coll Cardiol 1990; 15:119–127.

5. Henes CG, Bergmann SR, Perez JE, Sobel BE, Geltman EM. The time course of restoration of nutritive perfusion, myocardial oxygen consumption, and regional function after coronary thrombolysis. Coronary Artery Disease 1990; 1:687–696.

6. Bergmann SR, Herrero P, Markham J, Weinheimer CJ, Walsh MN. Noninvasive quantitation of myocardial blood flow in human subjects with oxygen-15-labeled water and positron emission tomography. J Am Coll Cardiol 1989; 14:639–652.

7. Rellas JS, Corbett JR, Kulkarni P, Morgan C, Devous MD Sr., Buja LM, Bush L, Parkey RW, Willerson JT, Lewis SE. Iodine-123 phenylpentadecanoic acid: Detection of acute myocardial infarction and injury in dogs using an iodinated fatty acid and single-photon emission tomography. Am J Cardiol 1983; 52:1326–1332.

8. Cannon RO III, Epstein SE. "Microvascular angina" as a cause of chest pain with angiographically normal coronary arteries. Am J Cardiol 1988; 61:1338–1343.

9. Wilson RF, Laughlin DE, Ackell PH, Chilian WM, Holida MD, Hartley CJ, Armstrong ML, Marcus ML, White CW. Transluminal, subselective measurement of coronary artery blood flow velocity and vasodilator reserve in man. Circulation 1985; 72:82–92.

10. Li Q-S, Solot G, Frank TL, Wagner HN,Jr., Becker LC. Myocardial redistribution of technetium-99m-methoxyisobutyl isonitrile (SESTAMIBI). J Nucl Med 1990; 31:1069–1076.

11. Shelton ME, Green MA, Mathias CJ, Welch MJ, Bergmann SR. Assessment of regional myocardial and renal blood flow with copper-PTSM and positron emission tomography. Circulation 1990; 82:990–997.

12. Krivokapich J, Smith GT, Huang S-C, Hoffman EJ, Ratib O, Phelps ME, Schelbert HR. ^{13}N ammonia myocardial imaging at rest and with exercise in normal volunteers. Quantification of absolute myocardial perfusion with dynamic positron emission tomography. Circulation 1989; 80:1328–1337.

13. Hutchins GD, Schwaiger M, Rosenspire KC, Krivokapich J, Schelbert H, Kuhl DE. Noninvasive quantification of regional blood flow in the human heart using N-13 ammonia and dynamic positron emission tomographic imaging. J Am Coll Cardiol 1990; 15:1032–1042.

14. Iida H, Kanno I, Takahashi, A., et al. Measurement of absolute myocardial blood flow with $H_2{}^{15}O$ and dynamic positron-emission tomography. Strategy for quantification in relation to the partial-volume effect. Circulation 1988; 78:104–115.

15. Kaul S, Newell JB, Chesler DA, Pohost GM, Okada RD, Boucher CA. Quantitative thallium imaging findings in patients with normal coronary angiographic findings and in clinically normal subjects. Am J Cardiol 1986; 57:509–512.

16. Geltman EM, Henes CG, Senneff MJ, Sobel BE, Bergmann SR. Increased myocardial perfusion at rest and diminished perfusion reserve in patients with angina and angiographically normal coronary arteries. J Am Coll Cardiol 1990; 16:586–595.

17. Uretsky BF, Murali S, Reddy S, Rabin B, Lee A, Griffith BP, Hardesty RL, Trento A, Bahnson HT. Development of coronary artery disease in cardiac transplant patients receiving immunosuppressive therapy with cyclosporine and prednisone. Circulation 1987; 76:827–834.

18. Nitenberg A, Tavolaro O, Benvenuti C, Loisance D, Foult J-M, Hittinger L, Castaigne A, Cachera J-P, Vernant P. Recovery of a normal coronary vascular reserve after rejection therapy in acute human cardiac allograft rejection. Circulation 1990; 81:1312–1318.

19. Nitenberg A, Tavolaro O, Loisance D, Foult J-M, Benhaiem N, Cachera J-P. Severe impairment of coronary reserve during rejection in patients with orthotopic heart transplant. Circulation 1989; 79:59–65.

20. Senneff MJ, Genton RE, Kenzora JL, Ludbrook PA, Courtois M, Sobel BE, Geltman EM, Bergmann SR. Altered myocardial perfusion in cardiac transplants. Circulation 1990; 82:III-714 (abstract).

21. Senneff MJ, Genton RE, Kenzora JL, Ludbrook PA, Geltman EM, Sobel BE, Bergmann SR. Perfusion abnormalities in cardiac allografts demonstrable with positron emission tomography (PET). J Nucl Med 1990; 31:841 (abstract).

22. Marcus ML, Doty DB, Hiratzka LF, Wright CB, Eastham CL. Decreased coronary reserve. N Engl J Med 1982; 307:1362–1367.

23. Goldstein RA, Haynie M. Limited myocardial perfusion reserve in patients with left ventricular hypertrophy. J Nucl Med 1990; 31:255–258.

24. Camici P, Chiriatti G, Lorenzoni R, Bellina RC, Gistri R, Italiani G, Parodi O, Salvadori PA, Nista N, Papi L. Coronary vasodilation is impaired in both hypertrophied and nonhypertrophied myocardium of patients with hypertrophic cardiomyopathy: a study with nitrogen-13 ammonia and positron emission tomography. J Am Coll Cardiol 1991; 17:879–886.

25. Scholl J-M, Chaitman BR, David PR, Dupras G, Brevers G, Val PG, Crepeau J, Lesperance J, Bourassa MG. Exercise electrocardiography and myocardial scintigraphy in the serial evaluation of the results of percutaneous transluminal coronary angioplasty. Circulation 1982; 66:380–390.

26. Brundage BH, Massie BM, Botvinick EH. Improved regional ventricular function after successful surgical revascularization. J Am Coll Cardiol 1984; 3:902–908.

27. Brundage BH, Lipton MJ, Herfkens RJ, Berninger WH, Redington RW, Chatterjee K, Carlsson E. Detection of patent coronary bypass grafts by computed tomography. A preliminary report. Circulation 1980; 61:826–831.

28. Daniel WG, Döhring W, Stender H-S, Lichtlen PR. Value and limitations of computed tomography in assessing aortocoronary bypass graft patency. Circulation 1983; 67:983–987.

29. Greenberg BH, Hart R, Botvinick EH, Werner JA, Brundage BH, Shames DM, Chatterjee K, Parmley WW. Thallium-201 myocardial perfusion scintigraphy to evaluate patients after coronary bypass surgery. Am J Cardiol 1978; 42:167–176.

30. Pfisterer M, Emmenegger H, Schmitt HE, Muller-Brand J, Hasse J, Gradel E, Laver MB, Burckhardt D, Burkart F. Accuracy of serial myocardial perfusion scintigraphy with thallium-201 for prediction of graft patency early and late after coronary artery bypass surgery. A controlled prospective study. Circulation 1982; 66:1017–1024.

31. Wijns W, Serruys PW, Reiber JHC, De Feyter PJ, Van Den Brand M, Simoons ML, Hugenholtz PG. Early detection of restenosis after successful percutaneous transluminal coronary angioplasty by exercise-redistribution thallium scintigraphy. Am J Cardiol 1985; 55:357–361.

32. Goldstein RA, Kirkeeide RL, Smalling RW, Nishikawa A, Merhige ME, Demer LL, Mullani NA, Gould KL. Changes in myocardial perfusion reserve after PTCA: Noninvasive assessment with positron tomography. J Nucl Med 1987; 28:1262–1267.

33. Ribeiro P, Shea M, Deanfield JE, Oakley CM, Sapsford R, Jones T, Walesby R, Selwyn AP. Different mechanisms for the relief of angina after coronary bypass surgery. Physiological versus anatomical assessment. Br Heart J 1984; 52:502–509.

34. Sobel BE. Coronary thrombolysis and the new biology. J Am Coll Cardiol 1989; 14:850–860.

35. Fry ETA, Sobel BE. Coronary thrombolysis. In: Zipes DP, Rowlands DJ, Eds. *Progress in Cardiology, Vol. 3/1.* Philadelphia: Lea & Febiger, 1990; 199–239.

36. Tiefenbrunn AJ, Sobel BE. The impact of coronary thrombolysis on myocardial infarction. Fibrinolysis 1989; 3:1–15.

37. Simoons ML, Serruys PW, van Den Brand M, Res J, Verheugt FWA, Krauss XH, Remme WJ, Bar F, De Zwaan C, Van Der Laarse A, Vermeer F, Lubsen J. Early thrombolysis in acute myocardial infarction: limitation of infarct size and improved survival. J Am Coll Cardiol 1986; 7:717–728.

38. Sheehan FH, Braunwald E, Canner P, Dodge HT, Gore J, Van Natta P, Passamani ER, Williams DO, Zaret B. The effect of intravenous thrombolytic therapy on left ventricular function: a report on tissue-plasminogen activator and streptokinase from the Thrombolysis in Myocardial Infarction (TIMI Phase I) Trial. Circulation 1987; 75:817–829.

39. Gruppo Italiano per lo Studio Della Streptochinasi Nell'infarto Miocardico (GISSI). Effectiveness of intravenous thrombolytic treatment in acute myocardial infarction. Lancet 1986; 1:397–402.

40. Laffel GL, Braunwald E. Thrombolytic therapy: A new strategy for the treatment of acute myocardial infarction (second of two parts). N Engl J Med 1984; 31:770–776.

41. Chesebro JH, Knatterud G, Roberts R, Borer J, Cohen LS, Dalen J, Dodge HT, Francis CK, Hillis D, Ludbrook P, Markis LE, Mueller H, Passamani ER, Powers ER, Rao AK, Robertson T, Ross A, Ryan TJ, Sobel BE, Willerson J. Thrombolysis in Myocardial Infarction (TIMI) Trial, Phase I: a comparison between intravenous tissue plasminogen activator and intravenous streptokinase. Circulation 1987; 76:142–154.

42. Bergmann SR, Lerch RA, Fox KAA, Ludbrook PA, Welch MJ, Ter-Pogossian MM, Sobel BE. Temporal dependence of beneficial effects of coronary thrombolysis characterized by positron tomography. Am J Med 1982; 73:573–581.

43. Granato JE, Watson DD, Flanagan TL, Gascho JA, Beller GA. Myocardial thallium-201 kinetics during coronary occlusion and reperfusion: influence of method of reflow and timing of thallium-201 administration. Circulation 1986; 73:150–160.

44. Beller GA. Role of myocardial perfusion imaging in evaluating thrombolytic therapy for acute myocardial infarction. J Am Coll Cardiol 1987; 9:661–668.

45. Santoro GM, Bisi G, Sciagrà R, Leoncini M, Fazzini PF, Meldolesi U. Single photon emission computed tomography with technetium-99m hexakis 2-methoxyisobutyl isonitrile in acute myocardial infarction before and after thrombolytic treatment: assessment of salvaged myocardium and prediction of late functional recovery. J Am Coll Cardiol 1990; 15:301–314.

46. White CW, Wright CB, Doty DB, Hiratza LF, Eastham CL, Harrison DG, Marcus ML. Does visual interpretation of the coronary arteriogram predict the physiologic importance of a coronary stenosis? N Engl J Med 1984; 310:819–824.

47. Ritchie JL, Trobaugh GB, Hamilton GW, Gould KL, Narahara KA, Murray JA, Williams DL. Myocardial imaging with thallium-201 at rest and during exercise. Comparison with coronary arteriography and resting and stress electrocardiography. Circulation 1977; 56:66–71.

48. Maddahi J, Garcia EV, Berman DS, Waxman A, Swan HJC, Forrester J. Improved noninvasive assessment of coronary artery disease by quantitative analysis of regional stress myocardial distribution and washout of thallium-201. Circulation 1981; 64:924–935.

49. Berger BC, Watson DD, Taylor GJ, Craddock GB, Martin RP, Teates CD, Beller GA. Quantitative thallium-201 exercise scintigraphy for detection of coronary artery disease. J Nucl Med 1981; 22:585–593.

50. Fintel DJ, Links JM, Brinker JA, Frank TL, Parker M, Becker LC. Improved diagnostic performance of exercise thallium-201 single photon emission computed tomography over planar imaging in the diagnosis of coronary artery disease: A receiver operating characteristic analysis. J Am Coll Cardiol 1989; 13:600–612.

51. Tamaki N, Yonekura Y, Mukai T, Kodama S, Kadotak, Kambara H, Kawai C, Torizuka K. Stress thallium-201 transaxial emission computed tomography: quantitative versus qualitative analysis for evaluation of coronary artery disease. J Am Coll Cardiol 1984; 4:1213–1221.

52. Kahn JK, McGhie I, Akers MS, Sills MN, Faber TL, Kulkarni PV, Willerson JT, Corbett JR. Quantitative rotational tomography with ^{201}Tl and [99m]Tc 2-methoxy-isobutyl-isonitrile. A direct comparison in normal individuals and patients with coronary artery disease. Circulation 1989; 79:1282–1293.

53. Rozanski A, Diamond GA, Berman D, Forrester JS, Morris D, Swan HJC. The declining specificity of exercise radionuclide ventriculography. N Engl J Med 1983; 309:518–522.

54. Robertson WS, Feigenbaum H, Armstrong WE, Dillon JC, O'Donnell J, McHenry PW. Exercise echocardiography: A clinically practical addition in the evaluation of coronary artery disease. J Am Coll Cardiol 1983; 2:1085–1091.

55. Gould KL, Goldstein RA, Mullani NA, Kirkeeide RL, Wong W-H, Tewson TJ, Berridge MS, Bolomey LA, Hartz RK, Smalling RW, Fuentes F, Nishikawa A. Noninvasive assessment of coronary stenoses by myocardial perfusion imaging during pharmacologic coronary vasodilation. VIII. Clinical feasibility of positron cardiac imaging without a cyclotron using generator-produced rubidium-82. J Am Coll Cardiol 1986; 7:775–789.

56. Stewart RE, Schwaiger M, Molina E, Popma J, Gacioch GM, Kalus M, Squicciarini S, Al-Aouarz ZR, Schork A, Kuhl DE. Comparison of rubidium-82, positron emission tomography, and thallium-201 SPECT imaging for detection of coronary artery disease. Am J Cardiol 1991; 67:1303–1310.

57. Schelbert HR, Wisenberg G, Phelps ME, Gould KL, Henze E, Hoffman EJ, Gomes A, Kuhl DE. Noninvasive assessment of coronary stenoses by myocardial imaging during pharmacologic coronary vasodilation. VI. Detection of coronary artery disease in human beings with intravenous N-13 ammonia and positron computer tomography. Am J Cardiol 1982; 49:1197–1207.

58. Tamaki N, Yonekura Y, Senda M, Yamashita K, Koide H, Saji H, Hashimoto T, Fudo T, Kambara H, Kawai C, Konishi J. Value and limitation of stress thallium-201 single photon emission computed tomography: Comparison with nitrogen-13 ammonia positron tomography. J Nucl Med 1988; 29:1181–1188.

59. Walsh NM, Bergmann SR, Steele RL, Kenzora JL, Ter-Pogossian MM, Sobel BE, Geltman EM. Delineation of impaired regional myocardial perfusion by positron emission tomography with $H_2^{15}O$. Circulation 1988; 78:612–620.

60. Proudfit WJ, Bruschke AVG, MacMillan JP, Williams GW, Sones Jr FM. Fifteen year survival study of patients with obstructive coronary artery disease. Circulation 1983; 68:986–997.

61. Mock MB, Ringqvist I, Fisher LD, Davis KB, Chaitman BR, Kouchoukos NT, Kiser GC, Alderman E, Ryan TJ, Russell RO,Jr., Mullin S, Fray D, and Killip T,III. Survival of medically treated patients in the Coronary Artery Surgery Study (CASS) registry. Circulation 1982; 66:562–568.

62. Martin CM, McConahay DR. Maximal treadmill exercise electrocardiography. Correlations with coronary arteriography and cardiac hemodynamics. Circulation 1972; 46:956–962.

63. Dash H, Massie BM, Botvinick EH, Brundage BH. The noninvasive identification of left main and three-vessel coronary artery disease by myocardial stress perfusion scintigraphy and treadmill exercise electrocardiography. Circulation 1979; 60:276–284.

64. Val PG, Chaitman BR, Waters DD, Bourassa MG, Scholl JM, Ferguson RJ, Wagniart P. Diagnostic accuracy of exercise ECG lead systems in clinical subsets of women. Circulation 1982; 65:1465–1474.

65. Gill JB, Ruddy TD, Newell JB, Finkelstein DM, Strauss HW, Boucher CA. Prognostic importance of thallium uptake by the lungs during exercise in coronary artery disease. N Engl J Med 1987; 317:1485–1489.

66. Gibson RS, Watson DD, Craddock GB, Crampton RS, Kaiser DL, Denny MJ, Beller GA. Prediction of cardiac events after uncomplicated myocardial infarction: a prospective study comparing predischarge exercise thallium-201 scintigraphy and coronary angiography. Circulation 1983; 68:321–336.

67. Demer LL, Gould KL, Goldstein RA, Kirkeeide RL, Mullani NA, Smalling RW, Nishikawa A, Merhige ME. Assessment of coronary artery disease severity by positron emission tomography. Comparison with quantitative arteriography in 193 patients. Circulation 1989; 79:825–835.

68. Píerard LA, DeLandsheere CM, Berthe C, Rigo P, Kulbertus HE. Identification of viable myocardium by echocardiography during dobutamine infusion in patients with myocardial infarction after thrombolytic therapy: comparison with positron emission tomography. J Am Coll Cardiol 1990; 15:1021–1031.

69. Lesser JR, Wilson RF, White CW. Can a physiologic assessment of coronary stenoses of intermediate severity facilitate patient selection for coronary angioplasty? Coronary Artery Dis 1990; 1:697–705.

70. Pasternak RC, Braunwald E, Sobel BE. Acute myocardial infarction. In: Braunwald E, Ed. *Heart Disease, Third Edition.*Philadelphia: W. B. Saunders Co., 1988; 1222–1313.

71. Myears DW, Sobel BE, Bergmann SR. Substrate use in ischemic and reperfused canine myocardium: quantitative considerations. Am J Physiol 1987; 253:H107-H114.

72. Buxton DB, Vaghaiwalla-Mody F, Krivokapich J, Phelps ME, Schelbert HR. Quantitative measurement of sustained metabolic abnormalities in reperfused canine myocardium. J Nucl Med 1990; 31:795 (abstract).

73. Weiss ES, Hoffman EJ, Phelps ME, Welch MJ, Henry PD, Ter-Pogossian MM, Sobel BE. External detection and visualization of myocardial ischemia with ^{11}C-substrates in vitro and in vivo. Circ Res 1976; 39:24–32.

74. Lerch RA, Ambos HD, Bergmann SR, Welch MJ, Ter-Pogossian MM, Sobel BE. Localization of viable, ischemic myocardium by positron-emission tomography with ^{11}C-palmitate. Circulation 1981; 64:689–699.

75. Sobel BE, Weiss ES, Welch MJ, Siegel BA, Ter-Pogossian MM. Detection of remote myocardial infarction in patients with positron emission transaxial tomography and intravenous ^{11}C-palmitate. Circulation 1977; 55:853–857.

76. Lerch RA, Bergmann SR, Ambos HD, Welch MJ, Ter-Pogossian MM, Sobel BE. Effect of flow-independent reduction of metabolism on regional myocardial clearance of ^{11}C-palmitate. Circulation 1982; 65:731–738.

77. Liedtke AJ. Alterations of carbohydrate and lipid metabolism in the acutely ischemic heart. Prog Cardiovasc Dis 1981; 23:321–336.

78. Fox, KAA, Abendschein DR, Ambos HD, Sobel BE, Bergmann SR. Efflux of metabolized and nonmetabolized fatty acid from canine myocardium. Implications for quantifying myocardial metabolism tomographically. Circ Res 1985; 57:232–243.

79. Tillisch J, Brunken R, Marshall R, Schwaiger M, Mandelkern M, Phelps M, Schelbert H. Reversibility of cardiac wall motion abnormalities predicted by positron tomography. N Engl J Med 1986; 314:884–888.

80. Neely JR, Morgan HE. Relationship between carbohydrate and lipid metabolism and the energy balance of heart muscle. Annu Rev Physiol 1974; 36:413–459.

81. Ratib O, Phelps ME, Huang S-C, Henze E, Selin CE, Schelbert HR. Positron tomography with deoxyglucose for estimating local myocardial glucose metabolism. J Nucl Med 1982; 23:577–586.

82. Gropler RJ, Siegel BA, Lee KJ, Moerlein SM, Perry DJ, Bergmann SR, Geltman EM. Nonuniformity in myocardial accumulation of F-18 fluorodeoxyglucose in normal fasted human. J Nucl Med 1990; 31:1749–1756.

83. Brown M, Marshall DR, Sobel BE, Bergmann SR. Delineation of myocardial oxygen utilization with carbon-11-labeled acetate. Circulation 1987; 76:687–696.

84. Brown MA, Myears DW, Bergmann SR. Noninvasive assessment of canine myocardial oxidative metabolism with carbon-11 acetate and positron emission tomography. J Am Coll Cardiol 1988; 12:1054–1063.

85. Brown MA, Myears DW, Bergmann SR. Validity of estimates of myocardial oxidative metabolism with carbon-11 acetate and positron emission tomography despite altered patterns of substrate utilization. J Nucl Med 1989; 30:187–193.

86. Walsh MN, Geltman EM, Brown MA, Henes CG, Weinheimer CJ, Sobel BE, Bergmann SR. Noninvasive estimation of regional myocardial oxygen consumption by positron emission tomography with carbon-11 acetate in patients with myocardial infarction. J Nucl Med 1989; 30:1798–1808.

87. Armbrecht JJ, Buxton DB, Schelbert HR. Validation of 1-^{11}C-acetate as a tracer

for noninvasive assessment of oxidative metabolism with positron emission tomography in normal, ischemic, postischemic, and hyperemic canine myocardium. Circulation 1990; 81:1594–1605.

88. Pohost GM, Reeves RC, Evanochko WT. Nuclear magnetic resonance: potential clinical relevance to the cardiovascular system. Circulation 1985; 72:IV-111–112.

89. Grover-McKay M, Schelbert HR, Schwaiger M, Sochor H, Guzy PM, Krivokapich J, Child JS, Phelps ME. Identification of impaired metabolic reserve by atrial pacing in patients with significant coronary artery stenosis. Circulation 1986; 74:281–292.

90. Camici P, Araujo LI, Spinks T, Lammertsma AA, Kaski JC, Shea MJ, Selwyn AP, Jones T, Maseri A. Increased uptake of F-18 fluorodeoxyglucose in postischemic myocardium of patients with exercise-induced angina. Circulation 1986; 74:81–88.

91. Araujo LI, Camici P, Spinks T, Jones T, Maseri A. Beneficial effect of nitrates on myocardial glucose utilization in unstable angina pectoris. Am J Cardiol 1987; 60:26H-30H.

92. Weiss ES, Ahmed SA, Welch MJ, Williamson JR, Ter-Pogossian MM, Sobel BE. Quantification of infarction in cross sections of canine myocardium in vivo with positron emission transaxial tomography and ^{11}C-palmitate. Circulation 1976; 55:66–73.

93. Ter-Pogossian MM, Klein MS, Markham J, Roberts R, Sobel BE. Regional assessment of myocardial metabolic integrity in vivo by positron-emission tomography with ^{11}C-labeled palmitate. Circulation 1980; 61:242–255.

94. Geltman EM, Biello D, Welch MJ, Ter-Pogossian MM, Roberts R, Sobel BE. Characterization of nontransmural myocardial infarction by positron emission tomography. Circulation 1982; 65:747–755.

95. Billadello JJ, Smith JL, Ludbrook PA, Tiefenbrunn AJ, Jaffe AS, Sobel BE, Geltman EM. Implications of "reciprocal" ST segment depression associated with acute myocardial infarction identified by positron tomography. J Am Coll Cardiol 1983; 2:616–624.

96. Sobel BE, Geltman EM, Tiefenbrunn AJ, Jaffe AS, Spadaro Jr. JJ, Ter-Pogossian MM, Collen D, Ludbrook PA. Improvement of regional myocardial metabolism after coronary thrombolysis induced with tissue-type plasminogen activator or streptokinase. Circulation 1984; 69:983–990.

97. Jaffe AS, Biello DR, Sobel BE, Geltman EM. Enhancement of metabolism of jeopardized myocardium by nifedipine. Int J Cardiol 1987; 15:77–89.

98. Marshall RC, Tillisch JH, Phelps ME, Huang SC, Carson R, Henze E, Schelbert HR. Identification and differentiation of resting myocardial ischemia and infarction in man with positron computed tomography, F-18-labeled fluorodeoxyglucose, and N-13 ammonia. Circulation 1983; 67:766–778.

99. Brunken R, Tillisch J, Schwaiger M, Child JS, Marshall R, Mandelkern M, Phelps ME, Schelbert HR. Regional perfusion, glucose metabolism and wall motion in patients with chronic electrocardiographic Q-wave infarctions. Evidence for persistence of viable tissue in some infarct regions by positron emission tomography. Circulation 1986; 73:951–963.

100. Hashimoto T, Kambara H, Fudo T, Hayashi M, Tamaki S, Tokunaga S, Tamaki N, Yonekura Y, Konishi J, Kawai C. Non-Q wave versus Q wave myocardial infarction: regional myocardial metabolism and blood flow assessed by positron emission tomography. J Am Coll Cardiol 1988; 12:88–93.

101. Kobayashi K, Neely JR. Control of maximum rates of glycolysis in rat cardiac muscle. Circ Res 1979; 44:166–175.

102. Braunwald E, Kloner RA. The stunned myocardium: Prolonged, postischemic ventricular dysfunction. Circulation 1982; 66:1146–1149.

103. Iskandrian AS, Heo J, Helfant RH, Segal BL. Chronic myocardial ischemia and left ventricular function. Ann Intern Med 1987; 107:925–927.

104. Dilsizian V, Rocco TP, Freedman MT, Leon MB, Bonow RO. Enhanced detection of ischemic but viable myocardium by the reinjection of thallium after stress-redistribution imaging. N Engl J Med 1990; 323:141–146.

105. Tamaki N, Yonekura Y, Yamashita K, Saji H, Magata Y, Senda M, Konishi Y, Hirata K, Ban T, Konishi J. Positron emission tomography using fluorine-18 deoxyglucose in evaluation of coronary artery bypass grafting. Am J Cardiol 1989; 64:860–865.
106. Brunken R, Schwaiger M, Grover-McKay M, Phelps ME, Tillisch J, Schelbert HR. Positron emission tomography detects tissue metabolic activity in myocardial segments with persistent thallium perfusion defects. J Am Coll Cardiol 1987; 10:557–567.
107. Gropler RJ, Geltman EM, Sampathkumaran K, Perez JF, Moerlein SM, Sobel BE, Bergmann SR, Siegel BA. Functional recovery after coronary revascularization for chronic coronary artery disease is dependent on maintenance of oxidative metabolism. J Am Coll Cardiol (in press).
108. Schwaiger M, Brunken R, Grover-McKay M, Krivokapich J, Child J, Tillisch JH, Phelps ME, Schelbert HR. Regional myocardial metabolism in patients with acute myocardial infarction assessed by positron emission tomography. J Am Coll Cardiol 1986; 8:800–808.
109. Eisenberg JD, Sobel BE, Geltman EM. Differentiation of ischemic from nonischemic cardiomyopathy with positron emission tomography. Am J Cardiol 1987; 59:1410–1414.
110. Grover-McKay M, Schwaiger M, Krivokapich HJ, Perloff JK, Phelps ME, Schelbert HR. Regional myocardial blood flow and metabolism at rest in mildly symptomatic patients with hypertrophic cardiomyopathy. J Am Coll Cardiol 1989; 13:317–324.
111. Perloff JK, Henze E, Schelbert HR. Alterations in regional myocardial metabolism, perfusion, and wall motion in Duchenne muscular dystrophy studied by radionuclide imaging. Circulation 1984; 69:33–42.
112. Sobel BE, Kjekshus JK, Roberts R. Enzymatic estimation of infarct size. In: Hearse DJ, DeLeiris J, Eds. *Enzymes in Cardiology: Diagnosis and Research.* Chichester: John Wiley and Sons Limited 1979; 257–289.
113. Coleman RE, Klein MS, Ahmed SA, Weiss ES, Buchholz WM, Sobel BE. Mechanisms contributing to myocardial accumulation of technetium-99m stannous pyrophosphate after coronary arterial occlusion. Am J Cardiol 1977; 39: 55–59.
114. Khaw B-A, Mattis JA, Melincoff G, Strauss HW, Gold HK, Haber E. Monoclonal antibody to cardiac myosin: Imaging of experimental myocardial infarction. Hybridoma 1984; 3:11.
115. Shelton ME, Dence CS, Hwang D-R, Welch MJ, Bergmann SR. Myocardial kinetics of fluorine-18 misonidazole: A marker of hypoxic myocardium. J Nucl Med 1989; 30:351–358.
116. Ter-Pogossian MM, Bergmann SE, Sobel BE. Influence of cardiac and respiratory motion on tomographic reconstructions of the heart: Implications for quantitative nuclear cardiology. J Comput Assist Tomogr 1982; 6:1148–1155.
117. Henes CG, Snyder AL, Bergmann SR, Geltman EM. Gating wall motion analysis with Fourier gated positron emission tomography (PET). J Nucl Med 1989; 30:771 (abstract).
118. Schwaiger M, Kalff V, Rosenspire K, Haka MS, Molina E, Hutchins GD, Deeb M, Wolfe Jr. E, Wieland DM. Noninvasive evaluation of sympathetic nervous system in human heart by positron emission tomography. Circulation 1990; 82:457–464.
119. Sobel BE, Shell WE. Jeopardized, blighted, and necrotic myocardium. Circulation 1973; 47:215–216.
120. Go RT, MacIntyre WJ, Go RT, Marwick TH, Saha GB, Neumann DR, Underwood DA, Simpfendorfer CC. Prospective comparison of rubidium-82 PET and thallium-201 SPECT myocardial perfusion imaging utilizing a single dipyridamole stress in the diagnosis of coronary artery disease. J Nucl Med 1990; 31:1899–1905.
121. Yonekura Y, Tamaki N, Senda M, Nohara R, Kambara H, Konishi Y, Koide H, Kureshi SA, Saji H, Ban T, Kawai C, Torizuka K. Detection of coronary artery disease with ^{13}N-ammonia and high-resolution positron-emission computed tomography. Am Heart J 1987; 13:645–654.

Color Figures

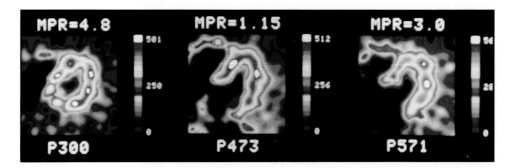

Color Figure 2. *Midventricular reconstructions obtained with PET and using ^{15}O-water after intravenous administration of dipyridamole to a normal subject (P300) and to 2 patients with chest pain and angiographically normal coronary arteries—1 with impaired myocardial perfusion reserve (MPR) (P473), and 1 with normal myocardial perfusion reserve (P571). In each subject, qualitative and quantitative assessment of myocardial perfusion indicated that perfusion was homogenous despite wide differences between patients in ability to increase flow after dipyridamole. Qualitative imaging by a static imaging protocol would not have permitted discrimination of the impaired flow reserve in P473. The orientation of the images is similar to that in Figure 5-7. (Reproduced from Geltman et al.,[65] with permission of the American College of Cardiology.)*

(See Chapter 5)

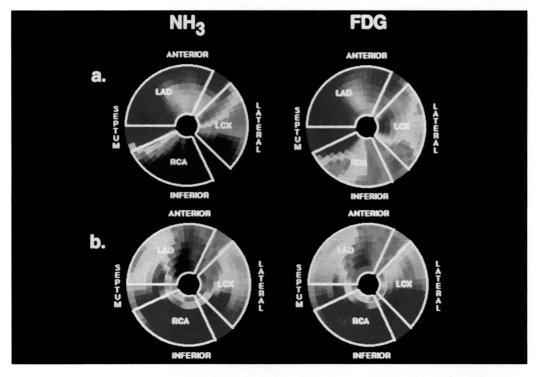

Color Figure 3. *Polar map display of reoriented short-axis PET images derived from transaxial images of myocardial perfusion and glucose metabolism depicted in Figures 7-3 and 7-4. A schematic outline of vascular territories is superimposed on each polar map.*

(See Chapter 7)

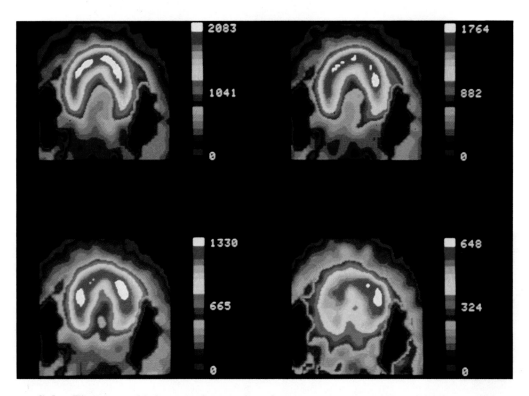

Color Figure 4. *Midventricular tomographic reconstructions obtained from a control study in an intact, anesthetized dog at 2 (upper left), 4 (upper right), 8 (lower left), and 18 minutes (lower right) after intravenous administration of* [11]*C-acetate. The left lateral ventricular wall is to the left, the anterior myocardium uppermost, the septum to the right, and the mitral valve plane (which is thin and not visualized) is lowermost. The color scale to the right of each image shows the counts per pixel before decay correction. Uptake of tracer is avid and uniform, and clearance from blood is rapid. Good contrast between myocardium, blood, and lung is present. Washout of* [11]*C from the myocardium is evident over time. (Reproduced with permission from Brown et al.[27])*

(See Chapter 9)

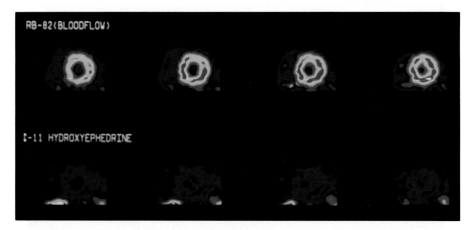

Color Figure 9. *Cross-sectional images obtained in a patient who had undergone transplantation. The blood flow images (*^{82}*Rb,top) show homogeneous perfusion throughout the left ventricle. *^{11}*C-HED retention is markedly reduced compared with that in the example shown in Color Figure 8, consistent with sympathetic denervation in patients with recent cardiac transplants. These data indicate very little nonspecific binding of *^{11}*C-HED in human heart.*

(See Chapter 10)

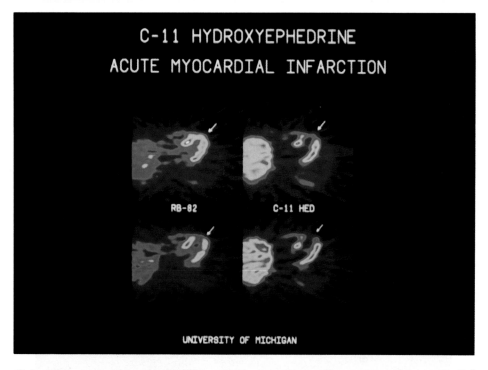

Color Figure 10. *Transaxial PET images from patients with recent anterior myocardial infarction and thrombolytic therapy. The blood flow images on the left show a small perfusion abnormality (*^{82}*Rb) in the anteroapical segments of the left ventricle. The images obtained after *^{11}*C-HED (right) show a marked reduction in regional uptake in the anterior wall, suggesting injury to sympathetic nerve terminals. Note that *^{11}*C-HED defects exceed the area of reduced perfusion, consistent with results of animal experiments indicating neuronal injury exceeding the area of infarction.*

(See Chapter 10)

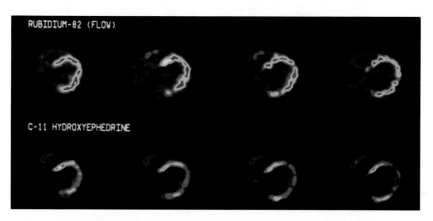

Color Figure 11. *Cross-sectional PET images obtained in a patient with congestive cardiomyopathy. ¹¹C-HED uptake is reduced in this dilated heart, with heterogeneous retention pattern and a gradient from the base to the apex.*

(See Chapter 10)

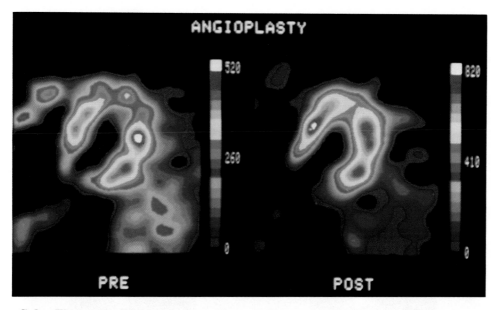

Color Figure 12. *Midventricular positron emission tomographic reconstructions of the relative distribution of $H_2{}^{15}O$ in the heart of a patient with obstruction of the left anterior descending coronary artery. The top of each image represents anterior myocardium; the right of each image corresponds to the patient's left side. Areas in white and red represent zones with the highest amount of radioactivity and areas in blue and violet represent those with the lowest amount of radioactivity. The image on the left was acquired before, and that on the right after, angioplasty. The discontinuity visible posteriorly is attributable to the mitral valve apparatus and the atria, which have dimensions below the spatial resolution of the instrument. The zone of decreased relative perfusion in the anterior wall resolved after angioplasty.*

(See Chapter 11)

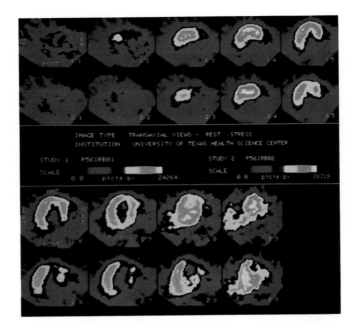

Color Figure 13. *Positron emission tomographic images of the heart acquired with* ^{82}Rb *from a patient with significant obstruction of the proximal left anterior descending coronary artery. Images at the top were acquired before and those at the bottom after the intravenous administration of dipyridamole, and handgrip stress. Views are oblique and semi-long-axis. They are displayed from the base (upper left) to the inferior wall (lower right). Each image is oriented with the anteroapical wall at the top and the lateral free wall to the left. White and red represent zones with the highest amounts of radioactivity and green and blue represent regions with the lowest amounts of radioactivity. A large anterior, septal, and apical defect is visualized after administration of dipyridamole in conjunction with handgrip stress. (Reproduced with permission from Demer et al.[67])*

(See Chapter 11)

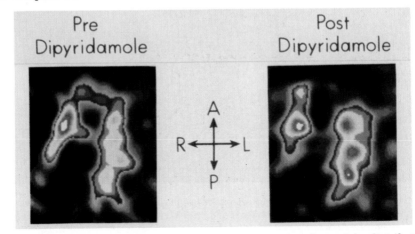

Color Figure 14. *Positron emission tomographic reconstructions of the distribution of relative perfusion acquired after the intravenous administration of* $H_2{}^{15}O$ *and administration by inhalation of* ^{15}O-*carbon monoxide to a patient with a high-grade stenosis of the left anterior descending coronary artery. Before dipyridamole, a subtle zone of decreased relative perfusion is seen in the anteroapical wall. It becomes markedly more prominent after dipyridamole. A = anterior, P = posterior, R = right, L = left. (Reproduced with permission from Walsh et al.[59])*

(See Chapter 11)

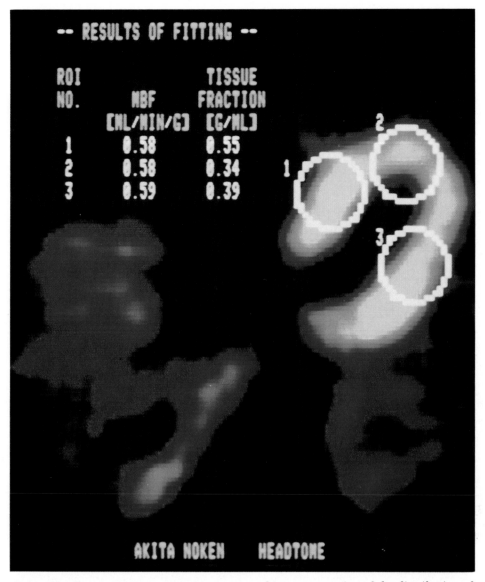

Color Figure 15. *Positron emission tomographic reconstruction of the distribution of relative perfusion at rest acquired after the intravenous administration of $H_2{}^{15}O$ and administration by inhalation of ^{15}O-carbon monoxide to a patient with trivessel coronary artery disease. Orientation within the image is septum to the left, anterior wall at the top, and lateral wall to the right. In the upper left are values for regional myocardial blood flow (MBF), in absolute terms, derived from dynamic $H_2{}^{15}O$ data, for circular regions of interest placed in septal, anterior, and lateral walls. The tissue fraction represents the difference between the amount of tracer per mass of tissue and the concentration of tracer within a specified volume defined by a region of interest. Relative perfusion is decreased only in the anterior wall. However, based on the quantitative measurements of MBF, regional perfusion is reduced diffusely when compared with that in normal subjects. (Courtesy of Hidehiro Iida, D.Sc.)*

(See Chapter 11)

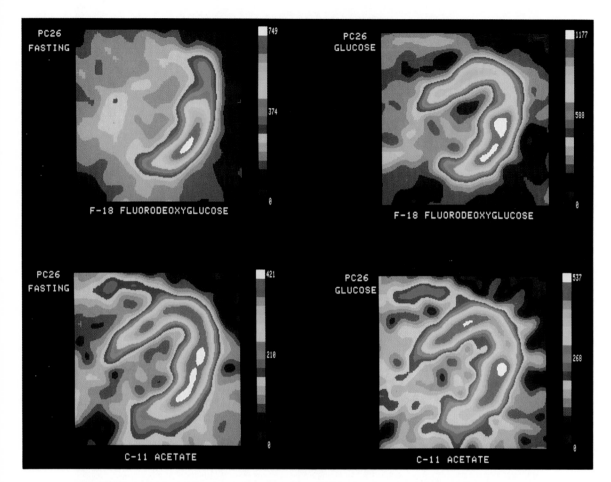

Color Figure 16. *Midventricular positron emission tomographic reconstructions from a normal subject. The tomograms depicted in the upper panels were obtained after the intravenous administration of ^{18}F-fluorodeoxyglucose. Those in the bottom panels were obtained after the intravenous administration of ^{11}C-acetate. The left-hand panel images were acquired after a 5 to 8 hour fast; those in the right-hand panels were acquired after administration of glucose. The subject's left is represented by the right side in the image. In the fasting state, marked heterogeneity of the accumulation of ^{18}FDG was evident. It was attenuated markedly after administration of glucose. Accumulation and clearance of ^{11}C-acetate were homogenous with both fasting and feeding. (Reproduced from Gropler et al,[82] with permission of the Society of Nuclear Medicine).*

(See Chapter 11)

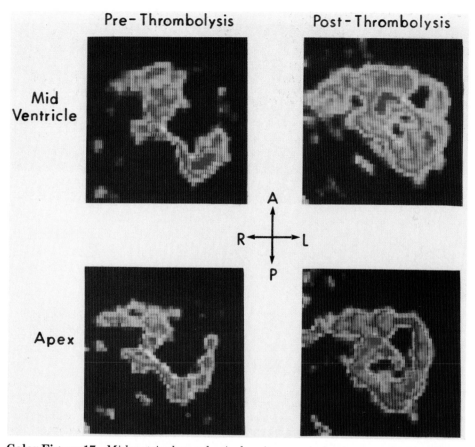

Color Figure 17. *Midventricular and apical positron-emission tomographic reconstructions obtained after the intravenous administration of ^{11}C-palmitate to a patient with successful thrombolysis of a completely occluded left anterior descending coronary artery. A large anterior defect was present on tomograms acquired before the initiation of thrombolysis (left), which demonstrated marked improvement 10 days later (right). (Reproduced with permission from Bergmann et al.[1])*

(See Chapter 11)

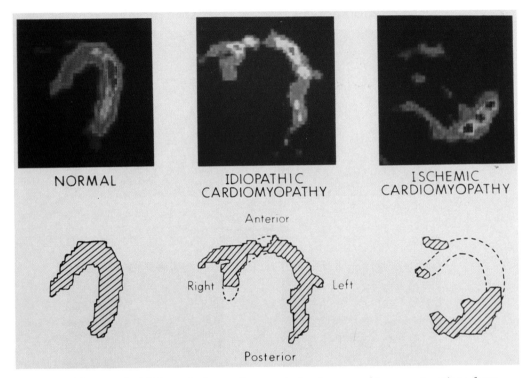

Color Figure 18. *Midventricular positron emission tomographic reconstructions from the heart of a normal subject, a patient with idiopathic dilated cardiomyopathy, and one with ischemic cardiomyopathy. The schematic shows zones of accumulation of tracer (slashed lines) and of expected outlines of ventricular walls at these levels (dashed lines). Hearts of patients with idiopathic dilated cardiomyopathy exhibited marked spatial heterogeneity of the accumulation of* ^{11}*C-palmitate. Those of patients with ischemic cardiomyopathy exhibited large, segmental zones with homogeneously depressed accumulation of* ^{11}*C-palmitate. (Reproduced with permission from Eisenberg et al.[109])*

(See Chapter 11)

Index

307